Physical Medicine and Rehabilitation

Neurologic and Orthopaedic Sequelae of Traumatic Brain Injury

Guest Editor:

Lance R. Stone, DO

Center for Brain Injury Rehabilitation
San Diego Rehabilitation Institute
San Diego, California

Volume 7/Number 3   October 1993
HANLEY & BELFUS, INC.   Philadelphia

STATE OF THE ART REVIEWS

Publisher: **HANLEY & BELFUS, INC.**
210 South 13th Street
Philadelphia, PA 19107
(215) 546-7293
(215) 730-9330 (Fax)

PHYSICAL MEDICINE AND REHABILITATION: State of the Art Reviews   (ISSN 0888-7357)
Volume 7, Number 3   (ISBN 1-56053-136-3)

PHYSICAL MEDICINE AND REHABILITATION: State of the Art Reviews is published triannually (three times per year) by Hanley & Belfus, Inc., 210 South 13th Street, Philadelphia, Pennsylvania 19107.

POSTMASTER: Send address changes to PHYSICAL MEDICINE AND REHABILITATION: State of the Art Reviews, Hanley & Belfus, Inc., 210 South 13th Street, Philadelphia, PA 19107.

The 1993 subscription price is $68.00 per year U.S., $80.00 outside U.S. (add $30.00 for air mail). Single copies $32.00 U.S., $36.00 outside U.S. (add $10.00 for single copy air mail).

Physical Medicine and Rehabilitation: State of the Art Reviews
Vol. 7, No. 3, October 1993

NEUROLOGIC AND ORTHOPAEDIC SEQUELAE OF
TRAUMATIC BRAIN INJURY
Lance R. Stone, DO, Editor

CONTENTS

Preface . . . .   **xi**
Lance R. Stone

Monitoring of Post-Traumatic Cerebral Sequelae **441**
Duncan Q. McBride and Aman B. Patel

Following head trauma, cellular damage often results from progressive hemorrhage, edema, or poor cerebral oxygenation due to elevated intracranial
pressure, anemia, hypotension, hypoxia, or seizure. Efforts to preserve neurologic
potential must be aimed at collecting data regarding cerebral function and
acting on this information. Cerebral monitoring methods currently in use are
described in this chapter, including radiologic methods, measurement of
intracranial pressure, cerebral blood flow, and cerebral metabolism, and
electrophysiologic methods.

Post-Traumatic Seizures **461**
Barry I. Ludwig

Post-traumatic epilepsy is a common sequela of traumatic brain injury that
further increases the patient's morbidity and social handicap and decreases his
or her quality of life. The overall incidence of post-traumatic epilepsy is
approximately 5%, but that percentage markedly rises with the severity of the
trauma. In this article, early and late seizures are differentiated, and preventive
and treatment strategies discussed.

Post-Traumatic Visual Disorders: Part I. Injuries and Mechanisms **475**
Alfredo A. Sadun

Trauma to any portion of the visual pathway results in some form of disturbance
in visual function. This article reviews the major types of injuries and their
mechanisms, including optic nerve atrophy, visual pathway's trauma, cortical
blindness, aberrant regeneration of the ocular motor nerve, and ophthalmoplegia.

**Post-Traumatic Visual Disorders: Part II. Management
and Rehabilitation** **485**
Don Liu

The clinical manifestations of a traumatized visual system vary greatly, and the
emergent care and rehabilitation of these patients must be highly individualized.

Rehabilitation entails preserving or restoring vision; but it also involves preserving or restoring *useful* vision function, ensuring comfort of the eye, and eradicating cosmetic disfigurement. Management approaches, including surgical treatment, are described for exposure keratitis, adnexal trauma, blow-out fractures of the orbit, retinal detachment, enucleation, and evisceration.

Peripheral Nerve Injury Following Traumatic Brain Injury 503
John L. Shen

Concomitant peripheral nerve injuries (PNIs) can coexist in the traumatic brain injury population, especially in patients with moderate to severe brain and polymusculoskeletal trauma, and these injuries frequently are detected during acute rehabilitation. PNI is commonly associated with long-bone fractures, but other risk factors include improper limb positioning, ill-fitting casts, nerve complications after surgery, and spasticity. Diagnosis and treatment of the various nerve injuries are detailed.

Post-Traumatic Movement Disorders 519
Mark F. Lew and Cheryl H. Waters

Cerebrospinal trauma may produce hyperkinetic or akinetic movement disorders. Delay between the injury and appearance of clinical symptoms often obscures a definitive cause-and-effect relationship. This review discusses reported cases in which trauma led to an excess of movement—dyskinesia (chorea and ballismus, dystonia, tics, tremor, myoclonus)—or a paucity of movement—parkinsonism.

**Management of Hypertonicity Using Chemical Denervation
Following Traumatic Brain Injury** 527
Lance R. Stone and Daniel Y. Shin

Clinicians treating traumatic brain injury patients should be familiar with the technical considerations of nerve blocks for management of hypertonicity. This chapter attempts to identify which patient group is likely to develop hypertonicity, then discusses the differential diagnosis of abnormal movement. The history of phenol as a therapeutic agent and specific clinical indications are presented. Botulinum toxin A is introduced as the newest and most selective treatment for hypertonicity.

Vestibular Deficits in the Head-Injured Patient 559
Susan J. Herdman and Janet O. Helminski

Persistent complaints of vertigo or of disequilibrium often indicate involvement of the vestibular system in patients with closed-head injury. Patients with head trauma can present with multiple vestibular deficits, including unilateral or bilateral vestibular loss, postconcussional Meniere's disease, benign paroxysmal positional vertigo, perilymphatic fistula, or central vertigo. Formal vestibular function studies and a clinical examination should be performed to identify the underlying cause of these complaints.

Post-Traumatic Neuroendocrine Disorders 569
James R. Hansen and Jennifer S. Cook

Endocrine abnormalities following head trauma are not commonly reported but may be overlooked. Appropriate screening studies to assess pituitary function are detailed here. Early recognition of hormone disturbances may promote the rehabilitation and recovery of head injury survivors.

Neurobehavioral Disorders Following Traumatic Brain Injury:
Part I. Neurobehavioral Sequelae in the Early Stages of Recovery **581**
Ronald E. Saul

Neurobehavioral sequelae of traumatic brain injury affect complex arrays of cognition, emotional expression, and behavior. These include attention and memory problems, cognitive and executive dysfunction, personality changes, anxiety and affective disorders, psychosis, irritability, and aggression. This chapter reviews recent literature on the subacute neurobehavioral sequelae of moderate to severe closed TBI, emphasizing the clinical features and syndromes associated with different stages of recovery, their precipitating biologic and psychosocial determinants, and appropriate intervention, including new pharmacologic approaches to treatment.

Neurobehavioral Disorders Following Traumatic Brain Injury:
Part II. Late Neurobehavioral Sequelae **593**
Ronald E. Saul

In patients with moderate to severe traumatic brain injury, disabling cognitive and behavioral problems often develop or become apparent months to a year or more after the trauma. These problems include cognitive impairment, aggression, affective disorders, and psychosis. A coordinated diagnostic evaluation of neurologic, cognitive, affective, and behavioral disturbances by the rehabilitation team is essential for appropriate management. Treatment measures generally include both behavioral approaches and pharmacotherapy.

Post-Traumatic Headache Syndrome **603**
Joel R. Saper

Typical symptoms of the post-traumatic headache syndrome are head, neck, or facial pain; sleep disturbance; cognitive symptoms; depression, anxiety, or other mood disturbances; and nonspecific dizziness with or without vertigo. Although once considered a psychological disturbance, increasing data now indicate the syndrome represents a neurologic, neuropsychiatric condition. The pathophysiology of these headaches is discussed, and principles of assessment and treatment outlined.

Heterotopic Ossification **611**
Douglas E. Garland

The majority of heterotopic bone formation associated with head injury is associated with joint trauma. Patients exhibiting marked hypertonicity, especially extensor rigidity, are most likely to develop this complication. Multiple sites are common in patients with marked neurologic compromise. Diagnosis and treatment strategies are discussed. Early detection may prevent joint ankylosis and long-term disability.

Surgical Management of Upper Extremity Deformities
Following Traumatic Brain Injury **623**
David J. Kolessar and Mary Ann E. Keenan

Surgical management of spastic upper extremity deformities following TBI are performed once neurologic recovery has plateaued. Preoperative evaluation combines a thorough physical examination with diagnostic nerve blocks and dynamic EMG testing. Surgical procedures to improve function at the elbow dynamic EMG testing. Surgical procedures to improve function at the elbow include proximal myotomy of the brachioradialis, Z-lengthening of the biceps tendon, and myotendinous lengthening of the brachialis muscle. Wrist and finger flexion deformities can be treated with fractional lengthenings of their respective tendons. Thumb-in-palm deformity can be corrected with thenar muscle releases, including adductor pollicis, Z-lengthening of flexor pollicis longus, and release of the first dorsal interosseous muscle. In the nonfunctional extremity, procedures are directed toward improving patient care and hygiene.

Lower Extremity Complications Following Traumatic Brain Injury 637
Michael S. Pinzur

Functional outcome in TBI patients is optimized when fracture care is approached with consideration given to rehabilitation, which will avoid leaving patients with long-term severe joint contractures that increase their disability and complicate their rehabilitation. Early intervention by a rehabilitation team is invaluable to ensure institution of appropriate therapies, including splinting, casting, positioning, and nerve blocks intended to maximize the potential for a good outcome. This chapter outlines the principles of fracture care, spasticity management, timing of functional orthopaedic interventions, patient evaluation, as well as surgical and nonsurgical treatments.

Nonsurgical Management of Upper Extremity Deformities After Traumatic Brain Injury: The Rancho Los Amigos Comprehensive Treatment Program 649
Eufrocina S. Tomas, Maureen Forte Undzis, Eileen A. Shores, and Marilyn R. Sidler

Abnormal muscle tone and hypertonicity are complications affecting the adult traumatic brain injury patient, posing significant obstacles to functional recovery. The occupational therapist should aim to maximize the patient's potential by facilitating upper-extremity control so the patient may once again participate in purposeful activities. In this chapter, key elements in the evaluation are highlighted, and a sequenced treatment progression is described through five phases to normalize upper-extremity tone and movement. This coordinated treatment approach discusses the timing and sequencing of serial casting, motor point or nerve blocks, and surgical procedures and how these are organized within a movement reintegration program.

Index 663

CONTRIBUTORS

Jennifer S. Cook, MD
Pediatric Endocrinologist, Blank Children's Hospital; and Iowa Physician's Clinic, Des Moines, Iowa

Douglas E. Garland, MD
Chief, Central Nervous System Division, Department of Surgery, Rancho Los Amigos Medical Center, Downey, California; and Clinical Professor, Department of Orthopaedics, University of Southern California, Los Angeles, California

James R. Hansen, MD
Pediatric Endocrinology and Diabetes, Emanuel Children's Hospital, Portland, Oregon

Janet O. Helminski, MS, PT
Institute for Neuroscience, Northwestern University, Chicago, Illinois

Susan J. Herdman, PhD, PT
Associate Professor, Department of Otolaryngology–Head and Neck Surgery, Johns Hopkins University, Baltimore, Maryland

Mary Ann E. Keenan, MD
Professor, Department of Orthopaedic Surgery, Albert Einstein Medical Center; Professor, Department of Physical Medicine and Rehabilitation, Temple University School of Medicine; and Chairman, Department of Orthopaedic Surgery, Albert Einstein Medical Center, Philadelphia, Pennsylvania

David J. Kolessar, MD
Special Fellow in Adult Reconstruction, Department of Orthopaedic Surgery, Mayo Clinic, Rochester, Minnesota; formerly, Department of Orthopaedic Surgery, Albert Einstein Medical Center, and Department of Physical Medicine and Rehabilitation, Temple University School of Medicine, Philadelphia, Pennsylvania

Mark F. Lew, MD
Assistant Professor of Neurology, Division of Movement Disorders, Department of Neurology, University of Southern California School of Medicine, Los Angeles, California

Don Liu, MD
Associate Professor, Department of Ophthalmology, Doheny Eye Institute, University of Southern California School of Medicine, Los Angeles, California

Barry I. Ludwig, MD
Associate Clinical Professor, Department of Neurology, University of California, Los Angeles, California; and Director, Brain Injury Unit, Daniel Freeman Memorial Hospital, Inglewood, California

Duncan Q. McBride, MD
Assistant Professor, Department of Surgery, UCLA Medical Center, Los Angeles, California; and Chief, Division of Neurosurgery, Harbor/UCLA Medical Center, Torrance, California

Aman B. Patel, MD
Department of Surgery, Division of Neurosurgery, UCLA Medical School, Los Angeles, California

Michael S. Pinzur, MD
Professor of Orthopaedic Surgery, and Director, Gait Analysis Laboratory, Loyola University Medical Center, Maywood, Illinois

Alfredo A. Sadun, MD, PhD
Professor, Departments of Ophthalmology and Neurosurgery, Doheny Eye Institute, and University of Southern California School of Medicine, Los Angeles, California

Joel R. Saper, MD
Director, Michigan Head-Pain and Neurological Institute, Ann Arbor, Michigan; Clinical Professor of Medicine, Department of Neurology, Michigan State University, East Lansing, Michigan; and Director, Head Pain Treatment Program, Chelsea Community Hospital, Chelsea, Michigan

Ronald E. Saul, MD
Associate Clinical Professor, Department of Neurology, UCLA School of Medicine, Los Angeles, California; Consultant, Adult Brain Injury Service, Rancho Los Amigos Medical Center, Downey, California; and Consultant, Traumatic Brain Injury Unit, Metropolitan State Hospital, Nowalk, California

John L. Shen, MD
Chief, Adult Brain Injury Service, Rancho Los Amigos Medical Center, Downey, California

Daniel Y. Shin, MD
Director, Electrodiagnostics Laboratory, Rancho Los Amigos Medical Center, Downey, California; Clinical Assistant Professor, Department of Physical Medicine and Rehabilitation, University of California at Irvine School of Medicine, Irvine, California; and Clinical Assistant Professor, Department of Neurology, University of Southern California School of Medicine, Los Angeles, California

Eileen A. Shores, BS, OTR
Supervisor I, Adult Brain Injury Occupational Therapy Department, Rancho Los Amigos Medical Center, Downey, California

Marilyn Ruth Sidler, MA, OTR
Occupational Therapist, Rancho Los Amigos Medical Center, Downey, California

Lance R. Stone, DO
Director, Center for Brain Injury Rehabilitation, San Diego Rehabilitation Institute, San Diego, California; Instructor, Department of Physical Medicine and Rehabilitation, University of California at Irvine School of Medicine, Irvine, California; and Clinical Assistant Professor, Department of Neurology, University of Southern California School of Medicine, Los Angeles, California

Eufrocina S. Thomas, OTR
Supervisor I, Adult Brain Injury Occupational Therapy Department, Rancho Los Amigos Medical Center, Downey, California

Maureen Forte Undzis, BS, OTR
Occupational Therapist and Assistant Director, Clinical Services, Rancho Los Amigos Medical Center, Downey, California

Cheryl H. Waters, MD, FRCPC
Assistant Professor and Chief, Division of Movement Disorders, Department of Neurology, University of Southern California School of Medicine, Los Angeles, California

PUBLISHED ISSUES 1987–1991
(available from the publisher)

Vol 1, No 2/1987   **A Primer on Management for Rehabilitation Medicine**
Edited by F. Patrick Maloney, MD, Little Rock, Arkansas

Vol 1, No 3/1987   **Medical Complications of Spinal Cord Injury**
Edited by Mark N. Ozer, MA, and James K. Schmitt, MD,
Richmond, Virginia

Vol 2, No 1/1988   **Joint, Soft Tissue, and Disk Disorders**
Edited by Robert L. Swezey, MD, Santa Monica, California

Vol 2, No 2/1988   **Rehabilitation of the Alcoholic**
Edited by Curtis Wright, MD, Baltimore, Maryland

Vol 2, No 3/1988   **Home Health Care and Rehabilitation**
Edited by Jay Portnow, MD, PhD, Norwell, Massachusetts

Vol 2, No 4/1988   **Rehabilitation of Neuromuscular Diseases**
Edited by William M. Fowler, Jr., MD, Davis, California

Vol 3, No 1/1989   **Traumatic Brain Injury**
Edited by Lawrence J. Horn, MD, Philadelphia, Pennsylvania,
and D. Nathan Cope, MD, Concord, California

Vol 3, No 2/1989   **Quantifying Neurologic Performance**
Edited by Ross David, MD, et al., VAMC, Togus, Maine

Vol 3, No 3/1989   **Medical Management of the Elderly Stroke Patient**
Edited by Roy V. Erickson, MD, Farmington, Connecticut

Vol 3, No 4/1989   **Clinical Electrophysiology**
Edited by Daniel Dumitru, MD, San Antonio, Texas

Vol 4, No 1/1990   **Rehabilitation of the Aging Population**
Edited by F. Patrick Maloney, MD, and Kevin M. Means, MD,
Little Rock, Arkansas

Vol 4, No 2/1990   **Neck and Back Pain**
Edited by Jeffrey A. Saal, MD, San Francisco, California

Vol 4, No 3/1990   **The Coma-Emerging Patient**
Edited by Elizabeth Sandel, MD, and David W. Ellis, PhD,
Camden, New Jersey

Vol 5, No 1/1991   **Rehabilitation of Chronic Pain**
Edited by Nicolas E. Walsh, MD, San Antonio, Texas

Vol 5, No 2/1991   **The Child with Physical Disability**
Edited by Gabriella Molnar, MD, Oakland, California

Vol 5, No 3/1991   **Musculoskeletal Pain**
Edited by Constance D. Schwab, MD, Chicago, Illinois

PUBLISHED ISSUES 1992–1993

Vol 6, No 1/1992   **Post-Concussive Disorders**
Edited by Lawrence J. Horn, MD, Houston, Texas
and Nathan D. Zasler, MD, Richmond, Virginia

Vol 6, No 2/1992   **Industrial Rehabilitation**
Edited by Chrisanne Gordon, MD, and Paul E. Kaplan, MD,
Columbus, Ohio

Vol 6, No 3/1992   **Neuropsychological Assessment**
Edited by Stephanie Hanson, PhD, Charlotte, North Carolina
and David Tucker, PhD, Austin, Texas

Vol 7, No 1/1993   **Long-term Consequences of Stroke**
Edited by Robert W. Teasell, MD, London, Ontario, Canada

Vol 7, No 2/1993   **Management for Rehabilitation Medicine II**
Edited by F. Patrick Maloney, MD, and Richard P. Gray, MD,
Little Rock, Arkansas

Vol 7, No 3/1993   **Neurologic and Orthopaedic Sequelae of Traumatic Brain Injury**
Edited by Lance R. Stone, DO, Downey, California

Vol 7, 1993   **HIV-Related Disability: Assessment and Management**
Special Issue   Edited by Michael W. O'Dell, MD, Cincinnati, Ohio

FUTURE ISSUES

1994   **Prosthetics**
Edited by Alberto Esquenazi, MD, Philadelphia, Pennsylvania

Cancer Rehabilitation
Edited by Fae H. Garden, MD, and Martin Grabois, MD,
Houston, Texas

Fracture Rehabilitation
Edited by Arun J. Mehta, MB, FRCPC, Sepulveda, California

Spasticity
Edited by Richard T. Katz, MD, St. Louis, Missouri

Subscriptions and single issues available from the publisher—Hanley & Belfus, Inc.,
Medical Publishers, 210 South 13th Street, Philadelphia, PA 19107 (215) 546-7293;
1-800-962-1892. Fax (215) 790-9330.

x

PREFACE

The burgeoning interest in traumatic brain injury (TBI) rehabilitation has generated a literature that is both impressive and bewildering in scope. The clinician questing for enhanced knowledge may find the reading lists necessary for adequate coverage of the subject to be unwieldy and the information provided in the reading difficult to integrate. In response to the latter difficulty, it is this editor's endeavor to provide a text that selectively discusses the major neurologic and orthopaedic sequelae. The content of the volume was chosen reflecting our bias that the purely physical and neurologic sequelae following severe TBI are well documented, but there is a real dearth of texts providing a comprehensive discussion for the interested clinician.

The result is that all aspects are treated in depth; indeed, each chapter is a review of the subject under discussion. Certain rehabilitation professionals may feel disappointed that some topics including hydrocephalus, fracture care, spinal cord injury, CSF fistulas, and neurovascular syndromes have been omitted. We have tried to include only the most common disorders or those not underscored in other texts. There is still general agreement and recognition that often the most prominent sequelae causing long-term morbidity after TBI are cognitive, behavioral, and psychosocial disturbances.

The gaps in knowledge are still large, but the recent advances are summarized in the volume by the authors, many of whom are authorities in areas of their special interest and all of whom have been intimately involved in the study of neurorehabilitation.

This volume will hopefully appeal and be a useful reference to various members of the interdisciplinary TBI team including allied health professionals as well as neurologists, neurosurgeons, traumatologists, orthopaedic surgeons, and physiatrists.

LANCE R. STONE, DO
GUEST EDITOR

DUNCAN Q. McBRIDE, MD
AMAN B. PATEL, MD

MONITORING OF POST-TRAUMATIC CEREBRAL SEQUELAE

From the
Division of Neurosurgery
UCLA Medical School
Harbor/UCLA Medical Center
Torrance, California

Correspondence to:
Duncan Q. McBride, MD
Division of Neurosurgery
Harbor/UCLA Medical Center
Box 424
1000 W. Carson Street
Torrance, CA 90509

Craniocerebral trauma is a leading cause of morbidity and mortality in our culture. Significant cerebral damage frequently occurs at the moment of impact in both open and closed injuries because of mechanical disruption of tissues, acute hemorrhage, elevation of intracranial pressure, and compromised cerebral perfusion. Subsequently, further cellular damage often results from progressive hemorrhage, edema, or poor cerebral oxygenation due to elevated intracranial pressure, anemia, hypotension, hypoxia, or seizure. Prevention of the latter, post-traumatic sequelae of acute brain injury is the principal thrust of current neurosurgical intensive care.

The system of rapid evacuation of victims to appropriate trauma hospitals, acute stabilization and resuscitation both in the field and emergency departments, and early and accurate diagnosis followed by appropriate surgical intervention has reached a high degree of efficiency in most communities in the United States and Europe. Therefore, future efforts to preserve neurologic potential must be aimed at collecting data regarding cerebral function and acting on this information. Cerebral monitoring methods currently in use are described in this chapter, but it is clear that the area of cerebral intensive care is in its infancy. New techniques and technologies are rapidly being developed that will further enhance our understanding of brain function. These include single-wire probes for analysis of tissue parameters, such as oxygenation, pH, lactate, CO_2 and other metabolites, plus microdialysis evaluation of injured tissue for a myriad of potentially important compounds. Clearly, the more information that we can obtain about the injured brain, the better our ability to preserve and recover neurologic function will become.

RADIOLOGY IN HEAD TRAUMA

Skull Films

The role of skull radiographs in the evaluation of head injury has become controversial.[30] These films have become less important with the advent of computed tomography (CT). However, they are rapid, safe, and relatively inexpensive and on occasion can be useful. In patients with head injury, anteroposterior and lateral views of the skull can be obtained at the same time as the cervical spine films with little additional effort. These and tangential views are particularly useful in the evaluation of depressed skull fractures. The selective use of plain skull radiogaphs, therefore, still has a place in the management of head injuries. Routine views also include Towne and Caldwell projections, but in most instances, the anteroposterior and lateral views will suffice. The latter are relatively sensitive in demonstrating vault fractures but will miss basilar fractures. Pneumocephalous or an air-fluid level may indicate the presence of a fracture in such cases.

Computed Tomography

Since its advent in 1972, CT has become the principal diagnostic tool in the evaluation of head injury and may have had the greatest positive effect on outcome of any single recent innovation.[22] During the acute period, it permits the rapid and safe detection and localization of intracranial hematomas, brain contusions, edema, and foreign bodies. In addition, serial CTs allow the diagnosis of subsequent developments. CT is also useful in the diagnosis and evaluation of skull fractures, particularly depressed skull fractures and basilar fractures.

All patients with head injury and altered level of consciousness, focal neurologic signs, disorientation, or history of loss of consciousness, seizure, or altered coagulation status, as well as all patients with depressed skull fractures or penetrating injuries should be scanned. A complete study, including the posterior fossa, should be performed and requires only 10 to 15 minutes. In critical circumstances, when the patient is rapidly deteriorating, a study limited to several slices can be obtained to detect intracranial pathology. In patients with multiple injuries, additional areas of the body can be scanned as well.

Movement of the patient's head will lead to artifacts, which can seriously degrade the quality of the image. These artifacts may obscure pathology or even resemble lesions. Therefore, the patient must be immobilized with restraints or neuromuscular blockade. In the acute period, scans without contrast suffice, and contrast studies are unnecessary in patients with hemorrhagic lesions. At times, however, contrast is helpful in delineating such lesions as chronic subdural hematomas, infarcts, subdural or intracerebral abscesses, and vascular lesions. Due to the progression of lesions and the appearance of delayed hematomas, serial scans are recommended in patients with head injury.[22]

Significant CT findings relate to mass effect on the brain and resultant compartmental herniation. In hemispheric and cerebellar lesions with mass effect, the cerebral ventricles become distorted or "effaced," and midline structures may be displaced to the opposite side. In addition, ventricular effacement of the perimesencephalic, suprasellar, or quadrigeminal cerebrospinal fluid cistern is indicative of active or pending brainstem compression.

Ventriculography

Ventriculostomy can be performed rapidly in patients with acute head injury and carries minimal risk to the patient.[4] It can provide two critical bits of information: the degree of supratentorial brain shift and the level of intracranial pressure. Prior to the advent of CT, this test and angiography were the most useful radiologic studies for patients who suffered severe head injury. These studies still have an important role in emergency diagnosis. If the hospital does not have CT immediately available, ventriculography should be used in patients unable to speak or follow commands. Other indications include patients with severe brain injuries who have other extracranial injuries that require immediate operation or that prevent the transfer to CT or angiography. In this procedure, a ventricular cannula is inserted via a frontal twist drill hole. Next, the intracranial pressure can be measured, and then approximately 7 mL of air or 1 to 2 mL of metrizamide contrast is carefully exchanged for cerebrospinal fluid. Then the head is tilted from side to side, and a brow-up anteroposterior skull film in the Towne projection is obtained.[4]

Angiography

Cerebral angiography remains an option in the diagnosis of traumatic mass lesions when CT is not available. The most important role of angiography in head injury is the definitive demonstration of traumatic vascular lesions. Injuries to the extracranial carotid vessels may result in dissection, aneurysm formation, or both, with subsequent occlusion or embolization. Injuries to the intracranial vessels may result in occlusion or the formation of a traumatic arteriovenous fistula or aneurysm.[46] Traumatic vasospasm may also be demonstrated. Subdural, epidural, and large parenchymal hemorrhages can be localized using angiography.

Angiography is indicated when neurologic deficit is out of proportion to CT findings, when penetrating injuries occur in the region of the major intracranial vessels, when CT or clinical evaluations suggest the presence of an arteriovenous fistula, or when subarachnoid hemorrhage occurs prior to or following head injury. With advances in interventional radiology, the angiographer may now treat as well as diagnose many of these lesions, particularly carotid-cavernous sinus fistula.

Magnetic Resonance Imaging

Experience with magnetic resonance imaging (MRI) is limited, and its role in the treatment of acute head trauma has yet to be determined.[43] A number of technical factors would appear to limit the usefulness of MRI during acute injury. The length of time required for the study, the problems with motion artifacts, and the inability to have metallic objects (such as ventilators) in proximity to the scanner are all problems. In addition, at low–magnetic-field strengths, acute hemorrhage gives a signal that is isointense with that of brain.[42] Therefore, CT is currently more useful in the diagnosis of acute hemorrhage. MRI has promise in the evaluation of head trauma in the post-acute phase, where parenchymal changes such as edema can be clearly defined.

INTRACRANIAL PRESSURE

Normal Physiology

Normal intracranial pressure in the relaxed patient who is not hypotensive, hypercarbic, or hypoxic is 10 mm Hg or less. Elevations above this level are abnormal. Although pressure in the range of 10 to 15 mm Hg may occur with minor shifts of intracranial volume, when the pressures exceed 15 mm Hg, a major intracranial alteration has occurred (Fig. 1).

Measurement and Control

A common sequela of head injury is increased intracranial pressure. Therefore, the measurement and control of intracranial pressure are of primary importance in the management of patients following head injury. It has been established that elevations of intracranial pressure to 40 mm Hg and above consistently result in decreased cerebral blood flow and abnormal electrical activity of the brain and correlate with poor outcome.[31] It has been found that at about 20 mm Hg, compression of capillary beds begins to compromise cerebral microcirculation. Thus, capillary circulation may approach zero flow in areas of focal compression, edema, or injury. Early and aggressive treatment of mild intracranial hypertension may prevent later harmful and uncontrollable elevations.[40] Clearly, marked intracranial hypertension requires treatment. In addition, because it cannot be accurately

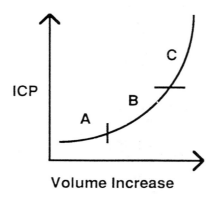

Volume Increase

FIGURE 1. An idealized depiction of the intracranial pressure–volume relationship showing the changes in intracranial pressure (ICP) occurring with the addition of volume (i.e., intravascular blood, cerebrospinal fluid (CSF), edematous brain, or hematoma) to the intracranial compartment. This curve defines the state of cerebral compliance. In segment *A,* following addition to intracranial volume, compensatory mechanisms, including displacement of CSF to the spinal compartment and collapse of intracranial venous channels, maintain intracranial pressure at near-normal levels. In segment *B,* the compensatory mechanisms begin to reach their limits, and there is inability to fully buffer even small additions of volume to the intracranial compartment. However, there is still some reserve because there can be further collapse of the venous channels and increased absorption of CSF. Segment *C* represents the final phase of decompensation with an elevated baseline intracranial pressure. The presence of progressive cerebrovascular vasomotor paralysis in this phase initially produces plateau waves associated with neurologic deterioration. Ultimately, sustained high elevations of intracranial pressure occur which are unresponsive to any treatment modality.

defined what a safe level is for a particular patient, even modest elevations should be treated.

Indications that intracranial pressure monitoring may be effective therapy arise from the improved outcome of patients with head injury treated at medical centers that monitor pressure, and a direct relationship has been demonstrated between highest level of intracranial pressure reached and mortality.[32,40] However, other clinicians have found that patients not monitored or patients that have received presumptive treatment with hyperventilation and periodic mannitol infusion irrespective of pressure readings have similar outcomes to those patients that are monitored.[45] Despite this ambiguity, it is well established that intracranial pressure monitoring is an important aid in the current management of head injury patients. Sole reliance on clinical deterioration to detect rising intracranial pressure is inadequate because of the variance between patients and delay in development of findings. Monitoring provides a means of detecting elevation early, and also criteria by which therapy can be employed and followed for patients who require it. Finally, intracranial pressure monitoring provides prognostic information because mortality correlates with the level of the intracranial pressure.[29]

Cerebral perfusion pressure (CPP) is defined as the difference between mean arterial blood pressure (^{m}ABP) and mean intracranial pressure (^{m}ICP):

$$CPP = {}^mABP - {}^mICP$$

This parameter describes the amount that the blood pressure exceeds the intracranial pressure and thus the perfusion pressure available to the brain. This pressure relates directly with cerebral blood flow. Recent clinical studies in multiple centers have defined a cerebral perfusion pressure of 60 to 70 mm Hg as the level that must be maintained for good outcome after head injury. Cell death begins at a cerebral perfusion pressure below about 40 mm Hg. Thus, both reduction of intracranial pressure and elevation or maintenance of arterial blood pressure can be used to achieve an adequate cerebral perfusion pressure.

Despite the importance of intracranial pressure monitoring, not all patients who are brought into the emergency room following head trauma should be monitored. This is because all of the available techniques to measure pressure are invasive and pose a certain risk. Therefore, criteria for selecting the patients at the greatest risk of developing intracranial hypertension should be established. One commonly employed method suggests that all adults with head injury and a score of 8 or less on the Glasgow Coma Scale should be monitored.[29] The most important contraindication to monitoring is the presence of abnormal hemostasis.

Techniques of Intracranial Pressure Monitoring

There are numerous devices available for the measurement of intracranial pressure. These are distinguished by the relative risks, reliability, sensitivity, cost, and the ease of insertion. For any device to be maximally effective, it must be able to make a hard copy of the pressure tracing. This allows one to detect trends and also to compare pressure at different periods of time.

The gold standard in terms of accuracy and sensitivity remains the ventricular catheter, which is coupled to a transducer or manometer. Other than occasionally becoming occluded, this technique is also very reliable. The catheter can be inserted at the bedside via a frontal twist drill hole.[29] The major advantage to this technique is that it allows drainage of cerebrospinal fluid from the ventricle for reduction of the intracranial-intraventricular pressure and also for analysis of the fluid. Fluid can also be removed from the ventricles to establish the compliance of the intracranial compartment, allowing one to plot the patient at a particular point on the intracranial pressure curve.[29] A drawback to this technique is the fact that it requires puncture of the brain. In addition, it may be difficult to insert the catheter into the ventricle if the ventricles are collapsed, shifted, or distorted. Despite these drawbacks, significant injury due to hemorrhage appears to be rare.[29] The most important risk of this method is the development of infection, which is seen with increasing frequency after a catheter has been left in place longer than 5 days.[1] Ventriculitis is the most likely infection, although meningitis and brain abscesses do occasionally occur. *Staphylococcus epidermidis* is the most common pathogen. However, many cases are due to gram-negative rods.[1] Insertion of the catheter under strict sterile technique reduces the incidence of infection, but prophylactic antibiotics have not been shown to be useful.[1]

Another method of measuring intracranial pressure is the subarachnoid bolt or screw. This device is usually placed into the subdural space via a twist-drill hole. This provides a fluid coupling from the brain surface, which acts as a sensing membrane, to a transducer.[49] This method avoids brain puncture and ventricular entrance, and therefore has a lower rate of hemorrhage and infection.[1] When infection does occur, it is superficial. Occlusion and inaccurate readings are the major difficulties with this method.[29] Sources of blockage include hemorrhage or an incompletely opened dura mater. Also, if the pia is lacerated, the brain can herniate into the bolt, causing occlusion. Inaccurate readings may arise when the bolt is not completely coplanar with the surface of the brain or if the bolt is inserted contralateral to the side of the lesion.

A third, and relatively new, device is the fiberoptic catheter (e.g., Camino catheter, Camino Laboratories, San Diego, CA). The tiny transducer head contains a membrane that, when distorted, causes the deflection of a mirror, attenuating a fiberoptically transmitted light beam.[3] This attenuation, detected by a sensor, provides a measure of the pressure on the transducer. This catheter is easily inserted via a small twist drill hole, and accurate readings are obtained regardless of whether the transducer is in the subdural space, brain parenchyma, or the ventricles. These catheters have the advantage that they do not require ventricular puncture, will not occlude, and are generally accurate. However, these devices are expensive, extremely fragile, and cannot be "zeroed" once in place, which can lead to incorrect intracranial pressure readings if the zero point drifts.

CEREBRAL BLOOD FLOW

Although relatively simple and inexpensive techniques are available for the determination of cerebral blood flow (CBF) and cerebral metabolism, these are not yet universally employed in monitoring patients following traumatic injury to the brain. Langfitt and Obrist[25] have defined several indications for clinical CBF studies. The first is to determine if CBF is adequate to meet the needs of cerebral metabolism. Although physiologic states such as coma can normally lead to a significant decrease in cerebral blood flow, there is still a certain amount of blood flow that must be maintained for the integrity of cells. Therefore, there is a threshold CBF for basic metabolism. These threshold values have not been exactly determined, and it is possible that the value is dependent on the individual circumstances. However, it seems that focal ischemia may occur immediately with a CBF of 7 mL/100 g/min, within 2 to 3 hours with a CBF of 10 to 12 mL/100 g/min, and with sustained CBF of 17 to 18 mL/100 g/min.[20]

A second indication for measuring CBF following severe head injury is to help predict outcome. The CBF, in addition to cerebral metabolic rate measurements and multimodality evoked potentials, seems to accurately predict outcome.[25]

CBF evaluations may also allow one to evaluate the responsiveness of the cerebral circulation by testing autoregulation and the responses to changing levels of the P_{CO_2} in the blood. One hypothesis suggests that these findings may be more indicative of outcome than the initial CBF measurements per se. Moreover, cerebrovascular reactivity may be closely linked to intracranial pressure changes.

Finally, CBF measurements may be used to evaluate various therapeutic regimens. If it is established that CBF is reduced to critical levels, certain therapeutic maneuvers (e.g., hypertensive therapy, volume expansion, and cerebral vasodilation) may be of benefit by increasing the CBF. These monitoring methods are more accurate than relying solely on the patient's neurologic status. It is likely that the beneficial therapy may have to be continued for a prolonged period before an improvement in clinical status is evident. Therefore, CBF monitoring may provide a basis for new interventions that will improve outcome after head trauma.

Normal Physiology

The intracranial arteries and their branches can be divided into the conduction system, resistance system, and exchange system. The conduction system consists of the large- and medium-sized arteries, most of which can be evaluated via angiography. Despite their name, these arteries constitute a larger portion of the vascular resistance to CBF than the other arterial systems. This stems from the fact that the cerebral arteries have long lengths compared to the lengths of the arterioles. The resistance system is formed by the arterioles, metarterioles, and thoroughfare channels. The arterioles function primarily in autoregulation because they have the ability to rapidly dilate and constrict. The metarterioles and thoroughfare channels contain the precapillary sphincters responsible for regulating the blood flow through the capillary beds. Vasomotion is an important physiologic property of these vessels. Vasomotion consists of regularly occurring series of partial constrictions and relaxations at intervals of 30 seconds to several minutes, which results in a waxing and waning of blood flow through capillary beds, producing complex hemodynamic changes in the microcirculation. Finally, the exchange of gases, nutrition, and metabolites takes place in the capillaries. Although capillaries are fairly numerous in the gray matter, they still pose a certain amount of resistance to flow due to their small size. Often, their diameter is less than the diameter of erythrocytes, thus requiring erythrocytes to deform while passing through the capillaries. Therefore, changes in erythrocyte deformability may result in resistance changes.

The maintenance of a disproportionately large and constant blood supply to the brain is essential because of the brain's high metabolic demand and its inability to store energy. Multiple mechanisms contribute to maintaining this blood supply. Global and regional CBF (reflecting both gray and white mater compartments) is about 50 to 55 mL/100 g brain tissue/min in the adult, with significantly higher values in those below 20 years of age and a decrease in those over 60 years.[19]

AUTOREGULATION

Metabolic autoregulation involves changes in vascular diameter produced by alteration in the energy demands of the cerebral tissue. Normally, there is a tight coupling between the demand of cerebral tissue for oxygen and glucose and the volume of blood flowing through that tissue, although for a number of years it was believed that the blood flow to the brain was stable under all conditions of activity. Measurement of CBF during a wide spectrum of activity, including intense mental activity, exercise, and sleep, has disclosed a remarkably stable level of blood flow. Only extreme changes in activity, such as those occurring in coma or seizure, produce appreciable changes in blood flow.[7] The introduction of techniques for the measurements of regional CBF in localized areas reveals a close relationship between regional blood flow and the activity of areas of the cerebral cortex. These methods provide convincing evidence that changes in activity of part of the brain are accompanied by appropriate changes in its blood flow.

The mechanisms by which metabolism influences CBF are still a matter of controversy. Although there is slight evidence that neuronal reflex mechanisms may be involved, it is more generally accepted that the release of vasodilating metabolites from the active nerve cell is responsible for the coupling between cerebral functional activity and metabolism on one hand, and cerebral vessel diameter and blood flow on the other. Promising candidates for responsible metabolites are adenosine and adenosine phosphorylated derivatives, potassium, hydrogen ion, calcium, and carbon dioxide. A reduction in tissue Po_2 may also contribute to vasodilation.

If the systemic arterial pressure is lowered or raised quickly, CBF falls or increases passively with changes in the arterial pressure, but blood flow normally returns to the control value within a few seconds. This ability to maintain a constant CBF over a wide physiologic range of arterial blood pressure is termed *autoregulation*. Below about 40 mm Hg diastolic, CBF will drop linearly with a drop in blood pressure because vasodilation is maximal. Above 140 mm Hg diastolic, CBF will rise because vasoconstriction is maximal (Fig. 2). When autoregulation is impaired but still present, the adjustment of blood flow is slower and less complete. When autoregulation is absent, blood flow passively follows changes in systemic arterial pressure. Thus, autoregulation is a quantitative, measurable variable in the control of the cerebral circulation and is not an all-or-nothing phenomenon.

Knowledge of the state of coupling or uncoupling between cerebral metabolism and CBF and an understanding of the mechanics of this coupling are important in the study and treatment of head injury. Vasodilation which can lead to increased intracranial pressure, may be metabolically appropriate, or may be physiologically unnecessary—the state known as hyperemia.

Methods for Measuring Cerebral Blood Flow

Intraarterial [133]Xe Method

The intraarterial (intracarotid) inert gas clearance method was introduced experimentally and elaborated for clinical application during the 1960s and 1970s. The introduction of ^{133}Xe, emitting high energies of γ-radiation enabled studies of CBF in humans under clinical conditions. Xenon is a freely diffusible tracer and as an inert gas does not take part in cerebral metabolism. When injected into an artery, it is eliminated very rapidly and almost completely through the lungs. Therefore, recirculation of the isotope and a second passage through the brain, which would influence the accuracy of measurement, can be disregarded.[23]

A bolus of the radioactive isotope ^{133}Xe is dissolved in saline and then injected through an indwelling catheter into the internal carotid artery. Ordinarily,

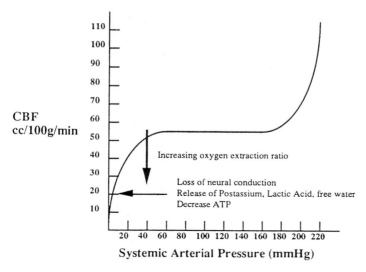

CBF cc/100g/min

Systemic Arterial Pressure (mmHg)

FIGURE 2. Cerebral blood flow (CBF) as a function of systemic arterial pressure. Maintenance of a constant CBF over a wide range of systemic arterial pressures is made possible by varying vessel caliber. Maximal vasoconstriction with precipitous rise in CBF occurs above 160 mm Hg. Maximal vasodilatation with precipitous drop in CBF and increasing O_2 extraction occurs below 40 to 50 mm Hg. ATP = adenosine triphosphate. (From Johnson DW, Stringer WA, Marks MP, et al: Stable xenon CT cerebral blood flow imaging: Rationale for and role in clinical decision making. *AJNR* 12:201–213, 1991; with permission.)

CBF studies are done on the hemisphere with the most evidence of brain damage. As the bolus of ^{133}Xe enters the intracranial circulation, the isotope diffuses rapidly throughout the brain tissue. Because the xenon is largely cleared from the body on circulation through the lungs, blood reaching the brain after the bolus injection is virtually free of the isotope. The clearance of ^{133}Xe from the cerebral tissue is recorded with multiple scintillation detectors mounted in a lead collimator block, which is placed adjacent to the patient's head.[23] The number of detectors can range from a few to more than 200, but 10 are commonly used.

When the isotope enters the cerebral circulation, there is an instantaneous rise in the γ-emission recorded by all detectors, and this constitutes the height of the CBF clearance curve. The number of counts diminishes over time, and the counts are recorded for an average of 10 to 15 minutes. CBF is then calculated as the ratio of height over area.[23] A good estimate of the blood flow can be obtained from the initial slope of the first 2 minutes of the clearance curve. Normally, the clearance curve contains two compartments, a fast-flow compartment, believed to represent blood flow to the gray matter, and a slow-flow compartment, thought to be blood flow to the white matter.[27] Toward the completion of the CBF study, the γ-emission from the brain approaches the background radioactivity in the study room, and another CBF study can be carried out, generally about half an hour after the initial study.

The major disadvantages of the intraarterial ^{133}Xe methodology are the need to cannulate the carotid artery to introduce the isotope and the fact that CBF is recorded from only one hemisphere. Because of the former, most investigators have concluded that CBF studies are justified only in patients who are undergoing carotid angiography for diagnostic purposes. However, with the advent of CT, the indications of cerebral angiography during the acute stages of injury have become limited. This means that the opportunities for measuring CBF with this technique have become extremely unusual. Fortunately, the development of noninvasive methodology for administering ^{133}Xe has permitted the continuation of studies of the cerebral circulation using this isotope.

Noninvasive Two-Dimensional [133]Xe Method

The noninvasive technique most widely used today is the inhalation methodology developed by Obrist et al.[36] and modified with introduction of the ^{133}Xe by intravenous injection, as recommended by Austin et al.[2] In the method of Muizelaar and Obrist,[33] a 30-mCi bolus of ^{133}Xe is injected intravenously or the patient is rebreathed during 1 minute with a gas mixture containing 10 mCi/L of ^{133}Xe, and then the radioactivity is monitored for 15 minutes by 16 scintillation detectors, 8 over each hemisphere.[33] Next, the clearance curves are subjected to a two-compartment computer analysis that corrects for the recirculation of the isotope based on the concentration of the isotope in the expired gas. This provides estimates of blood flow from fast-clearing and slow-clearing compartments.

Due to the instability of this compartmental analysis in patients with severe intracranial pathology, a second blood index (CBF_{15} or $CBF_{infinity}$) is also calculated.[33] This second blood index is relatively insensitive to compartmental shifts that occur following severe head injury. CBF_{15} and CBF_{inf} are mathematically equivalent to the height over area method of calculating blood flow in the intracarotid method. The difference between the CBF_{15} and the CBF_{inf} methods is that the former cuts off the tail of the washout curve at 15 minutes, thus neglecting the slowest clearing or recirculating compartments. The CBF_{15} method is more accurate at very high flows because the contribution of the very slow compartments becomes negligible. The CBF_{inf} method can be inaccurate at high flows because it may include the contribution of skin blood flow into its analysis. However, this method is very accurate at low flows.

Three-Dimensional Stable Xenon Technique

In addition to anatomic detail, cranial CT can be used to delineate brain function. The inhalation of a diffusible indicator, nonradioactive xenon, followed by CT scans obtained at approximately 1-minute intervals has been used to quantitate regional cerebral blood flow. Nonradioactive, or stable, xenon is an inert inorganic gas that freely moves across the blood brain barrier. There is a rapid entry and clearance of xenon from the brain that has been well characterized using radioactive xenon.[36] Because the atomic number of xenon is 54, and hence it is in the same group of elements on the periodic table as iodine, the density of the brain substance as monitored by CT scanning will increase if xenon is present in a sufficient concentration. Due to the fact that CT scanning is employed, this method has excellent anatomic specificity. The technique is also rapid, easily repeated, and, perhaps most importantly, widely available.

Like other methods that indirectly measure CBF, the stable xenon technique uses Kety's application of the Fick principle of indicator dilution, which relates the concentration of a freely diffusible nonmetabolized indicator absorbed in the tissue per unit time as the difference between the arterial and venous concentrations of the indicator.[19,21] In the case of stable xenon, one can directly quantitate the concentration in the brain by the CT scanner due to the element's radiodensity, making measurement of the venous concentration unnecessary. The brain xenon concentration at a given time is dependent on the arterial concentration of xenon, the brain blood flow, and the duration of exposure to xenon. These factors combine to determine the total amount of xenon presented to the brain. The amount of xenon in the brain is also dependent on the brain's affinity for xenon, which is measured by the blood-brain partition coefficient, lambda (λ).[19] This reflects the concentration of xenon in the blood and the brain at equilibrium.

Using these principles with many complicated computerized calculations, an image is obtained that is a map of CBF values with a full width at half-maximum resolution of about 4 mm. Depiction of the CBF map uses a gray scale of 0 to 100 mL/100 g/min.[19] Numeric values of flow can be obtained by placing voxels on the CBF map to obtain mean and standard deviations of flow. Owing to the inherent noise of the system, caution must be used in relying on numeric values from too small a voxel.

The main advantage of stable xenon CT is that it noninvasively provides relatively high-resolution, quantitative local CBF data coupled to CT anatomy. CBF studies can be repeated at 20-minute intervals, allowing for the evaluation of hemodynamic states as well as the response to therapeutic interventions. In addition, the widespread availability of CT scanners decreases the cost in implementing this technique. Current reconstruction time makes the information available for review within a short enough interval that therapeutic decisions can be made while the patient is still in the scanner.[19]

The radiation dose, pharmacologic effects of xenon gas, and limitations of area surveyed are three disadvantages of the xenon CT CBF technique. With current risk estimates, the amount of absorbed radiation yields a lifetime risk of from 1×10^{-4} to 1×10^{-5} that a member of the general population who undergoes this procedure will develop a radiation-related brain tumor.[19] Although this is a clinically acceptable level, the patient receives a dose of radiation that is not insignificant.

The pharmacologic properties of xenon are associated with a few problems. Xenon alters the sensorium of most individuals and may induce patient movement, but this can be minimized by careful prestudy positioning. Xenon has also been associated with minimal respiratory suppression.

SINGLE-PHOTON EMISSION COMPUTED TOMOGRAPHY (SPECT)

The SPECT method is based on single-photon tomography using a rotating γ-camera and ^{133}Xe inhalation. ^{33}Xe tomography for CBF measurement is based on the principles pioneered by Kuhl et al. in 1976.[24] The instrument used was developed with the specific aim of allowing dynamic studies, i.e., to record a series of 1-minute images of the isotope distribution in slices of brain tissue. It consists of four γ-cameras rotating at a fairly rapid speed close to the head. The instrument rotates at a constant speed and collects data in brief time intervals ($\frac{1}{8}$ second). Thus, in each time interval all four cameras record a projection of the isotope distribution in a 2-cm-thick slice of brain tissue.[26] Three slices of brain tissue are recorded simultaneously. Conventional filtering and back-projection techniques are used for reconstructing the isotope distribution in each slice. The ^{133}Xe is administered in a closed respiratory system of approximately 5 L in volume.

The raw data from a study consist of the lung curve (this curve is used to record the shape of the arterial input curve to the brain) and the three sequences

of tomographic images taken. Each sequence comprises four images averaging the
^{133}Xe concentration over the time intervals 0 to 1.5 minutes, 1.5 to 2.5 minutes,
2.5 to 3.5 minutes, and 3.5 to 4.5 minutes. The sum of the first two pictures is
called the "early picture."

CBF is calculated as described by Celsis et al. in 1981.[9] The calculation is
essentially the same as that used by Kety[21] in developing the autoradiographic
method for calculating CBF. In essence, many complicated calculations are
performed by the computer in order to form the final CBF map. There can be
error in this CBF map due to the Compton effect of photo scattering.[9]

An advantage to this method is that it is relatively atraumatic to the patient
and is easy to perform. In the routine clinical setting, the low cost of ^{133}Xe is
attractive. The cost per investigation is at the same level as performing routine CT
scans, due to the recycling of the radioactive substance.[26] As the instrument is
programmed for function, it can be run by a medical doctor or nurse after a brief
training period. The short duration of the study (4.5 minutes) is also advantageous.
Potential disadvantages include the effect of the xenon pharmacologically, the risk
of the radioactivity, the danger of Compton scattering, and the ability to obtain
only three image slices. Various studies have also been conducted using other
radioactive tracers, such as ^{123}I and ^{99m}Tc-hexametazime (HM-PAO).[38]

Transcranial Doppler Monitoring

Ultrasonic methods are of use in assessing the hemodynamics and morphology
of the blood vessels that supply the brain, where direct information on the circulation in the brain itself is not obtained. Ultrasound waves sent into the body are
reflected at interfaces, with arterial walls being particularly strong reflecting
interfaces. The reflections from the blood cells are significantly smaller than the
reflections from the walls, making it possible to depict the vessel walls as an image.
Two different methods are available to obtain information from the reflected
ultrasound: the pulse echo method for imaging vessels, and the Doppler method
for evaluating flow.

With the pulse echo method, short trains of pulses are sent in rapid sequence,
and in the intervals, the intensity and transit time of the reflected signals are
measured. The return time is a measure of the depth from which the signal is
reflected. A reflection is shown as a spot with varying brightness according to the
intensity of the reflection. Thus, this reflection provides a method for observing
structures such as vessels.

With the Doppler method, it is not the transit time of the reflected ultrasound
but the speed of the reflector in relation to the transmitter that is measured by
using the Doppler effect. If the reflector is approaching the transmitter-receiver,
then the received frequency is higher than the transmitted frequency. The
difference between the two is the Doppler frequency or shift, which is proportional
to the velocity of the blood cells and is dependent on the angle of insonation.[48]
This method can also be broken down into the continuous-wave and pulsed
Doppler method. With continuous-wave Doppler, the tip of the probe contains
separate transmitting and receiving crystals, which continuously transmit and
receive.[48] All particles that move contribute to the resulting sonogram measurement.
Thus, these measurements give no indication of the depth at which the measurement
is made. With pulsed Doppler, the instrument acts as a receiver during the
intervals between transmissions. With this method, the position and size of the
sample volume can be selected by means of electronic gating.[48]

Cervical Doppler ultrasonography has been used for some time to estimate intracranial circulatory arrest in brain death.[41] Recently, attempts have been made to apply transcranial Doppler in the confirmation of brain death.[34] However, these results are inconclusive: some patients exhibit the same pattern before and after brain death.[37] Also, the relationships between intracranial and extracranial arterial flow patterns on Doppler ultrasonograms of severely brain-damaged patients have not been clarified. Recent data suggest that post-traumatic cerebral vasospasm may contribute to cerebral dysfunction by inappropriately lowering CBF. This hypothesis is currently being studied.

Conclusions

Results from CBF measurements after severe head injury have been confusing in the past. Data now emerging reveal that the status of the cerebral vasculature can change quickly, especially shortly after the injury; therefore, every effort must be made to measure CBF consistently early and to state exactly when the measurements were performed. Furthermore, post-traumatic CBF and cerebral vascular activity may be more important than has been believed, especially because various forms of therapy have a great impact on CBF and cerebral blood volume. Simultaneous measuremens of cerebral O_2 metabolism (see later discussion) greatly help in understanding the underlying pathophysiologic measurements. However, there remains a need for measurements of brainstem blood flow, and new techniques must be developed for this.

CEREBRAL METABOLISM

Arteriovenous Oxygen Difference

Cerebral metabolism can be estimated by the measurement of the difference in oxygen content between cerebral arterial and venous blood. This can be determined by placing a catheter in jugular bulb, simultaneously sampling systemic arterial and jugular venous blood, and determining their oxygen contents.[35] It is possible to calculate the oxygen content by measuring the hemoglobin concentration and the O_2 saturation of the blood specimen. Then according to the Fick equation:

$$CMRO_2 = CBF \times AVDO_2$$

where $CMRO_2$ = cerebral metabolic rate for oxygen, CBF = cerebral blood flow, and $AVDO_2$ = cerebral arteriovenous oxygen difference.

Therefore, $AVDO_2$ reflects the adequacy of CBF relative to the metabolic requirements. As CBF falls below or rises above metabolic demands, the O_2 difference widens or narrows, respectively. The normal value of the $AVDO_2$ is 1.2 to 6.3 mL $O_2/100$ mL of blood.[14] Thus, knowing the $AVDO_2$ is more important than knowing the CBF alone because it indicates whether a particular level of CBF is adequate, excessive, or inadequate. This measurement provides information on the adequacy of cerebral metabolism. An additional advantage to this method is the ease with which it is performed. Furthermore, this technique has been refined with the advent of fiberoptic oximeter catheters to measure the O_2 content of the jugular venous and arterial blood directly and continuously.[11] Thus, with this method one can continuously monitor the CBF and adequacy of the flow for cerebral metabolism.

A limitation of these techniques is that they provide global measurement of cerebral O_2 extraction, and thus may not detect regional mismatch of flow and metabolism. However, clinical experience indicates that with diffuse injury, global, rather than regional, changes in CBF are more important.[35] Also, focal areas of ischemia or infarction may actually lead to a widening of cerebral $AVDO_2$. Another problem is that some areas, such as the brainstem and cerebellum, do not contribute to the venous drainage in the jugular bulb. Therefore, the $AVDO_2$ does not indicate the blood flow in those particular regions. Finally, the readings obtained for $AVDO_2$ with systemic alkalosis or acidosis are less reliable because of shifts in the oxyhemoglobin dissociation curve.[35]

Arteriovenous Glucose Difference

It is well documented that under physiologic conditions the brain oxidizes only glucose to obtain energy. When glucose has passed the blood-brain barrier, it is glycolytically metabolized to form pyruvate, 7% of which is normally converted to lactate, which is then released into the venous blood. Pyruvate is one of two precursors for acetylcholine synthesis.[18] Thus, the total amount of glucose taken up by the brain relates directly to the activity of glycolysis. In addition, the amount of lactate and pyruvate formation and the lactate-glucose index provide information on pyruvate oxidation. This information can be summated by the calculation of the glucose oxidation ratio, which may be calculated by[18]:

$$\frac{\text{Glucose} - \text{Lactate}}{\text{Oxygen}}$$

The uptake of glucose can be determined by measuring the difference in glucose concentration between the arterial blood and jugular venous blood. In addition, one can measure the lactate and pyruvate concentration in the venous blood. If the uptake of glucose is reduced but the metabolic rate of oxygen is still normal, it would be of great interest to investigate which substrates other than glucose are used oxidatively by the brain. Ketone bodies, amino acids, free fatty acids, and endogenous brain substrates are possible sources of energy metabolism (Table 1).

POSITRON-EMISSION TOMOGRAPHY

Positron-emission tomography (PET) allows the imaging of the spatial distribution of a radiolabeled pharmaceutical agent within the human brain and other organs.[8] The goal of PET is to provide insights into the biologic function of the imaged organ. Thus, PET strategies hinge on choosing radiolabeled compounds capable of tracing specific biologic processes, as well as appropriate mathematical

TABLE 1. Mean values $\pm$ SD of Some Cerebral Metabolic Measurements*

Cerebral blood flow (CBF)	52.9 $\pm$ 4.9 mL/100 g/min
Cerebral metabolic rate of oxygen ($CMRO_2$)	3.54 $\pm$ 0.42 mL/100 g/min
Cerebral metabolic rate of CO_2	3.77 $\pm$ 0.51 mL/100 g/min
Cerebral metabolic rate of glucose	4.97 $\pm$ 0.75 mL/100 g/min
Cerebral metabolic rate of lactate	0.36 $\pm$ 0.22 mL/100 g/min
Cerebral respiratory quotient	1.06 $\pm$ 0.09
Lactate/glucose index	0.07 $\pm$ 0.01
Glucose oxidation ratio	1.34 $\pm$ 0.17

* Adapted from Hoyer S: The young adult and normally aged brain: Its blood flow and oxidative metabolism: A review part I. *Arch Gerontol Geriatr* 1:195–207, 1982.

models with which to interpret the quantitative behavior of tracers in physiologic terms. Thus, although PET yields tomographic images, it is not primarily an anatomic but rather a physiologic method. PET derives its particular powers from (1) the nature of the labeled compounds that may be employed and (2) the advantages afforded to tomographic reconstruction. Labeled fluorodeoxyglucose (^{18}FDG) which traces cerebral glucose distribution has been the most commonly employed PET marker, giving data on regional blood flow and glucose metabolism.

To date, the greatest value of PET lies in the capacity of this technique to make regional measurements of multiple physiologic variables in the human brain. The ^{15}O-steady-state technique is a well-established method for measuring regional CBF, oxygen extraction ratio, and cerebral oxygen metabolic rate by PET. Reliable quantitation requires attenuation correction by means of a ring source transmission scan and correction of the oxygen extraction ratio data for the effects of unextracted $^{15}O_2$ in the blood volume compartment.[15] The technique is not difficult to apply but requires cooperative patients and considerable attention to detail at all stages. Analysis of the relationships between different variables has consistently provided more valuable information than their absolute values considered in isolation.

ELECTROPHYSIOLOGIC MONITORING

Since the development of the clinical electroencephalogram (EEG), neurophysiologic techniques have been used for multiple purposes in the post-traumatic head-injured population. Initial expectations of the EEG for prognostic information were not met because studies failed to show significant correlations between the routine EEG and outcome of post-traumatic coma. With the advent of CT scanning, the usefulness of the routine EEG in acute stages further decreased. However, new methods of analyzing the EEG and other neurophysiologic techniques have been developed. Long-term monitoring, computer-aided EEG analysis using compressed spectral arrays and other display techniques, and evoked potentials (EPs) have demonstrated significant value in the management and prognostication of head-injured patients. With the development of more sophisticated tests, as well as new uses for those already established, clinical neurophysiologic testing will have increasing utility in the head-injured population.

Electroencephalography

There have been several reviews of the routine EEG in traumatic brain injury.[44] The EEG in the acute post-traumatic period shows greater correlation with the clinical state than it does in the chronic phase,[44] with changes observed in the acute stages after head injury divided into focal and generalized abnormalities.

Focal EEG abnormalities consist of slowing, voltage attenuation, and various types of paroxysmal activity, including paroxysmal lateralized epileptiform discharges.[44] Focal abnormalities may be transient and insignificant or secondary to structural brain injury. Whereas focal brain lesions usually produce an abnormal EEG pattern, it has no etiologic specificity. For example, EEG patients with subdural hematomas may show no EEG changes, generalized slowing, focal slowing, or focal voltage attenuation so that the EEG is of little use in ruling out this entity.[44] Therefore, in the CT scan era, the EEG is of little value in the diagnosis of focal brain injuries, unless complicated by seizures.

Generalized EEG abnormalities found in the acute post-traumatic state can be divided according to the predominant frequencies, voltages, and the degree of variability in the EEG. The most common findings are voltage reduction or slowing, both of which are nonspecific concomitants of brain injury. Voltage reduction is frequently found in patients who have a concussion.[44] Slowing of the EEG, like voltage attenuation, is usually seen after head trauma and does not reflect the degree of permanent cerebral damage. Age is also a consideration; for example, children often develop more marked changes in their EEG than adults after head injury of similar severity.[44]

Another generalized pattern occasionally seen is the "burst-suppression" EEG, whose presence in the traumatically brain-injured group usually implies coexisting hypoxic brain damage or drug intoxication.[44] If there are no drugs present, the occurrence of this pattern connotes a poor prognosis because of the associated diffuse anoxic encephalopathy.[39]

The routine EEG is useful in detecting both focal and generalized paroxysmal activity. Clinical seizures, although unusual in the immediate post-traumatic period, probably occur in 5% of the cases.[5] The presence of seizure activity, including status epilepticus, is generally associated with severe cerebral injury and carries a worsened prognosis except in children.[44] Subclinical, purely electroencephalographic seizures may also occur, although less frequently, and may imply an even worse prognosis.[39] With the advent of monitoring in neurologic intensive care units and the increasing use of muscle relaxants, the apparent incidence of subclinical seizures appears to be rising. Monitoring patients for the presence of these seizures, and then treating them when recognized is important because they may cause further neural injury directly or indirectly by causing a rise in intracranial pressure or an increased metabolic demand.[28] Although the EEG may be important for identifying seizures in the acute period, it has little value in predicting which patient will develop post-traumatic epilepsy.[28]

With the large amount of data involved in long-term monitoring, and the need for presentation of the data in a readable format, the use of computer-assisted analysis, using the compressed spectral array and other similar techniques has been necessitated. This recording method has been shown to be of some value as a prognostic device. In one study, approximately 95% of patients whose compressed spectral arrays were slow and monotonous had unfavorable outcomes, as contrasted with 30% of patients with changeable compressed spectral arrays.[6] The compressed spectral arrays can also assess the dominant EEG frequencies and their distribution better than a conventional study, and these may have some prognostic value. Bricolo et al. found worse outcomes among patients who had significant interhemispheric amplitude asymmetries using compressed spectral arrays.[6]

Evoked Potentials

Over the past 10 years, evoked potentials have demonstrated significant clinical value as a neurophysiologic method for assessing multiple sensory pathways. Short-latency evoked potentials are useful because of the close relationship between the evoked potential waveforms and specific anatomic structures. This specificity allows localization of conduction defects to within a few centimeters. Neurophysiologic assessment of sensory pathways is important in the head-injured patient because of the loss of subjective responses, either because of coma or the use of muscle relaxants or barbiturates. In addition, these evoked potentials are very resistant to alteration by anything other than structural pathology in the sensory pathways. For example, barbiturate doses sufficient to cause the EEG to go flat do not significantly affect short-latency evoked potentials.

Thus, short-latency evoked potentials are effacious in the post-traumatic brain-injured population, where they can be used for physiologic monitoring of comatose patients, for locating the lesions more precisely, and for helping determine prognosis.

BRAINSTEM AUDITORY EVOKED POTENTIALS

Brainstem auditory evoked potentials (BAEPs) consist of up to seven scalp-recorded waves occurring within the first 10 ms after a brief intra-aural click stimulus. The first five waves are generated in the brainstem auditory structures from the eighth nerve up to the inferior colliculus. The last two waves are presumed to arise from more rostral levels. Brainstem auditory evoked potentials are thus capable of localizing brainstem pathology.[10] In head-injured patients, BAEPs also have been helpful in predicting outcome, and BAEP abnormalities correlate with the level of the coma determined clinically.[47] Normal or mildly abnormal BAEPs have less prognostic significance than markedly abnormal ones. In one study, all patients had unfavorable outcomes if their BAEP contained only one wave or no waves in the absence of a peripheral auditory lesion.[47] One difficulty with using the BAEPs following head injury is that peripheral auditory structures may be damaged in serious head injury.

SOMATOSENSORY EVOKED POTENTIALS

Somatosensory evoked potentials (SSEPs) are elicited following electrical stimulation of a large peripheral nerve, usually the median nerve. The waveforms recorded within the first 25 ms after stimulation are generated in the brachial plexus, lower medulla, thalamus, and primary sensory cortex. Because SSEPs are elicited by peripheral nerve stimulation, it is essential to ensure that the stimulus is reaching the brainstem in order to eliminate a peripheral nerve or spinal cord lesion as the cause of the abnormal SSEP. De la Torre et al.[12] attempted to correlate the SSEPs with outcome from post-traumatic coma in 17 patients. The 4 patients who had good outcomes had eight defined peaks within 300 ms following the stimulus, whereas the 12 patients with poor outcomes had fewer than six SSEP peaks within 500 ms. Therefore, SSEPs seem to have some value in predicting outcome following brain injury.

VISUAL EVOKED POTENTIALS

The visual evoked potential (VEPs) produced by strobe stimulation contains poorly reproducible waves that presumably arise from the visual cortex. Strobe-evoked VEPs have not been studied as much as BAEPs and SSEPs in the head-injured population, in part due to the variability of the response. Although VEPs may not be as helpful as the other tests in predicting the outcome of the post-traumatic patient, Feinsod and Auerbach[13] have stated that this is a good method of assessing visual system continuity in a comatose patient. They used a combination of electroretinograms and VEPs, and found the localization of the visual pathway defect thus obtained to be helpful in predicting visual function and potentially helpful in patient management.

MULTI-MODALITY EVOKED POTENTIALS

Multimodality evoked potentials pool the results of all three evoked potentials to create an overall grading system. Some researchers have attempted to improve on the prognostic abilities of the evoked potentials by combining the results of each of the single-modality evoked potentials and obtaining an overall rating value. Greenberg et al.[16] used the VEP, SSEP, BAEP, and auditory evoked potentials. Each evoked potential of 51 comatose head-injured patients was graded into four levels, depending on the degree of abnormality (I, almost normal to IV, most abnormal with no waves originating within or above the level of the brainstem). This was determined primarily by counting the number of waveforms in the first 200 ms poststimulus for the SSEP, the first 300 ms for the VEP, and the first 400 ms for the auditory evoked potential. Among all patients who had grade I or II multimodality evoked potentials (MMEPs), 80% became responsive within 30 days. Seventy-six percent of the patients graded into groups III and IV had a severe disability, remained in a vegetative state, or died. All of the patients in group IV had a poor outcome[17] Overall MMEP grades, obtained by taking the poorest grade of the four individual ones, correctly predicted outcome at 1 year in 80% of the patients. This was slightly better than all the other clinical factors, and the accuracy could be slightly improved by combining the MMEP results with those factors or by eliminating from the analysis patients who died from non-CNS causes. Another conclusion was that the time to ultimate recovery correlated with the MMEPs. Patients who had grade I responses reached maximum recovery within 3 to 6 months, whereas patients who had grade II to III responses did not reach maximum recovery for up to 1 year. Therefore, the MMEPs appear to be an effective prognostic tool following head injury.

CONCLUSIONS

Clinical neurophysiology has a significant though not yet completely defined role in the post-traumatic head-injured population. The three potential uses are as (1) an aid to diagnosis and localization of CNS injuries; (2) a tool for monitoring CNS function in the unresponsive patients, both acutely and chronically; and (3) a factor to help in predicting the overall outcome and modality-specific outcome.

REFERENCES

1. Aucoin PJ, Kotilainen HR, Gantz NM, et al: Intracranial pressure monitors: Epidemiologic study of risk factors and infection. Am J Med 80:369–376, 1986.
2. Austin G, Horn N, Rouhe S, et al: Description and early results of an intravenous radioisotope technique for measuring regional cerebral blood flow in man. Eur Neurol 8:43–51, 1972.
3. Becker DP, Gade GF, Young HF, Feuerman TF: Diagnosis and treatment of head injury in adults. In Youmans JR (ed): Neurological Surgery, 3rd ed. Philadelphia, WB Saunders, 1990, pp 2017–2148.
4. Becker DP, Vries JK, Sakalas R, et al: Early prognosis in head injury based on motor posturing, oculocephalic reflexes and intracranial pressure. In McLaurin RL (ed): Head Injuries: Second Symposium on Neural Trauma. New York, Grune & Stratton, 1976, pp 27–30.
5. Bricolo A: Electroencephalography in neurotraumatology. Clin Electroencephalogr 7:184–197, 1976.
6. Bricolo A, Turazzi S, Faccioli F, et al: Clinical application of compressed spectral array in long term EEG monitoring of comatose patients. Electroencephalogr Clin Neurophysiol 45:211–225, 1978.
7. Brodersen P, Paulson OB, Bolwig TG, et al: Cerebral hyperemia in electrically induced epileptic seizures. Arch Neurol 28:334–338, 1973.
8. Brownell GL, Budinger TF, Lauterbur PL, McGeer PL: Positron tomography and nuclear magnetic resonance imaging. Science 215:619–626, 1982.
9. Celsis P, Goldman T, Henriksen L, et al: A method for calculating regional cerebral blood flow from emission computed tomography of inert gas concentrations. J Comput Assist Tomogr 5:641–645, 1981.
10. Chiappa KH, Ropper AH: Evoked potential in clinical medicine. N Engl J Med 306:1140–1150; 1205–1211, 1982.

11. Cruz J, Miner ME: Modulating cerebral oxygen delivery and extraction in acute traumatic coma. In Miner ME, Wagner KA (eds): Neurotrauma: Treatment, Rehabilitation, and Related Issues. Boston, Butterworth, 1986, pp 55–72.
12. De La Torre JC, Trimble JL, Beard RT, et al: Somatosensory evoked potentials for the prognosis of coma in humans. Exp Neurol 60:304–317, 1978.
13. Feinsod M, Auerbach E: Electrophysiological examinations of the visual system in the acute phase after head injury. Eur Neurol 9:56–64, 1973.
14. Finnerty FA, Witkin L, Fazekas J: Cerebral hemodynamics during cerebral ischemia induced by acute hypotension. J Clin Invest 33:1227–1237, 1954.
15. Frackowiak RSJ, Lenzi GL, Jones T, Heather JD: Quantitative measurement of regional cerebral blood flow and oxygen metabolism in man using ISO and positron emission tomography: Theory, procedure, and normal values. J Comput Assist Tomogr 4:727–736, 1980.
16. Greenberg RP, Mayer DJ, Becker DP, Miller JD: Evaluations of brain function in severe human head trauma with multimodality evoked potentials: Part 1 and Part 2. J Neurosurg 47:150–177, 1977.
17. Greenberg RP, Newlon PG, Hyatt MS, et al: Prognostic implications of the early multimodality evoked potentials in severely head injured patients. J Neurosurg 55:227–236, 1981.
18. Hoyer S: The young adult and normally aged brain: Its blood flow and oxidative metabolism. A review part I. Arch Geront Geriatr 1:195–207, 1982.
19. Johnson DW, Stringer WA, Marks MP, et al: Stable xenon CT cerebral blood flow imaging: Rationale for and role in clinical decision making. Am J Neuroradiol 12:201–213, 1991.
20. Jones TH, Morawetz RB, Cromwell RM, et al: Threshold of focal cerebral ischemia in awake monkeys. J Neurosurg 54:773–782, 1981.
21. Kety SS: The theory and applications of the exchange of inert gas at the lungs and tissues. Pharmacol Rev 3:1–41, 1951.
22. Kobayashi S, Nakazawa S, Otsuka T: Clinical value of serial computed tomography with severe head injury. Surg Neurol 20:25–29, 1983.
23. Kohlmeyer K: The intraarterial xenon-133 method: Principles and clinical application. In Hartmann A, Hoyer S (eds): Cerebral Blood Flow and Metabolism Measurement. New York, Springer-Verlag, 1985, pp 1–18.
24. Kuhl DE, Edwards RQ, Ricci AR: The Mark IV system for radionuclide computed tomography of the brain. Radiology 121:405–413, 1976.
25. Langfitt TW, Obrist WD: Cerebral blood flow and metabolism after intracranial trauma. Prog Neurol Surg 10:14–48, 1981.
26. Lassen NA: Cerebral blood flow tomography using xenon-133 inhalation—methodological considerations. In Hartmann A, Hoya S (eds): Cerebral Blood Flow and Metabolism Measurements. New York, Springer-Verlag, 1985, pp 224–233.
27. Laurent JP, Lawner P, Simeone FA, et al: Pentobarbital changes compartmental contribution to cerebral blood flow. J Neurosurg 56:504–510, 1982.
28. Marierme J, Robert G, Bagnat E: Post-traumatic acute rise of ICP related to subclinical epileptic seizures. Acta Neurochir Suppl 28:89–92, 1979.
29. Marshall LF, Marshall SB: Medical management of intracranial pressure. In Cooper PR (ed): Head Injury, 2nd ed. Baltimore, Williams & Wilkins, 1987, pp 177–196.
30. Masters SJ, McClean PM, Arcarese JS, et al: Skull x-ray examinations after head trauma: Recommendations by a multidisciplinary panel and validation study. N Engl J Med 316:87–91, 1987.
31. Miller JD, Becker DP, Ward JD, et al: Significance of intracranial hypertension in severe head injury. J Neurosurg 47:501–516, 1977.
32. Miller JD, Butterworth JF, Gudeman SK, et al: Further experience in the management of severe head injury. J Neurosurg 54:289–299, 1981.
33. Muizelaar JP, Obrist WD: Cerebral blood flow and brain metabolism with brain injury. In Becker DP, Povlishock JT (eds): Central Nervous System Trauma: Status Report. Bethesda, MD, National Institute of Communicative Disorders and Stroke, 1985, pp 123–138.
34. Newell DW, Grady MS, Sirotta P, Winn HR: Evaluation of brain death using transcranial Doppler. Neurosurgery 24:509–513, 1989.
35. Obrist WD, Langfitt TW, Jaggi JL, et al: Cerebral blood flow measurement and metabolism in comatose patients with acute brain injury: Relationship to intracranial hypertension. J Neurosurg 61:241–253, 1984.
36. Obrist WD, Thompson HK, Wang HS, et al: Regional cerebral blood flow estimated by [133]xenon inhalation. Stroke 6:245–256, 1975.
37. Powers AD, Graeber MC, Smith RR: Transcranial ultrasonography in the determination of brain death. Neurosurgery 24:884–889, 1989.

38. Roper SN, Mena I, King WA, et al: An analysis of cerebral blood flow in acute closed-head injury using technetium-99m-HMPAO SPECT and computed tomography. J Nucl Med 32:1684–1687, 1991.
39. Rumpl E: Cranio-cerebral trauma. In Niedermeyer E, Lopes da Silva F (eds): Electroencephalography: Basic Principles, Clinical Application and Related Fields. Baltimore, Urban & Schwarzenberg, 1982, pp 291–304.
40. Saul TG, Ducker TB: Effect of intracranial pressure monitoring and aggressive treatment on mortality in severe head injury. J Neurosurg 50:498–503, 1982.
41. Shiogai T, Sato E, Tokitsu M, et al: Transcranial Doppler monitoring in severe brain damage: Relationships between intracranial haemodynamics, brain dysfunction and outcome. Neurol Res 12:205–213, 1990.
42. Sippomen JT, Sippomen RE, Sivula A: Nuclear magnetic resonance imaging of intracerebral hemorrhage in the acute and resolving phase. J Comput Assist Tomogr 7:954–959, 1983.
43. Snow RB, Zimmerman RE, Gandy SE, Deck MD: Comparison of magnetic resonance imaging and computed tomography in the evaluation of head injury. Neurosurgery 18:45–52, 1986.
44. Stockard JJ, Bickford RG, Aung MH: The electroencephalogram in traumatic brain injury. In Vinken PJ, Bruyn GW (eds): Handbook of Clinical Neurology: Vol 23. Injuries of the Brain and Skull. New York, Elsevier, 1975, pp 317–367.
45. Stuart GG, Merry GS, Smith JA, Yelland JDM: Severe head injury managed without intracranial pressure monitoring. J Neurosurg 59:601–605, 1983.
46. Tsai FY, Teal JS, Hieshima GB: Neuroradiology of Head Trauma. Baltimore, University Park Press, 1984, pp 201–242.
47. Uziel A, Benezech J, Lorenzo S, et al: Clinical applications of brain stem auditory evoked potentials in comatose patients. In Courjon J, Mauguiere F, Revol M (eds): Clinical Applications of Evoked Potentials in Neurology. New York, Raven Press, 1982, pp 195–202.
48. von Reuter GM, Kapp H: The capabilities of ultrasonic diagnostic procedures in cerebrovascular disease. In Hartman A, Hoyer S (eds): Cerebral Blood Flow and Metabolism Measurement. New York, Springer-Verlag, 1985, pp 546–555.
49. Vries JK, Becker DP, Young HF: A subarachnoid screw for monitoring intracranial pressure: Technical note. J Neurosurg 39:416–419, 1973.

BARRY I. LUDWIG, MD

POST-TRAUMATIC SEIZURES

From the
Brain Injury Unit
Daniel Freeman Memorial Hospital
Inglewood, California

Correspondence to:
Barry I. Ludwig, MD
301 N. Prairie Avenue
Inglewood, CA 90301

Traumatic brain injury (TBI) is a major cause of neurologic impairment and disability and causes about 500,000 individuals to be hospitalized yearly in the United States.[16,37,38] About 15% of these injuries are severe,[16] and most are associated with varying degrees and combinations of physical, cognitive, psychological, and behavioral disorders. Post-traumatic epilepsy (PTE) is a common sequela of TBI that further increases the patient's morbidity and social handicap and decreases his or her quality of life. Many individuals who make otherwise good or excellent recoveries may be rendered severely disabled due to PTE. The overall incidence of PTE is approximately 5%, but that percentage markedly rises commensurate with the severity of the trauma. It is estimated that between 5,000 and 30,000 individuals with head injuries develop PTE each year in the United States[2,27,28,35]; however, in attempting to ascertain precise incidence figures, one encounters a bewildering array of statistics arising from the variable populations studied (civilian versus military), inconsistent definitions of head trauma and seizures, especially in the older literature, varied duration of follow-up, and inconstant hospital admission criteria and study inclusion parameters. Therefore, wide variations in these figures abound.

Regarding the classification of post-traumatic seizures, there is a general consensus that *early* seizures, or those commencing within the first post-traumatic week, should be differentiated from those beginning sometime thereafter, or *late* seizures, because their prognoses differ.

EARLY SEIZURES

In both civilian and military studies, seizures following a TBI are much more frequent in the first post-traumatic week than in any subsequent week.[36] These early attacks result from an acute, localized cerebral insult or disruption, or from the highly irritating effect that blood has on the cerebral cortex. An early attack is regarded as a reaction to the acute lesion but does not necessarily denote a chronic disorder and should correctly not be considered a form of epilepsy.

In civilian studies, *early* seizures are reported to occur in 1.5 to 15% of brain-injured patients,[42,48] this marked disparity resulting from variable case selection and definitions. In the community-based study of Annegers et al.,[2] which followed a cohort of 2,747 patients for 28,176 person-years, early seizures occurred in 2.1%. With a severe head injury, the risk rose to 30.5% in children and 10.3% in adults. Jennett and Teasdale[36] found the rate to be 5% in those admitted to a hospital with a nonmissile head injury, and that figure is essentially the same in military studies, which comprise a large proportion of cases with penetrating wounds.[14]

Fifty percent of early attacks occur in the first 24 hours, and, of these, one-half occur in the first post-traumatic hour.[35] About two-thirds of those who have seizures have more than one early episode, and 10% develop status epilepticus.[35] Early seizures are more commonly observed in children than in adults, and the younger the child, the more likely the occurrence.[26] In fact, in young children, seizures may follow a relatively trivial traumatic event.[10,36] In one study, the overall frequency of early seizures was 5% in those aged 15 years or younger, 7% in those younger than 5 years, and 17% in those with a TBI in the first year of life.[29] Status epilepticus is more common in children as well, especially in those younger than 5 years, in whom the incidence approaches 20%.[36]

Factors that place one at risk for the development of an early seizure are presented in Table 1. These are generally considered to include presence of an intracranial hematoma, focal neurologic signs, post-traumatic amnesia for more than 24 hours, depressed skull fracture, and injury before the age of 5.[34]

The major implication of an early seizure is its correlation with the development of late epilepsy, particularly in adults with moderate or severe injuries. This does not appear to be the case in children, however. In fact, most authors believe that a child who experiences an early seizure, without manifesting other risk factors, is in no or little danger of developing late epilepsy.[2,10,21,29,36,48]

LATE SEIZURES

Late seizures follow a dormant period of variable duration during which structural and physiologic changes occur at both a cellular and regional level. These epileptogenic alterations seem to occur most readily if the pathologic process destroys some neurons while leaving others intact.[21] Structural reorganization and synaptic integration within the disrupted neuronal aggregate ensues, and inhibitory mechanisms may be locally disrupted. This predisposes the patient to neuronal hyperexcitability and synchronization of firing that ultimately leads to spontaneous and recurrent ictal events or *epilepsy.*

TABLE 1.   Risk Factors for Early Seizures

Intracranial hematoma	Depressed skull fracture
Focal neurologic signs	Injury before age 5
Post-traumatic amnesia >24 hours	Penetrating head injury

The exact incidence of late seizures varies generally from 5% in civilian studies to 33 to 50% in military studies,[53,63] the latter figures reflecting a larger percentage of severe injuries. About 5 to 15% of patients with closed-head injuries (nonpenetrating) in military studies develop late epilepsy.[39]

In the report of Annegers et al.,[2] the risk of developing late seizures after a severe injury was 7.1% at 1 year and 11.5% at 5 years. The risk after a moderate head injury, at 1 and 5 years, was 0.7% and 1.6%, and that for a minor injury was 0.1% and 0.6%, respectively. Those statistics for minor injuries are, therefore, no different from the uninjured population at large.

It is important to recognize that a first late spontaneous seizure may occur up to 10 years or longer after a closed-head injury[34]; however, the annual risk decreases dramatically after the first year. In Jennett's seminal study of subjects with nonmissile injuries,[34] 56% of all who were to experience PTE did so in the first year, with about half of these beginning within the first 3 months. That percentage increased to 69% at the end of the second post-traumatic year, 77% at the end of the third year, and 85% at the conclusion of the fifth year. A similar study by Caveness et al.[14] found that 80% of those developing PTE did so by the end of the second post-traumatic year. Anneger et al.[2] established that by the fifth post-traumatic year, the annual incidence of PTE was the same as in the general population.

In military studies, the cumulative incidence of PTE has remained at about 33% during World War I, World War II, and the Korean and Vietnam conflicts,[31,48] despite clearly improved early care of open injuries, a decreased rate of infection,[36] and the use of prophylactic anticonvulsants in Vietnam.[14] The incidence of PTE in Israeli soldiers injured in the Labanese conflict and followed up for 6 years was somewhat lower, at 22%.[7] This may reflect less aggressive debridement techniques or a methodologic artifact. In another study of 421 veterans who had sustained a penetrating brain wound, 53% had seizures (including early and late attacks— about 50% late), and in 57% of those, attacks began within 1 year of injury.[53] In over 18% (8.3% of all with penetrating wounds), the first attack occurred more than 5 years after the injury, and 7% of those who were to develop PTE had their first episode 10 or more years following the inciting injury.[53] Weiss et al.,[62] reporting on the same cohort numbering 520, acknowledged that patients were at increased risk up to 10 to 15 years after the traumatic event, but noted that by using a predictive formula, based on time elapsed after injury and presence or absence of specific clinical and computed tomographic risk factors, most could be 95% certain of avoiding epilepsy if they had been seizure free for 3 years after the trauma.

Factors that predispose one to *late* epilepsy and their approximate cumulative risk are shown in Table 2. These factors include penetrating head injuries (33 to 50%)[36,53,62] and intracranial hematoma (25–35%), with intracerebral clots being more significant than subdural hematomas, and these, in turn, being more causally related to seizures than epidural clots.[33,36] Additional risk factors are early seizure (25%) and depressed skull fracture (15%), with the precise risk of the latter varying from 3 to 70%, depending on the presence, absence, or combinations of early epilepsy, focal findings, dural tear, or post-traumatic amnesia for more than 24 hours.[36] Whether the duration of coma or post-traumatic amnesia is an independent variable is less certain. Jennett and Teasdale[36] note that post-traumatic amnesia of more than 24 hours is of importance only if there is an associated early seizure; otherwise, the risk of late epilepsy is on the order of 1.5%. Similarly, De Santis et al.[17a] believe that alteration of consciousness, even if prolonged and severe, is

TABLE 2.   Risk Factors for Late Seizures

Penetrating head injury (33–50%)*
Intracranial hematoma (25–35%)
Early seizure (25%)
Depressed skull fracture (3–70%)[†]
     Early seizure
     Focal deficit
     Dural tear
     Post-traumatic amnesia >24 hours
Prolonged coma or post-traumatic amnesia (35%)[‡]

* Percentages in parentheses represent approximate cumulative risk for developing post-traumatic seizures.
[†] Precise risk varies with presence, absence, or combinations of the additional four factors.
[‡] Possibly only a significant risk factor if associated with an early seizure or focal lesion.

not a risk factor unless it is associated with a focal lesion. Guidice,[25] on the other hand, observed a direct correlation between occurrence of PTE and duration of coma, the incidence being 35% among individuals in coma for 3 weeks or longer.

Other factors that play a probable role in the genesis of PTE include the extent and location of the lesion or lesions.[13,21] Salazar et al.[53] noted that the risk of epilepsy in an individual sustaining a gunshot wound to the head was directly related to total brain volume loss, as seen on computed tomographic scanning, as well as early evidence of hematoma and retained metal fragments. They also noted that specific clinical features, such as hemiparesis, aphasia, organic mental disorder, or visual field loss correlated with PTE, and, in fact, the incidence of PTE was as high as 86% in those with residual aphasia. Others have demonstrated that damage to regions adjacent to the central sulcus or to more than one lobe of the brain increases the likelihood of seizures.[36,48] Russell and Whitty[52] have emphasized the particular importance of injury to the parietal lobe in this regard. The presence of bone fragments within lacerated brain tissue may also be an important etiologic factor.[4] Genetic predisposition may play an important contributory role as well, in that the incidence of a family history of epilepsy in those with late post-traumatic seizures is 6 to 17%, as contrasted with only 3 to 4% of those without ictal episodes.[34]

POST-TRAUMATIC SEIZURE TYPES

Seizures are classified according to the scheme established by the International League against Epilepsy,[15] and a condensed version of this is presented in Table 3. In essence, they are divided into two major types: partial and generalized. The former originate within a localized area of one hemisphere and are accompanied by focal electroencephalographic (EEG) abnormalities, whereas generalized seizures are characterized by clinical and EEG evidence of bilateral, simultaneous involvement of all or large portions of both cerebral hemispheres from the onset. Partial seizures can be further subdivided into simple and complex forms, the distinguishing feature being the clouding of consciousness that accompanies partial complex attacks. Simple partial seizures may have associated motor, sensory, autonomic or psychic symptoms, and depending on the pattern of electrical spread, may evolve into partial complex or secondarily generalized (grand mal) patterns. Generalized seizures are subclassified into absence, myoclonic, clonic, tonic, atonic, and tonic-clonic varieties, depending on the presence or absence of different varieties of convulsive movements. Generalized tonic-clonic (grand mal type) seizures may thus be generalized from the onset (primary generalized) or

TABLE 3.   Classification of Seizures

Partial seizures
   Simple partial seizures (consciousness preserved)
      With motor signs (jacksonian, adversive)
      With somatosensory or special sensory symptoms
      With autonomic symptoms or signs
      With psychic symptoms
   Complex partial seizures (consciousness impaired)
      Simple partial onset followed by impaired consciousness
      Impaired consciousness at onset
   Secondarily generalized seizures
      Simple partial seizures evolving to generalized tonic-clonic seizures
      Complex partial seizures evolving to generalized tonic-clonic seizures
      Simple partial seizures evolving to complex partial seizures, then
         to generalized tonic-clonic seizures

Generalized-onset seizures
   Tonic-clonic seizures
   Absence seizures
   Atypical absence seizures
   Myoclonic seizures
   Tonic seizures
   Clonic seizures
   Atonic seizures

may result from a focal epileptogenic process, which begins locally and then rapidly engages both hemispheres (partial with secondary generalization).

The types of seizures that follow TBI are protean, and the precise frequency of each specific type varies dramatically among different series. Jennett[35] found that about half of *early* seizures had partial features, most (75%) focal motor. The other 50% of early seizures had generalized attacks, being either partial at onset with secondary spread or primarily generalized. On the other hand, in Lee and Lui's recent series[40] of 4,232 adult patients with head injuries considered to be mild (yet included cases with intracranial hemorrhage), 84% had generalized tonic-clonic attacks.

Approximately 50 to 70% of *late* seizures with closed-head trauma and 30% with penetrating wounds have generalized tonic-clonic seizures without a focal component.[14,36] Most of these generalized attacks are likely of frontal lobe origin,[5] or are secondarily generalized from a clinically silent focus. Some may bespeak individuals with a genetic predisposition whose primarily generalized attacks are activated by the traumatic event. In civilian series, about 40% of late post-traumatic seizures have focal features. Jennett and Teasdale[36] found that 20% had partial complex seizures, but these were rare in the series of Walker and Erculei.[61] Clearly, from Jennett's extensive work in a civilian population, it would appear as if partial seizures with motor symptoms are less commonly seen following late than early seizures, whereas attacks with loss of consciousness, whether primarily or secondarily generalized, are more commonly a manifestation of late seizures. Caveness,[13,14] in his military studies, indicates that one-quarter of late ictal attacks are focal (partial), one-half are focal with secondary generalization, and one-quarter are primarily generalized.

Although in the earlier literature absence and myoclonic types of seizures were supposedly encountered and were reported to carry a particularly poor prognosis,[29] most investigators have stated that "petit mal" seizures, presumably typical absence attacks with three-per-second spike-and-wave discharges, are not a sequela of head trauma.[14,36,61]

SEIZURE PREVENTION AND PROPHYLAXIS

Although the overall incidence of early post-traumatic seizures is low, in individuals with a severe brain injury, or with significant risk factors, the likelihood of having an attack would seem to be sufficiently high to warrant *prophylactic* intervention. Also, given the deleterious impact that seizures can have on individuals already suffering the aftermath of TBI, it would seem that *prevention of epileptogenesis and late epilepsy* would be appropriate, if it could be accomplished reliably without further adverse effects. *Early* seizures and their associated postictal depression of mental status may obscure important changes in the neurologic assessment. Postictal focal deficits may interfere with the accurate monitoring of the acutely head-injured patient. Status epilepticus, with its adverse effect on cerebral metabolism and its potential for producing significant morbidity and mortality, may also directly follow a TBI.

Until recently, there have been few data to corroborate the contention that antiepileptic medication is efficacious in preventing either an initial seizure following a TBI or late epilepsy, and early optimism regarding the prophylactic use of phenytoin[47,54,65] waned with the presentation of less auspicious data.[41,49,66,67] With the results of the well-designed study of Temkin et al.,[56] however, it appears as if prophylactic treatment with phenytoin is effective in suppressing *early* reactive seizures but not in inhibiting the development of *late* epilepsy. In this study, patients with moderate-to-severe brain injuries were either treated with phenytoin at a dose of 20 mg/kg within the first 24 hours of the traumatic event or given placebo. Between drug loading and day seven, the phenytoin group had a cumulative seizure rate of $3.6 \pm 1.3\%$, as opposed to the $14.2 \pm 2.6\%$ in the placebo group ($p < 0.001$). No such protective effect was detected between day eight and the end of the second post-traumatic year. That is, phenytoin does not appear to be an effective antiepileptogenic agent, and its use beyond the first post-traumatic week cannot be generally espoused. This is not to say that it is not an effective antiepileptic drug once a chronic epileptic focus has been established and recurrent clinical ictal attacks occur. Whether other drugs would prove to possess greater antiepileptogenic properties remains to be ascertained.

The ease and speed with which phenytoin can be loaded, its efficacy, and its relatively low frequency of serious side effects would seem to make it the agent of choice for preventing *early* attacks. Phenobarbital can be readily loaded as well; however, its sedative effects vitiate its value. The lack of parenteral forms of valproic acid and carbamazepine makes their use less appealing in the acute setting.

After the first post-traumatic week, when the irritative effects of the acute injury have diminished and the beneficial effects of phenytoin have waned, it is less certain how to proceed. If one could predict with relative certainty, perhaps with an objective neurophysiologic measure, which patients will develop PTE, it would be critical to attempt to prevent epileptogenesis. Unfortunately, neurophysiologic studies, including standard EEG, do not seem to provide sufficient information in this circumstance. In individuals with severe brain injuries, EEGs are virtually always abnormal acutely; however, even the presence of epileptiform discharges does not necessarily correlate with the emergence of PTE. In fact, at least 2% of the population[68] and 3% of children[12] have epileptiform abnormalities in their EEGs without ever having a seizure. In one large retrospective study of Vietnam veterans, studied 12 to 16 years after a penetrating injury, all individuals with either anterior temporal or central spike foci had PTE.[32] On the other hand, in a study of 80 patients on whom serial EEGs were performed, 40% of those who developed post-traumatic seizures had a normal EEG before their first attack.[17] Jennett and others[36,42] have therefore concluded that routine EEG is not helpful in predicting the development of late epilepsy. Cassette ambulatory EEG recording is at least two and a half times more likely to detect paroxysmal abnormalities than is routine EEG,[8] potentially making its predictive use more valuable; however, a well-designed prospective study of its efficacy in this setting has not been carried out.

Risk-factor analysis, therefore, remains the primary manner by which the relative likelihood that PTE will emerge is determined. A mathematical approach to the prediction of PTE that is based on these various factors and time since injury has been adapted for computer use and has been found to be useful by some clinicians.[23] Using this type of analysis, it becomes clear that there are some individuals with multiple risk factors who surely seem destined to develop PTE, and prophylactic intervention would seem appropriate if an agent with sufficiently minimal deleterious effects were available.

Experimental models of epileptogenesis have provided us with additional possible preventive treatment strategies.[27] Blood extravasated into the cerebral parenchyma is highly irritative to cortex, and iron is capable of producing a chronic epileptic condition.[64] Intrinsic chelating agents within the brain generally are sufficient to counteract the effects of minor traumatic events; however, they are presumably overwhelmed by the larger amounts of blood that may accompany more severe injuries. Deposition of heme-containing compounds initiates a sequence of reactions that generate various free radicals leading to peroxidation of lipids and disruption of neuronal membranes. Steroids (methylprednisolone), tocopherol, and selenium effectively prevent tissue injury initiated by iron salts and heme compounds,[63] and treatment with hydroxyl radical scavengers following injection of hemoglobin or iron salts inhibits epileptic discharges in the rat.[46] The value of antiperoxidants and chelators in human subjects remains to be established.

Following central nervous system trauma, there are also marked elevations in extracellular levels of excitatory amino acids which are believed to contribute both to delayed tissue damage and to epileptogenesis.[10a,48a,49a] N-methyl-D-aspartate (NMDA)-type glutamate receptor antagonists have been shown to possess anticonvulsant activity in animal seizure models, yet their utility in humans remains uncertain at present given the variety of serious adverse affects with which they have been associated.[49a]

Kindling is another paradigm that is useful in studying epileptogenesis.[24] It entails repetitive, low-intensity stimulation of cerebral neurons that ultimately leads to an independent epileptic focus and spontaneous seizures. Oral or intra-peritoneal administration of phenytoin or carbamazepine is ineffective in inhibiting kindling, but valproic acid, benzodiazepines, and phenobarbital do suppress the process. In a recent study by Silver et al.,[55] phenobarbital, carbamazepine, and valproic acid were all used to prevent the development of kindling in rats. Again, valproic acid, and to a lesser extent, phenobarbital were particularly effective antiepileptogenic agents. Thus, these studies lead one to conclude that valproic acid might be effective for post-traumatic seizure prophylaxis in patients in high-risk categories, but this inference requires corroboration by further clinical trials.

A current recommendation is that one might consider phenytoin prophy-laxis for a period of 3 months post-injury, followed by a 6-week taper.[63a] That recommendation notwithstanding, it remains uncertain whether a period of antiepileptic prophylaxis, with any of the currently available agents, exceeding 1 week can be genuinely justified.

TREATMENT OF POST-TRAUMATIC EPILEPSY

Epilepsy is defined as the occurrence of two or more unprovoked seizures. Therefore, definitive treatment is frequently withheld until a second attack occurs. However, in individuals with a presumed or known cause for ictal attacks, the risk of a recurrence, once a first late episode has occurred, is quite high.[3,6] Annegers et al.[3] found that in patients who had an initial seizure, thought to be related to a postneonatal insult to the central nervous system, such as a TBI, the recurrence rate was 56% after 1 year, and 77% by 5 years. In the study by Salazar et al.[53] of veterans with penetrating head wounds, 92% had more than one seizure. Therefore, once a patient suffers a first late post-traumatic seizure, definitive therapy should generally be initiated. It must be remembered that an epileptic seizure is a symptom of an underlying problem, and although a prior TBI may be the most likely cause, other etiologic processes must be considered, especially if the traumatic event was mild or remote. A review of other diagnostic possibilities and their evaluation is beyond the scope of this review.

In managing an existing seizure disorder, the drug that is selected must be appropriate for the seizure type. Because most post-traumatic seizures are generalized tonic-clonic, partial motor, or complex partial, they may be treated rationally with either carbamazepine or phenytoin. Myoclonic, absence, and other generalized nonconvulsive seizures, traditionally treated with valproic acid, ethosuximide, or clonazepam, are not usually sequelae of brain injury (although myoclonic attacks may follow an associated hypoxic encephalopathy). In individuals with generalized tonic-clonic seizures, especially those with a genetic predisposition, valproic acid might also be used. In a number of controlled trials, carbamazepine and phenytoin have been found to be equally effective for partial and secondarily generalized seizures.[43,44,50] Therefore, in choosing among them, one must assess other criteria (expense, side effects, pharmacokinetic properties) to make an appropriate selection in an individual case. Table 4 includes data regarding usual adult dosage, plasma half life, therapeutic range, and various potential adverse effects of five of the more commonly used antiepileptic agents.

Several new antiepileptic drugs including felbamate, vigabatrin, gabapentin, and lamotrigine are currently in the final stages of clinical testing and likely to be released soon by the FDA. All will probably play some role in the treatment of patients with refractory seizures. Felbamate, in particular, has demonstrated efficacy in treating individuals with partial onset seizures.[22a,52a]

Neurobehavioral Effects of Antiepileptic Drugs

Few clinical studies have dealt with the neurobehavioral effects of antiepileptic drugs in the TBI population, and no study comparing the various antiepileptic agents and their cognitive ill effects in this group exists. Most of the relevant literature on this subject is based on patients with epilepsy or on normal individuals. The studies based on normal control subjects generally involve the short-term use of drugs, usually at doses lower than those employed in clinical populations.[18,43,57] Generalizing these results to a brain-injured population is hazardous given the differential effects that specific drugs may have on damaged brains.

TABLE 4. Information on Five Common Antiepileptic Drugs

Drug	Usual Adult Dosage (mg/d)	Usual Adult Dosage (mg/kg/d)	Half-Life (h)	Therapeutic Range* (µg/mL)	Side Effects
Carbamazepine	800–1600	15–25	11–22[†]	8–12	Drowsiness, blurred vision, diplopia, dysequilibrium, leukopenia, hepatic failure
Phenytoin	300–400	3–8	22[‡]	10–20	Ataxia, dysarthria, gingival hypertrophy, hirsutism, acneiform, eruption, hepatic failure, osteomalacia
Phenobarbital	90–180	2–4	100	15–35	Sedation, depression, loss of concentration, mental dulling, hyperactivity
Primidone	750–1250	10–20	5–15	5–12	Sedation, dizziness, nausea, ataxia, depression
Valproate	1000–3000	15–60	15–20	50–120	Gastrointestinal upset, weight gain, hair loss, tremor, thrombocytopenia, liver failure, pancreatitis

* May be lower in the elderly and in patients on multiple drugs.
† The half-life of carbamazepine is considerably longer when the drug is first administered than it is after several weeks when autoinduction of its metabolism takes place.
‡ The half-life of phenytoin is dose-dependent, being 22–24 hours when the plasma concentration is between 10–20 mg/mL but increases to about 36 hours at higher concentrations.

Dikmen et al.[18] evaluated the use of phenytoin in moderately to severely brain-injured individuals and found significant negative cognitive effects on severely injured individuals at 1 month after injury, as compared with their untreated counterparts. Furthermore, those whose phenytoin was stopped between the first and second post-traumatic years improved more than the corresponding control cases on several cognitive measures, when tested at 2 years after injury. The authors correctly point out that their findings do not indicate that phenytoin's detrimental effects are necessarily worse than those of other antiepileptic drugs.

Phenobarbital, despite its recognized effectiveness as an anticonvulsant, is not considered a first-line drug in the brain-injured population given its well-known propensity to affect cognitive functioning adversely even in the therapeutic range.[9,22] Phenytoin, carbamazepine, and valproic acid all appear to exert some lesser injurious effect on cognitive abilities in epileptic patients, and these impairments worsen with increasing plasma levels.[43] Phenytoin has been thought to decrease attention, concentration, motor speed, and mental processing more than carbamazepine and valproic acid,[1,1a,19,30,59] although this issue has not been completely resolved,[20,45,45a,60] and certainly individual patients may be particularly sensitive to the untoward effects of one particular drug and not another. Clearly, the use of antiepileptic polypharmacy should be rigorously avoided if at all possible.[51,57,58]

LONG-TERM OUTLOOK FOR SEIZURE CONTROL

Military and civilian studies both demonstrate that PTE can be a serious long-term problem. In one study of war veterans,[13] 56% had persistent seizures after 4 years, and, of those having more than three seizures in the first year, two-thirds continued to have attacks 8 years after injury. In another study of veterans with penetrating wounds,[53] persistent seizures, defined as more than one attack in the prior 2 years, were recorded in 53%. Of those with refractory seizures, 66% were taking anticonvulsant medication at the time of the last seizure, but plasma levels had not been recorded. Unrelenting seizures were more common in patients with partial seizures.[53] Jennett[35] found that 80% had recurrent seizures when followed for 2 to 5 years, and more than one-third of these individuals had "frequent fits." Even remissions of 2 or more years were commonly followed by recurrences. Complex partial seizures often persisted, as did epilepsy that was delayed in onset for more than 2 years after injury.[35]

On the other hand, in some prolonged follow-up studies of individuals with PTE, there appears to be a natural remission rate, perhaps irrespective of anticonvulsant usage.[42] In one military series with follow-up for at least 15 years, approximately 50% had had no seizures for at least 5 years.[61] In another,[14] 53% had a seizure-free interval of 2 years, with no difference between missile and non-missile injuries.

In these reports citing rates of remission, it is generally unclear whether patients were taking antiepileptic drugs, and if so, if plasma levels were available or in the therapeutic range. There are no studies specifically addressing the safety of withdrawal of anticonvulsant drugs in individuals free of post-traumatic seizures. Using the available data on withdrawal of antiepileptic drugs in the general seizure populations, there is a variable rate of remission. For example, the remission rate for generalized seizures may be as high as 80%, whereas that for complex partial seizures may be as low as 20%. Engel[21] notes that actual figures for remission have not changed appreciably throughout this century, suggesting that they may reflect the natural history of epilepsy rather than the influence of antiepileptic drugs. The type of seizure, number of attacks prior to control, type of treatment withdrawn, and EEG patterns all influence outcome,[11] although the predictive role of EEG has been questioned.[42] In general, it would seem rational to consider withdrawing antiepileptic medication from a patient who has been seizure free for 2 or more years, whose attacks were few and easily brought under control with monotherapy.

CONCLUSIONS

The incidence of *early* seizures in individuals hospitalized following a TBI is approximately 5%, as is the cumulative incidence of *late* epilepsy. Specific factors exist that can be used to estimate the relative risk of having either. Generally, the more severe the injury, the more likely it is that one will develop PTE. In those individuals with one or more risk factors, immediate post-trauma treatment with phenytoin seems prudent to prevent an early seizure. After the first week, anti-epileptic treatment may be continued in the hope that epileptogenesis can be averted. Whether it indeed should be continued depends on the patient's specific risk and the physician's and family's assessment of the risk/benefit ratio. No specific therapeutic agent can be endorsed at this time, although current available evidence in humans suggests that phenytoin is ineffective in addressing epileptogenesis, and experimental models indicate that valproic acid shows promise in inhibiting late epilepsy. Given the potential adverse cognitive effects of all antiepileptic agents, one cannot justify prolonged prophylaxis at this time with any specific agent.

A single *late* post-traumatic seizure, occurring in patients with one or more risk factors, generally indicates the presence of a chronic epileptic condition and should be treated. Ictal episodes that occur are either elementary partial, partial with secondary generalization, generalized without obvious focal onset, or occasionally complex partial and may be managed with phenytoin, carbamazepine or valproic acid. Therapy should continue until the patient has been seizure free for at least 2 years, after which the need for continued therapy should be reassessed.

REFERENCES

1. Andrewes DG, Bullen JG, Tomlinson L, et al: A comparative study of the cognitive effects of phenytoin and carbamazepine in new referrals with epilepsy. Epilepsia 27:128–134, 1986.
1a. Aldenkamp AP, Alpherts WLJ, Blennow G, et al: Withdrawal of antiepileptic medication in children—Effects on cognitive function: The multicenter Holmfrid study. Neurology 43:41–50, 1993.
2. Annegers JF, Grabow JD, Groover RV, et al: Seizures after head trauma: A population study. Neurology 30:683–689, 1980.
3. Annegers JF, Shirts SB, Hauser WA, Kurland LT: Risk of recurrence after an initial unprovoked seizure. Epilepsia 27:43–50, 1986.
4. Askenasy JJ: Association of intracerebral bone fragments and epilepsy in missile head injuries. Acta Neurol Scand 79:47–52, 1989.
5. Bancaud J, Talairach J, Morel P, et al: "Generalized" epileptic seizures elicited by electrical stimulation of the frontal lobe in man. Electroencephalogr Clin Neurophysiol 37:275–282, 1974.
6. Berg AT, Shinnar S: The risk of seizure recurrence following a first unprovoked seizure: A quantitative review. Neurology 41:965–972, 1991.
7. Brandvold B, Levi L, Feinsod M, George ED: Penetrating craniocerebral injuries in the Israeli involvement in the Lebanese conflict, 1982–1985. J Neurosurg 72:15–21, 1990.
8. Bridgers SL, Ebersole JS: The clinical utility of ambulatory cassette EEG. Neurology 35:166–173, 1985.
9. Brown ER: Interictal cognitive changes in epilepsy. Semin Neurol 11:167–174, 1991.
10. Bruce DA: Head injuries in the pediatric population. Curr Probl Pediatr 20:61–107, 1990.
10a. Bullock R, Kuroda Y, Teasdale GM, et al: Prevention of post-traumatic excitotoxic brain damage with NMDA antagonist drugs: A new strategy for the nineties. Acta Neurochir Suppl (Wien) 55:49–55, 1992.
11. Callaghan N, Garrett A, Goggin T: Withdrawal of anticonvulsant drugs in patients free of seizures for two years. N Engl J Med 318:942–946, 1988.
12. Cavazzuti GB, Capella L, Nalin A: Longitudinal study of epileptiform EEG patterns in normal children. Epilepsia 21:43–55, 1980.
13. Caveness WF: Onset and cessation of fits following craniocerebral trauma. J Neurosurg 20:570–583, 1963.
14. Caveness WF, Meirowsky AM, Rish BL, et al: The nature of post-traumatic epilepsy. J Neurosurg 50:545–553, 1979.
15. Commission on Classification and Terminology of the International League Against Epilepsy. Proposal for revised clinical and electroencephalographic classification of epileptic seizures. Epilepsia 22:489–501, 1981.
16. Cooper KD, Tabaddor K, Hauser WA, et al: The epidemiology of head injury in the Bronx. Neuroepidemiology 2:70–88, 1983.
17. Courjan J: A longitudinal electroclinical study of 80 cases of post-traumatic epilepsy observed from the time of original trauma. Epilepsia 11:39, 1970.
17a. De Santis A, Sganzerla E, Spanoli D, et al: Risk factors for late post traumatic epilepsy. Acta Neurochir Suppl (Wein) 55:64–67, 1992.
18. Dikmen SS, Temkin NR, Miller B, et al: Neurobehavioral effects of phenytoin prophylaxis of post-traumatic seizures. JAMA 265:1271–1277, 1991.
19. Dodrill CB, Troupin AS: Psychotropic effects of carbamazepine in epilepsy: A double-blind comparison with phenytoin. Neurology 27:1023–1028, 1977.
20. Dodrill CB, Troupin AS: Neuropsychological effects of carbamazepine and phenytoin: A reanalysis. Neurology 41:141–143, 1991.
21. Engel J: Seizures and Epilepsy. Philadelphia, FA Davis, 1989, pp 221–229.
22. Farwell JR, Lee YJ, Hirtz DG, et al: Phenobarbital for febrile seizures—Effects on intelligence and on seizure recurrence. N Engl J Med 322:364–369, 1990.

22a. Faught E, Sachdeo RC, Remler MP, et al: Felbamate monotherapy for partial-onset seizures: An active-control trial. Neurology 43:688–692, 1993.
23. Feeney DM, Walker AE: The prediction of post-traumatic epilepsy. Arch Neurol 36:8–12, 1979.
24. Goddard CV, McIntyre DC, Leech CK: A permanent change in brain function resulting from daily electrical stimulation. Exp Neurol 25:295–330, 1969.
25. Guidice MA, Berchou RC: Post-traumatic epilepsy following head injury. Brain Inj 1:61–64, 1987.
26. Hahn YS, Chyung C, Barthel MJ, et al: Head injuries in children under 36 months of age. Childs Nerv Syst 4:34–40, 1988.
27. Hauser WA: Prevention of post-traumatic epilepsy. N Engl J Med 323:540–541, 1990.
28. Hauser WA, Kurland LT: The epidemiology of epilepsy in Rochester, Minnesota 1935 through 1967. Epilepsia 16:1–66, 1975.
29. Hendrick EB, Harris L: Post-traumatic epilepsy in children. J Trauma 8:547–556, 1968.
30. Hirtz DG, Nelson KB: Cognitive effects of antiepileptic drugs. In Pedley TA, Meldrum BS (eds): Recent Advances in Epilepsy, II. New York, Churchill Livingstone, 1988, pp 161–181.
31. Hughes JR: Post-traumatic epilepsy in the military. Mil Med 151:416–419, 1986.
32. Jabbari B, Vengrow MI, Salazar AM, et al: Clinical and radiological correlates of EEG in the late phase of head injury: A study of 515 Vietnam veterans. Electroencephalogr Clin Neurophysiol 64:285–293, 1986.
33. Jamjoon AB, Kane N, Sanderman D, Cummins B: Epilepsy related to traumatic extradural hematomas. BMJ 302:448, 1991.
34. Jennett B: Epilepsy after Non-missile Head Injuries, 2nd ed. Chicago, William Heinemann, 1975, p 179.
35. Jennett B: Post-traumatic epilepsy. In Thompson RA, Green JR (eds): Advances in Neurology. New York, Raven Press, 1979, pp 137–147.
36. Jennett B, Teasdale G: Management of Head Injuries. Philadelphia, FA Davis, 1981, pp 236–238; 281–288.
37. Kalsbeek WD, McLaurin RL, Harris BSH, et al: The National Head and Spinal Cord Injury Survey: Major findings. J Neurosurg 53(suppl):19–31, 1980.
38. Kraus JF: Epidemiology of head injury. In Cooper PR (ed): Head Injury. Baltimore, Williams & Wilkins, 1987, pp 1–19.
39. Kuhl DA, Boucher BA, Muhlbauer MS: Prophylaxis of posttraumatic seizures. Ann Pharmacother 24:227–285, 1990.
40. Lee ST, Lui TN: Early seizures after mild closed head injury. J Neurosurg 76:435–439, 1992.
41. McQueen JK, Blackwood DH, Harris P, et al: Low risk of late post-traumatic seizures following severe head injury: Implications for clinical trials of prophylaxis. J Neuro Neurosurg Psychiatry 46:899–904, 1983.
42. Marsden CD, Reynolds EH: Seizures in adults. In Laidlaw J, Richens A, Oxley J (eds): A Textbook of Epilepsy. Edinburgh, Churchill Livingstone, 1988, pp 163–167.
43. Massagli TL: Neurobehavioral effects of phenytoin, carbamazepine and valproic acid: Implications for use in traumatic brain injury. Arch Phys Med Rehabil 72:219–226, 1991.
44. Mattson RH, Cramer JA, Collins JF, et al: Comparison of carbamazepine, phenobarbital, phenytoin and primidone in partial and secondarily generalized tonic-clonic seizures. N Engl J Med 313:145–151, 1985.
45. Meador KJ, Loring DW, Huh K, et al: Comparative cognitive effects of anticonvulsants. Neurology 40:391–394, 1990.
45a. Meador KJ, Loring DW, Abney OL, et al: Effects of carbamazepine and phenytoin on EEG and memory in healthy adults. Epilepsia 34(1):153–157, 1993.
46. Mori A, Hiramatsu M, Yokoi I, Edamatsu R: Biochemical pathogenesis of post-traumatic epilepsy. Pav J Biol Sci 25:54–62, 1990.
47. North JB, Penhall RK, Hanieh A, et al: Phenytoin and postoperative epilepsy. J Neurosurg 58:672–677, 1983.
48. Pacult A, Gudeman SK: Medical management of head injuries. In Becker DP, Gudeman SK (eds): Textbook of Head Injury. Philadelphia, WB Saunders, 1989, pp 206–209.
48a. Pellegrini JW, Lipton SA: Delayed administration of memantine prevents N-methyl-D-aspartate receptor-mediated neurotoxicity. Ann Neurol 33:403–407, 1993.
49. Penry JK, White BG, Brackett CE: A controlled prospective study of the pharmacologic prophylaxis of posttraumatic epilepsy. Neurology 29:600–601, 1979.
49a. Porter RJ, Rogawski MA: New antiepileptic drugs: From serendipity to rationale discovery. Epilepsia 33(suppl 1):51–56, 1992.
50. Ramsay RE, Wilder BJ, Berger JR, Bruni J: A double-blind study comparing carbamazepine with phenytoin as initial seizure therapy in adults. Neurology 33:904–910, 1983.

51. Reynolds EH, Trimble MR: Adverse neuropsychiatric effects of anticonvulsant drugs. Drugs 29:570–581, 1985.

52. Russel WR, Whitty CWM: Studies in traumatic epilepsy: Factors influencing incidence of epilepsy after brain wounds. J Neurol Neurosurg Psychiatry 15:93–98, 1952.

52a. Sachdeo R, Kramer LD, Rosenberg A, et al: Felbamate monotherapy: Controlled trial in patients with partial onset seizures. Ann Neurol 32:386–392, 1992.

53. Salazar AM, Jabbari B, Vance SC, et al: Epilepsy after penetrating head injury. I. Clinical correlates: A report of the Vietnam Head Injury Study. Neurology 35:1406–1414, 1985.

54. Servit Z, Musil F: Prophylactic treatment of post traumatic epilepsy: Results of a long-term follow-up in Czechoslovakia. Epilepsia 22:315–320, 1981.

55. Silver JM, Shin C, McNamara JO: Antiepileptogenic effects of conventional anticonvulsants in the kindling model of epilepsy. Ann Neurol 29:356–363, 1991.

56. Temkin NR, Dikmen SS, Wilensky AJ, et al: A randomized, double blind study of phenytoin for the prevention of post-traumatic seizures. N Engl J Med 323:497–502, 1990.

57. Thompson PJ, Huppert FA, Trimble MR: Phenytoin and cognitive functions: Effects on normal volunteers. Br J Soc Psychol 20:155–162, 1981.

58. Thompson PJ, Trimble MR: Anticonvulsant drugs and cognitive functions. Epilepsia 23:531–544, 1982.

59. Trimble MR: Anticonvulsant drugs and cognitive function: A review of the literature. Epilepsia 28(suppl 3):S37–S45, 1987.

60. Trimble MR: Cognitive effects of anticonvulsants. Neurology 41:1326, 1991.

61. Walker AE, Erculei F: Post-traumatic epilepsy 15 years later. Epilepsia 11:17–26, 1970.

62. Weiss GH, Salazar AM, Vance SC, et al: Predicting post-traumatic epilepsy in penetrating head injury. Arch Neurol 43:771–773, 1986.

63. Willmore LJ: Post-traumatic epilepsy: Cellular mechanisms and implications for treatment. Epilepsia 31(suppl 3):S67–S73, 1990.

64. Willmore LJ, Sypert GW, Munson JB: Recurrent seizures induced by cortical iron injection: A model of posttraumatic epilepsy. Ann Neurol 4:329–336, 1978.

65. Wohns RA, Wyler AR: Prophylactic phenytoin in severe head injuries. J Neurosurg 5:507–509, 1979.

66. Young B, Rapp RP, Norton JA, et al: Failure of prophylactically administered phenytoin to prevent early post-traumatic seizures. J Neurosurg 58:231–235, 1983.

67. Young B, Rapp RP, Norton JA, et al: Failure of prophylactically administered phenytoin to prevent late post-traumatic seizures. J Neurosurg 58:236–241, 1983.

68. Zivin L, Ajmone Marsan C: Incidence and prognostic significance of "epileptiform" activity in the EEG of nonepileptic subjects. Brain 91:751–778, 1968.

ALFREDO A. SADUN, MD, PHD

POST-TRAUMATIC VISUAL DISORDERS:

Part I. Injuries and Mechanisms

From the
Departments of Ophthalmology
  and Neurosurgery
Doheny Eye Institute
University of Southern California
  School of Medicine
Los Angeles, California

Correspondence to:
Alfredo A. Sadun, MD, PhD
Doheny Eye Institute
1450 San Pablo Street
Los Angeles, CA 90033-4667

OPTIC NERVE ATROPHY

Optic atrophy is not a diagnosis; it is a clinically observable endpoint that reflects loss of axons in the optic nerve and an associated dropout of ganglion cells in the retina. Because of anterograde and retrograde degeneration, a lesion involving any part of the visual system, from the retina to the retinal ganglion cell axon terminations in the lateral geniculate nucleus, can cause optic atrophy. Optic atrophy secondary to trauma is usually due to injury of the optic nerve.

Primary optic atrophy should be distinguished from *secondary* optic atrophy. The former is sometimes called "simple" optic atrophy and follows the course of most diseases of the optic nerve. Secondary optic atrophy occurs when there is axonal loss associated with severe disc edema (such as that due to increased intracranial pressure) or inflammation. Blunt head trauma resulting in a sphenoid fracture will lead to primary optic atrophy through one of three mechanisms:

1. Displaced fracture of the sphenoid may cut the optic nerve;

2. A smaller hairline fracture may lead to bleeding that accumulates in the subperiosteal space within the narrow confines of the optic canal as well as subsequent optic nerve compression; and

3. Even in the absence of a fracture of the sphenoid bone, shearing forces may directly contuse the optic nerve or tear the many small traversing blood vessels that feed it at the level of the optic canal.

In all of these circumstances, primary optic atrophy, in its severe form, is seen funduscopically as a white optic disc with sharp margins. No gray or fuzzy gliotic reaction is seen overlying the disc or at its margins. In subtotal optic atrophy, there is optic disc pallor or an absence of the pink or rose color of the normal disc.

The absence of color in the optic disc reflects decreased blood perfusion. This is thought to be due primarily to capillary dropout, although others have hypothesized that columns of optic nerve axons normally act as light pipes that conduct the red color of capillaries to the surface.[8]

Optic disc atrophy can be slight, moderate, or severe and can be diffuse or confined to single sector of the optic nerve head. For example, trauma can produce shearing at the level of the optic chiasm, which affects only the decussating fibers. Hence, ganglion cell axons emanating from the retina nasal to the fovea are involved primarily, and atrophy will be seen in both temporal (but nasal to fovea) and nasal portions of the optic disc, but with sparing of the superior and inferior regions, which remain pink.

Once optic atrophy has developed, the structural integrity of the disc has been compromised. At this point, further damage from even relatively normal intraocular pressure may continue. Hence, low-tension glaucoma often develops in patients who once had primary optic atrophy due to an injury. The diagnosis is difficult and requires serial disc photographs and serial visual fields. This type of glaucoma is particularly difficult to treat because the intraocular pressures have to be kept even lower than normal.

Secondary optic atrophy has an entirely different appearance in that there is disorganization of the nerve fiber layer as it enters the optic nerve. In addition, there is marked gliosis within and overlying the optic nerve head. Secondary optic atrophy is seen usually in cases of severe disc edema (most often papilledema) but may be seen also in ocular inflammation. The essence of secondary optic atrophy is that the axons do not die quietly; in their swollen or inflamed state, a great deal of fibrosis develops.

Histopathologically, secondary optic atrophy is characterized by gliosis overlying and at the edges of the optic disc. Astrocytes are seen throughout the optic nerve head as well as heaped up anteriorly on it. Trauma that produces significant increases in intracranial pressure (such as that occurring in association with venous sinus thrombosis or cerebral edema) often leads to secondary optic atrophy. Secondary optic atrophy may be less dramatic in appearance than is primary optic atrophy and is therefore subject to being overlooked on funduscopic examinations. Nonetheless, because of the risk of low-tension glaucoma, and as a marker of previous papilledema or inflammation, it is very important to identify secondary optic atrophy.

VISUAL PATHWAYS

The human visual pathways are often divided into anterior and posterior components. The anterior visual pathway begins with the approximately 1.5 million retinal ganglion cells in each eye that contribute their axons to form the optic nerves. At the optic chiasm, there is a partial decussation (approximately 54% of the fibers cross), and these axons continue to form the optic tracts. They do not synapse until the primary visual nuclei.[2]

Although conventional teaching describes all of these fibers as going to the lateral geniculate nuclei, there are at least seven other primary visual nuclei in the brain. Retinal ganglion cell axons terminate in the pretectal nuclei, superior colliculus, accessory optic system, pulvinar, and three nuclei of the hypothalamus. However, for what we regard as high-resolution, conscious vision, the major projection is that to the lateral geniculate nucleus.

The lateral geniculate nucleus consists of six layers. Layers one and two are the magnocellular layers, which are thought to subserve contrast sensitivity of low spatial frequencies, motion detections, and stereopsis (the most important cue for depth perception). Layers three, four, five, and six are composed of smaller cells (parvocellular) that are thought to subserve color vision and fine-form resolution. Layers two, three, and five receive input from the ipsilateral eye, whereas layers one, four, and six receive a contralateral projection. There is a synapse at the level of the lateral geniculate nucleus, after neurons from each of the six layers contribute axons to form the optic radiations.

The posterior visual pathway begins with the optic radiations from the lateral geniculate nucleus. Approximately half of the fibers fan out dorsally through the parietal lobe to the occipital cortex; the other half traverse the temporal lobe, first swinging anteriorly (Myer's loop) and then coursing posteriorly toward the occipital cortex. Fibers that form the optic radiation synapse in layers of the primary visual cortex (striate cortex or area 17 or area V1). There are further projections from V1 to V2 to V3, as well as projections to V4 and to the medial temporal lobe cortex; all of these projections can be considered part of the posterior visual pathway.

Trauma

Trauma to either the anterior or posterior visual pathway can produce significant visual impairments, the nature of which depends largely on the level of the visual pathway that is interrupted and on the degree of vulnerability of each of these levels. Depending on the type and severity, trauma can affect any or all of the ocular structures. Trauma to the eye can produce damage at the level of the retinal ganglion cells per se or can damage its axons at the optic nerve head. Retinal detachments can occur directly or indirectly as a consequence of traction exerted by adhesions produced by the trauma or by the attempt to repair the trauma. The blood supply to the eye may be impaired, particularly at the level of the optic nerve head. Furthermore, infection following trauma can produce devastating injury to the retina or to the optic nerve head.

The optic nerve itself is highly vulnerable to various traumatic insults. Retrobulbar injections associated with ocular surgery can cause optic nerve injury if the needle pierces the optic nerve or the subarachnoid space. Injection under pressure of an anesthetic or epinephrine can have many untoward consequences, including hemorrhage, spasm of the ophthalmic artery (Fig. 1), ischemia from compression, and effects of the anesthetic on the central nervous system.

Penetrating injuries to the orbit, such as from knives or screw drivers, often lead to irreversible damage to the optic nerve, particularly if the penetration is from an anterior-inferior direction. The optic nerve may be transected directly, or the damage may be a consequence of an interruption in its blood supply. Retro-orbital hemorrhages may lead to compression of the optic nerve and, subsequently, to ischemia. Infections of the orbit can also cause damage to the optic nerve. Surgical trauma, especially during operations on the ethmoid sinus, is not uncommon.

Blunt trauma to the orbit can lead to optic nerve injury by one of four mechanisms. Contusion of the optic nerve occurs in many such cases. Fortunately,

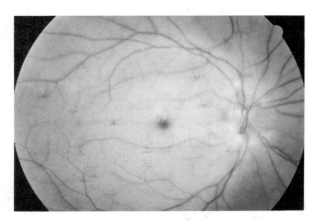

FIGURE 1. Fundus photograph of the right eye in a patient in whom a retrobulbar injection led to a blind eye. About 8 hours after the injection, the arterials were noted to be very attenuated and there was marked retinal edema leaving only the avascular and the thinnest portion of the retina as pink (foveal cherry-red spot). This central retinal artery occlusion was probably due to vasospasm of the ophthalmic artery, produced by the inadvertent positioning of the retrobulbar needle.

this often causes only a temporary loss of function, and many of these patients regain good vision over several days. This return of visual acuity may be assisted by the use of systemic steroids.

A retrobulbar hemorrhage can act as a space-occupying lesion in the orbit and may lead to an increase in intraorbital and intraocular pressure. Eventually, there may be ischemia to the optic nerve due to either direct compression or to spasm of the ophthalmic artery.

Although this is very rare, the optic nerve may be evulsed from its attachment to the optic disc.

Finally, blunt trauma may lead to blindness through damage to the optic nerve at the level of the optic canal. This damage is thought to occur through one of three mechanisms.[10] There may be a fracture of the sphenoid wing, which can shear across the optic nerve, resulting in an immediate loss of vision. A second mechanism is through spasm of the ophthalmic artery, either a direct consequence of trauma or secondary to a retrobulbar hemorrhage. Loss of vision generally occurs very quickly (seconds or minutes) after the trauma. Third, blood may accumulate in the sub-periosteal space of the sphenoid bone adjacent to the optic canal. This accumulation can lead to compression of the optic nerve within the canal and to subsequent ischemia. Visual loss in these circumstances may develop over a period of hours.

Treatment of optic nerve impairment following blunt trauma at the level of the optic canal remains controversial. We generally use high-dose steroids, although recent evidence suggests that decompression of the optic nerve at the level of the optic canal may be of benefit in selected cases. To be successful, this decompression probably needs to be performed within a couple of days of the trauma.

The optic nerve may also be injured in the intracranial space due to a contrecoup type contusion to the nerve at the intracranial entrance of the optic canal. At this site, there is a fold of dura that descends dorsally, and this fold may also lead to notching of the superior half of the optic nerve in the setting of generalized brain swelling, which in turn produces an inferior visual field defect.

Although rare, there have been descriptions of shearing of the optic chiasm due to blunt head trauma,[9] and the resultant binasal field defect may be indistinguishable from that due to other chiasm syndromes, such as pituitary adenoma.[11] The mechanism for the shearing is thought to be related to the fact that decussating fibers are under greater "stretch" than are nondecussating ipsilateral fibers.

Traumatic injury to the optic tract is extremely rare, but this can occur secondary to uncal herniation. The ischemia to the optic tract and lateral geniculate nucleus area can be on the side ipsilateral or contralateral to the uncal herniation.

Trauma to the optic nerve *anterior* to the optic chiasm generally results in at least some variation of a centrocecal scotoma, which leads to a loss of acuity that can range from mild to very profound. Lesions *posterior* to the optic chiasm, however, at least when they are ipsilateral, should not produce any change in visual acuity; a hemifield is suffcient for 20/20 vision.

Trauma to the posterior visual pathways produces, in addition to visual impairment, numerous other neurologic signs and symptoms. Generally speaking, when lesions in the parietal or temporal cortex are sufficient to produce significant visual field defects, there will be other extensive neurologic problems. Trauma to the tips of the temporal lobes can lead to characteristic superior visual field defects termed *pie in the sky* visual field impairments. Lesions anywhere along the optic radiations will produce visual field defects that appear similar for both eyes. However, because the optic radiations are not fully sorted out at this level, these field defects tend to be noncongruous (unless there is a complete homonymous hemianopia).[15]

It is important to keep in mind that the optic radiations fan out rather widely over the temporal and parietal lobes, and thus, only wide-scale injury leads to any significant visual field defect. However, the optic radiations converge again as they approach the occipital cortex. At the level of the calcarine cortex, relatively discrete lesions may produce significant visual field loss without other associated neurologic signs and symptoms.

Cerebral concussion may rarely produce a temporary visual field defect. Other visual impairments, such as finger agnosia, alexia, or agraphia, can also occur with injury of the cerebral cortex. These other impairments may be temporary or permanent.

CORTICAL BLINDNESS

Some authors reserve the term *cortical blindness* or *cerebral blindness* for individuals who are completely blind due to damage to the occipital cortex. However, we prefer to apply these terms whenever injury to the cerebral cortex leads to a loss of visual acuity. Unilateral lesions never impair visual acuity; thus, this term applies only to bilateral cortical lesions. The anatomy of the cerebral hemispheres is such that injury usually occurs at the occipital tip, where both hemispheres lie together. Lesions that do not involve both occipital tips may still produce visual impairments such as visual field loss (e.g., homonymous hemianopsia).

Cortical blindness may occur as a direct or indirect consequence of trauma. For example, penetrating injury to the back of the head (such as from a bullet) may lead to congruous visual field defects and loss of central visual field, associated with poor visual acuity. However, blunt head injury may also cause cortical blindness through various other mechanisms. For example, severe head injury can lead to generalized brain swelling that can cause occlusion of the posterior cerebral arteries as they pass the tentorium, which may lead to an infarction of the occipital cortex. In the setting of vascular hypotension, infarcts of the occipital cortex occur often in the watershed area. This watershed area usually involves the very tips of the occiptial lobes, which subserve macular vision. Similarly, patients may suffer watershed due to hypotension or cerebral edema infarctions secondary to surgical interventions associated with traumatic injury. Cortical blindness has also been associated with the ictal and postictal states, which may be consequent to previous head trauma.[4]

Several interesting features characterize cortical blindness. The pupils continue to react to light, and there should be no afferent pupillary defect, unless there is injury to the anterior visual pathways as well. Funduscopic examination will not reveal any optic atrophy. The visual evoked response (flash, not pattern) may remain robust, even in complete cortical blindness.[14] Not surprisingly, the pattern-evoked visual response will be diminished in proportion to the loss of visual acuity. The paradoxical sparing of the flash visual evoked response is thought to reflect the electrophysiology of visual pathways that bypass the lateral geniculate nucleus (in particular, projections from the eye to the superior colliculus and pulvinar, which are then relayed onto secondary areas of the visual cortex).

It has often been noted that there is a tendency for partial or complete sparing of vision within 5 to 10° from fixation. Various theories have been proposed on the mechanism of this macular sparing, which is seen more often in cases of cortical blindness due to infarction than in those due to the direct effects of trauma. As much as 5° around fixation may be spared in an otherwise complete homonymous hemianopia. Extensive cortical representation of the central 5° of visual field, a dual blood supply, and an uncrossed projection are possible explanations for this phenomenon.

At times, there may appear to be a remarkable dissociation between various forms of visual impairment due to cortical blindness from trauma. For example, in patients in whom there is relative sparing of visual acuity, there is often a profound loss of stereopsis, color vision, or the recognition of faces (prosopagnosia). Dissociated visual loss provides clinical evidence of parallel visual processing.

This concept of dissociation of visual functions in the setting of cortical blindness, taken to the extreme, leads to the subject of blindsight. Animal experiments have demonstrated that subcortical pathways may provide important information, particularly for visual motor responses. For example, hamsters in which the visual cortex was bilaterally ablated still performed well on certain visual tasks, provided that the superior colliculus was also uninjured.[12] Monkeys in which the visual cortex has been destroyed have demonstrated subsequent recovery to the point where they could learn to discriminate simple shapes.[7] Weiskrantz,[16] in 1986, published an extensive report of one patient with blindsight. In essence, he demonstrated that this patient (who had residual visual acuity) could, in his partially blind field, detect movement (Riddoch's phenomenon) and discriminate bar orientation out of proportion to the residual visual acuity. It is important to keep in mind that blindsight represents a coarse residual function in selected patients with cortical blindness that is unexpected in view of the level of their visual acuity. However, this visual information is very crude and is apparently available only at a subconscious level; it is thought to be mediated by nongeniculostriate pathways.

Patients with cortical blindness may also describe positive visual phenomena. Thus, these patients not only do not see what is there (negative visual phenomena) but they also do see what is not there. These positive visual phenomena vary from simple phosphenes (glowing lights) to structured photopsias (solid or scintillating jagged visual patterns) to simple figures (which often have a schematic nature) to a complete and detailed scene (usually described as a visual hallucination). All types of positive visual phenomena are apt to occur soon after the onset of visual loss and may in fact be seen with bilateral anterior lesions (and even bilateral ocular occlusion). At least part of this syndrome is thought to occur as a "release phenomenon" that is consequent to the disinhibiton brought on by deafferentation. This phenomenon is distinct from positive visual phenomena that occur as a consequence of abnormal excitation from pathologic discharges. In Anton's syndrome, the patient denies his blindness and confabulates a visual scene.

Various more complex clinical symptoms also may appear after bilateral lesions of the occiptial cortex. Perceptive visual agnosias can be described as the inability to recognize familiar images due to the loss of some fundamental visual components, such as movement perception, color perception, or stereopsis. Aperceptive visual agnosias occur usually in the occipital-parietal and occipital-temporal areas and are more global. Associative visual agnosias represent the inability to recognize distinct categories of familiar objects, despite the ability to comprehend the underlying shapes (such as prosopagnosia). In Balint's syndrome, the patient may perceive components of the visual world but cannot integrate these into a whole. This inability may contribute to an oculomotor apraxia, in which the patient cannot willfully shift gaze onto a target, despite normal reflex eye movements. In addition, there may be other general types of agnosias, such as confusions and spatial disorientations.[3]

ABERRANT REGENERATION

The oculomotor misdirection syndrome was originally described by Gowers in 1879. Many years later, Bielschowsky proposed that this syndrome was caused by aberrant regeneration of fibers of the third cranial nerve. In 1938, Bender and Fulton sectioned the ocular motor nerves in chimpanzees and found that regenerated fibers were indiscriminantly reinnervating all of the extraocular muscles. Breinin, in 1955, used electromyography in a patient to demonstrate that the misdirection syndrome was caused by the simultaneous stimulation of all of the extraocular muscles receiving third-nerve innervation, regardless of the direction of the gaze.

These and similar corroborating investigations led to the general acceptance that aberrant regeneration is, in fact, the mechanism underlying oculomotor misdirection. Aneurysm and trauma are the most common causes of aberrant regeneration of the ocular motor system. Rarely, a tumor, syphilis, or meningitis can cause a similar syndrome.

The most common manifestations of aberrant regeneration of the ocular motor nerve are in the form of pseudo–von Graefe's and pseudo–Argyll Robertson signs. The first is adduction that occurs on attempted vertical gaze and is relatively uncommon. Pseudo–Argyll Robertson sign is pupillary constriction on infraduction and, more commonly, an attempted adduction of the eye. This is a clinical manifestation of a remarkable rewiring in which smooth muscle is reinnervated by nerve that normally subserves striated muscle.

Until recently, there has been considerable controversy regarding the etiology of aberrant regeneration. The studies of Sibony et al.[13] and of Fernandez et al.[1]

have demonstrated in cat and rat that following sectioning of the third nerve, there is first degeneration and then regeneration. Neither ephaptic transmission nor central synaptic reorganization accounts for the error in circuitry.

Unfortunately, it is extremely difficult to manage the double vision produced by the ophthalmoplegia seen in aberrant regeneration. Standard or even special strabismus techniques are generally not effective. Regarding the cosmetic problems of ptosis or lid retraction that are produced by the aberrant regeneration, plastic surgery is sometimes helpful; however, here, too, the results are almost always suboptimal.

OPHTHALMOPLEGIA

Injury to the efferent (or motor) system has the potential to produce oculomotor paresis (ophthalmoplegia). Such injury may affect the efferent system at any level from proximal to distal. Beginning distally, there may be damage to one or more of the six muscles that control each eye's movements. These muscles can be ruptured, disinserted from their attachment to the sclera, inflamed, contused, develop hematomas, or become entrapped by either fibrous tissue or through bony defects of the orbit.

Blow-out fractures are a common injury from blunt trauma to the eyeball. Hydraulic effects cause the eye to expand in each direction, and the weakest wall of the orbit may "blow out." The injury most often affects the medial wall but is more likely to produce symptoms of diplopia when it affects the inferior wall, where either the inferior oblique or inferior rectus muscles can become entrapped.

The third cranial nerve supplies four extraocular muscles. Traumatic injuries to the third nerve usually occur with frontal head injury. The nerve is most vulnerable to damage at or near the orbital apex. It has been estimated that approximately 1% of all head injuries result in a third-nerve palsy.[6] In most cases, the blunt trauma required to produce ocular motor palsy is quite severe and is associated with a skull fracture.

Occasionally, a third-nerve palsy is seen with relatively minor head trauma. In these cases, neuroimaging frequently demonstrates an intracranial mass. The explanation is that these patients either misattributed their diplopia to unrelated trauma, or that perhaps the intracranial mass causes stretching of the third nerve so that it becomes far more vulnerable to relatively minor trama.

There may be some recovery of function following ocular motor paresis due to trauma. This generally occurs 2 to 3 months after the injury, although there may be continuous improvement for up to 6 months after the injury. For this reason, strabismus surgery should be deferred for at least 6 months following injury. In cases of a residual partial third-nerve palsy, ocular alignment can usually be restored, although the limited ductions may result in diplopia on lateral gaze. Traumatic injury to the third nerve is one of the most common causes of ocular motor synkinesis or aberrant regeneration.

The fourth (trochlear) cranial nerve subserves only the superior oblique muscle. This nerve is very thin and pursues a long course as it crosses in the medullary velum beneath the cerebellum on the dorsum of the brainstem. This characteristic makes it quite susceptible to trauma; indeed, the fourth cranial nerve is the only nerve for which the most frequent cause of paresis is trauma. A fourth-nerve palsy may be unilateral or bilateral, and it may occur with relatively minor trauma to the top (vertex) of the head.[5]

Fourth-nerve palsies are less likely to show recovery than is any other cranial nerve palsy, and if recovery does occur, it takes place by the sixth month. In patients with residual diplopia due to a traumatic fourth-nerve palsy, strabismus surgery is indicated. Several excellent techniques for restoring ocular alignment are available.

The sixth cranial nerve subserves ocular abduction. A cranial nerve palsy involving the sixth nerve may also be due to blunt trauma. Frontal or temporal injury can lead to a basal skull fracture along the petrous pyramid area that damages the sixth nerve as it passes under the petroclinoid ligament. However, general brain swelling, increased intracranial pressure, and shifts of the brain can all lead to a sixth-nerve palsy because the attachments of the sixth nerve are under the petroclinoid ligament. Hence, sixth-nerve palsy is relatively nonlocalizing.

There may be recovery from sixth-nerve palsy for up to 6 months after injury, but thereafter, specialized surgical techniques are required to restore not only ocular alignment but also some abduction potential. Two techniques in particular involve muscle transposition procedures that permit abduction even following total sixth-nerve palsies.

Combinations of third-, fourth-, and sixth-nerve palsies may result from injury at the level of the orbital apex or the superior orbital fissure. Trauma to the cavernous sinus can produce these types of ophthalmoplegias in addition to facial hypesthesia secondary to injury of the fifth nerve. Trauma can lead to a carotid-cavernous fistula or, in a less severe form, to a dural shunt fistula. In both of these cases, the trauma leads to a tear between the arterial and venous sides. This leads to a rise in intravenous pressure that is manifest by ocular injection, proptosis, increased intraocular pressure, and numerous other ocular conditions. In most cases, however, the patient is distressed most by the diplopia that occurs. The diagnosis is often facilitated by listening to the orbit for a bruit.

Less commonly, trauma leads to injury at the level of the brainstem itself, which can lead to nuclear or supranuclear disorders of ocular motility. Such injuries are usually the consequence of infarctions. For example, an intranuclear ophthalmoplegia may be due to brainstem strokes that involve the posterior circulation. Nuclear, intranuclear, and supranuclear disorders of oculomotility may be self-limiting or permanent. If permanent, these eye movement disorders are not usually amenable to prism use or surgical intervention.

REFERENCES

1. Fernandez E, Pallini R, Gangitano C, et al: Oculomotor nerve regeneration in rats: Functional, histological, and neuroanatomical studies. J Neurosurg 67:428–437, 1987.
2. Glaser JS, Sadun AA: Anatomy of the visual sensory system. In Glaser JS (ed): Neuro-Ophthalmology, 2nd ed. Philadelphia, JB Lippincott, 1990, pp 61–82.
3. Grusser OJ, Landis T: Visual Agnosias and Other Disturbances of Visual Perception and Cognition. Boca Raton, FL, CRC Press, 1991, pp 1–24.
4. Lessell S, Lessell IM, Glaser JS: Topical diagnosis: Retrochiasmal visual pathways and higher cortical function. In Glaser JS (ed): Neuro-Ophthalmology, 2nd ed. Philadelphia, JB Lippincott, 1990, pp 213–238.
5. Lindenberg R: Significance of the tentorium in head injuries from blunt forces. Clin Neurosurg 12:129–142, 1966.
6. Memon MY, Paine KWE: Direct injury of the oculomotor nerve in craniocerebral trauma. J Neurosurg 35:461–464, 1971.
7. Pasik T, Pasik P: The visual world of monkeys deprived to striate cortex: Effective stimulus parameters and the importance of the accessory optic system. Vision Res (suppl 3):419–435, 1971.
8. Quigley HA, Anderson DR: The histologic basis of optic disk pallor in experimental optic atrophy. Am J Ophthalmol 83:709–717, 1977.

9. Savino PJ, Glaser JS, Schatz NJ: Traumatic chiasmal syndrome. Neurology 30:963–970, 1980.
10. Savino PJ, Harbour R: Neuro-ophthalmic manifestations of trauma. In Smith BC, Della Rocca RC, Nesi FA, et al (eds): Ophthalmic Plastic and Reconstructive Surgery. St. Louis, CV Mosby, 1987, pp 311–326.
11. Schatz NJ, Schlezinger NS: Noncompressive causes of chiasmal disease. In Symposium on Neuro-Ophthalmology: Transactions of the New Orleans Academy of Ophthalmology. St. Louis, CV Mosby, 1976, pp 90–07.
12. Schneider GE: Two visual systems: Brain mechanisms for localization and discrimination are dissociated by tectal and cortical lesions. Science 163:895–902, 1969.
13. Sibony PA, Evinger C, Lessell S: Retrograde horseradish peroxidase transport after oculomotor nerve injury. Invest Ophthalmol Vis Sci 27:975–980, 1986.
14. Spehlmann R, Gross RA, Ho SU, et al: Visual evoked potentials and postmortem findings in a case of cortical blindness. Trans Am Neurol Assoc 102:157–160, 1977.
15. Trobe JD, Lorber ML, Schlezinger NS: Isolated homonymous hemianopia: A review of 104 cases. Arch Ophthalmol 89:377–381, 1973.
16. Weiskrantz L: Blindsight: A Case Study and Implications. Oxford, Oxford University Press, 1986.

DON LIU, MD

POST-TRAUMATIC VISUAL DISORDERS:

Part II. Management and Rehabilitation

From the
Department of Ophthalmology
Doheny Eye Institute
University of Southern California
    School of Medicine
Los Angeles, California

Correspondence to:
Don Liu, MD
Doheny Eye Institute
1450 San Pablo Street
Los Angeles, CA 90033-4667

Rehabilitation of traumatic brain injury patients who have trauma-induced visual impairment can be complex and challenging. The clinical manifestations of a traumatized visual system vary greatly, and the emergent care and rehabilitation of these patients must be highly individualized. The visual pathway includes the cornea, lens, vitreous body, retina, optic nerve and chiasm, lateral geniculate body, optic radiation, and occipital cortex. Trauma to any portion of this pathway results in some form of disturbance in visual function. Furthermore, trauma to the adnexa, such as the eyelids, extraocular muscles, and lacrimal gland, can also result in serious disturbances in visual function. For the convenience of discussion, trauma to the visual system can be classified etiologically as blunt or sharp trauma, and anatomically as anterior or posterior segment trauma; or it can be classified in terms of its effect as sensory system trauma or motor system trauma (Figs. 1 and 2).

A patient who sustains a penetrating injury (sharp trauma) to the cornea suffers a severe decrease in visual acuity (sensory trauma) but experiences no diplopia (motor system disturbance). Accordingly, the specific management and rehabilitation of such a patient are quite different from those which would be appropriate for a patient who sustained a sharp injury to an extraocular muscle, who would have good vision (intact sensory system) but debilitating diplopia (motor system problem). A patient who has a ptotic or paralyzed eyelid as a result of a sharp

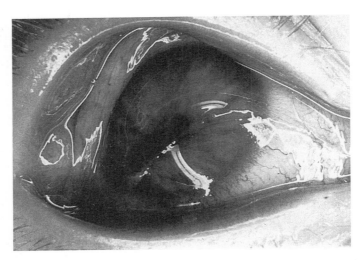

FIGURE 1. Sharp penetrating injury to the globe. The cornea is lacerated, and the anterior chamber is collapsed. Visual acuity is threatened, but there is no disturbance to the motor system.

injury to the lid may have intact visual acuity, but visual function can be compromised if the ptotic eyelid causes deprivation of normal single binocular vision or affects depth perception; in addition, injuries or their sequelae that mar

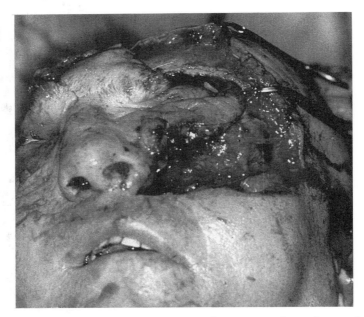

FIGURE 2. Severe facial trauma. Both the anterior and posterior pathways of the visual system are involved. Disturbance in the motor and sensory systems is evident.

appearance can affect the patient's self-image. Furthermore, if the eyelid is paralyzed, discomfort and eventual damage to the cornea can ensue.

Even blunt trauma to the orbital region can affect both sensory and motor functions of the visual system. For example, a fist blow to the orbital region may result in traumatic hyphema, a dislocated lens, vitreous hemorrhage, retina detachment, or even a ruptured globe, which would affect the sensory system. On the other hand, such a blow may result in a blow-out fracture of the orbit, with extraocular muscle entrapment, which would affect the motor function. A knife injury may damage the lids, extraocular muscles, globe and the optic nerve, and can thus result in both sensory and motor disturbances. A patient with cortical blindness (posterior visual pathway) has an intact motor system, and the management and rehabilitation of such a patient is far different from that of a patient with, for example, a retinal detachment (anterior visual pathway). Furthermore, almost all of these injuries cause cosmetic blemish, and many patients suffer from psychological trauma secondary to an altered self-image.

Rehabilitation of a patient with a traumatized visual system thus entails more than merely preserving or restoring vision per se; it also involves preserving or restoring *useful* vision function, ensuring comfort of the eye, and eradicating, at least as much as possible, any cosmetic disfigurement. In some patients, rehabilitation will involve retraining or teaching new skills that will enable the patient to function independently and that will assist the patient in adjusting socially and psychologically to any residual deficit in vision.

EXPOSURE KERATITIS

When proper eyelid closure is compromised, the cornea becomes dry, irritated, and, eventually, damaged; the health of the cornea is adversely affected also when blinking is decreased or incomplete.[24,38] If the eyelid problem is not promptly and adequately treated, exposure keratitis can lead to corneal abrasion, ulceration, opacification, or perforation (Fig. 3). Exposure keratitis can occur in patients with traumatic loss of an eyelid, chemical or thermal burn injury to the

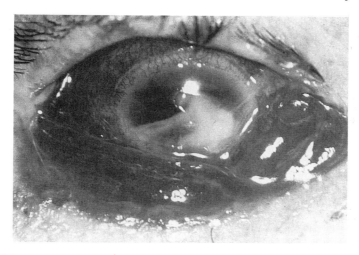

FIGURE 3. The devastating effect of exposure keratitis. The cornea is ulcerated, and the conjunctiva is chemotic and injected.

eyelids, traumatically paralyzed eyelids, and dysthyroid ophthalmopathy. The signs of exposure keratitis, regardless of etiology, are injection or chemosis of the conjunctiva and a watery discharge; symptoms include photophobia, irritation, or pain in the eye, and a slight decrease in visual acuity. The cornea shows varying degrees of staining with fluorescein. When there is traumatic loss of an eyelid, an ophthalmic plastic surgeon should be consulted; in addition to assessing the patient's visual status, an oculoplastic specialist can tailor management of the acute injury to facilitate eventual reconstructive surgery.

Protecting the cornea is the foremost concern in both the acute and rehabilitation stages. In the acute stage, constant lubrication with a bland ointment or an antibiotic preparation and a moisture chamber are used to ensure preservation of vision and comfort of the eye. A bland lubricant such as Lacri-Lube (Allergan) or Refresh PM (Allergan) can be used in small amounts from as little as twice daily to as frequently as every other hour, depending on the patient's clinical findings and responses. Antibiotic preparations such as Polysporin (Burroughs-Wellcome), Neosporin (Burroughs-Wellcome), or gentamicin are necessary when keratitis is evident or infection is present. These antibiotic preparations also can be used from twice a day to as frequently as every other hour. The frequency of antibiotic application is usually decreased when antibiotics are used in conjunction with a moisture chamber. Moisture chambers of various designs are available commercially, but a simple and inexpensive way to accomplish the same goal is to use plastic wrap: petrolatum is first applied to the periorbital region, then a sheet of plastic wrap, cut to the appropriate size, is placed over this region and sealed with petrolatum.

A traumatic defect of the lid can be reconstructed by various techniques, depending on the exact nature of the injury, extent of tissue loss, and size and location of the defect.[3] In principle, missing conjunctiva can be replaced by conjunctiva from the fellow eye or by the use of buccal mucosa; missing tarsal plate can be replaced with tarsus from a fellow eyelid or auricular or nasal cartilage; missing eyelid skin can be replaced by a local flap of skin grafted from the fellow eyelid or by skin from elsewhere (Fig. 4). Care is taken so that only the mucosal surface is in contact with the cornea, and lashes or hair are directed away from it. In general, because of the rich vascularity in this region, these grafts take very well, and the infection rate is low. When reconstructing an upper eyelid, the levator muscle or aponeurosis must be properly identified and repaired to ensure normal opening and closing of the lid. Both medial and lateral canthal tendons need to be reattached in order to achieve proper lacrimal drainage function and good cosmesis.

For burn patients, management during the acute stage consists of protecting the cornea by the use of lubricants, antibiotics, and a moisture chamber. Because of the severe cicatricial contracture of the soft tissues secondary to burn injury, these patients develop progressive retraction or ectropion of the eyelid, with secondary exposure keratitis and tearing problems. Fortunately, these problems can be corrected surgically. In principle, correction is accomplished by excising the scar tissues, releasing the cicatricial bands, and applying skin or mucosa grafts. This often needs to be done in several stages, and both split-thickness and full-thickness grafts are used.[14,23,32]

Paralyzed eyelids can be surgically corrected in several ways, including muscle transplantations and nerve cross-overs,[3,4,46,49] but these are complex procedures that have a relatively high morbidity and low success rate. In general,

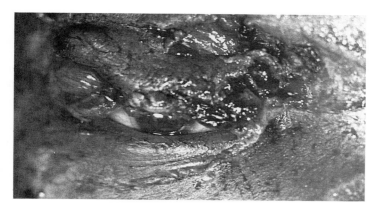

FIGURE 4. This patient's eyelid needs to be properly reconstructed; otherwise, his visual acuity may be threatened. Ptosis or tearing may be a sequela. The upper eyelid levator needs to be identified and repaired. The surgeon needs to make sure that the lacrimal gland is not damaged, the medial canthal tendon is reinserted, and the tear drainage duct is functioning.

these are not suitable for traumatic brain injury patients. Some of the simpler techniques include tarsorrhaphy, the use of a silicone encircling band,[2,27] a gold weight implantation,[29,47] and the insertion of palpebral springs[28,37]; each of these procedures or devices has its own advantages and disadvantages. All of these devices are available commercially, and all of these procedures can be performed under local anesthesia. However, all of these procedures require a certain degree of patient cooperation in order to achieve the best result. Tarsorrhaphy, requiring the least amount of patient cooperation, may be performed at bedside with a few instruments. When performed properly, this procedure can be reversed, and other procedures can be considered at a later time without fear of distorting the eyelid cosmetically.

Tarsorrhaphy. In general, a good lateral tarsorrhaphy alone is sufficient to protect the globe; only rarely is a medial tarsorrhaphy necessary. To perform a medial tarsorrhaphy, one needs to take into consideration the lacrimal drainage system so that these structures are not inadvertently injured. A lateral tarsorrhaphy can be performed at bedside during the acute stage following the trauma, but it can also be performed later if the patient is not tolerating the regimen of constant lubrication or the use of moisture chamber. Although the patient's cooperation is helpful, it is not necessary in achieving the desired results when performing a tarsorrhaphy.

The surgeon can first estimate the desired effect by bringing both the upper and lower eyelids together at various positions. Moving from laterally to medially, one can estimate the protection that will be rendered for the globe once the lids are sewn together. Therefore, the surgeon may decide to do a tarsorrhaphy that involves the lateral third, or half, or three-quarters of the entire eyelid as the clinical situation dictates. A small amount of 2% lidocaine with epinephrine is then injected along the posterior edge of both the upper and lower eyelids. The eyelids are prepared and draped, and the posterior edges of the eyelids are excised and denuded. A 4.0 chromic suture is first anchored in the skin laterally. This needle is then inserted into the tarsal plate of the upper eyelid to emerge from the denuded wound. This same needle is then inserted into the tarsal plate of the lower eyelid via the denuded wound, to emerge more medially. Moving more medially, this needle goes continuously between the upper and lower eyelid tarsal plate, closing the denuded wound. It finally reaches the medial end of the tarsorrhaphy, and the needle emerges out of the skin and is anchored there. This continuous suture with the denuded lid edge will form a strong bond, and protection of the globe is achieved. However, when necessary this procedure may be easily reversed by severing the eyelids at this very edge.

When the patient is more alert and cooperative, or when both cosmetic and functional considerations require a more sophisticated procedure, a silicone encircling band, gold weight implantation, or a palpebral spring may be considered at a later stage.

Silicone Encircling Band.   For insertion of a silicone encircling band, small incisions are made in the medial and the lateral canthal areas. With the aid of an inserter, the silicone band is positioned between the orbicularis muscle and the tarsal plate near the lid margin, so as to encircle the entire eyelid. The band is anchored to the medial and the lateral canthal tendons with sutures, and tension in the band is adjusted so that complete lid closure is achieved when the patient is instructed to close the eyelids. The incisions are then closed. Silicone bands are readily available commercially, and the procedure is fairly simple to perform. When properly inserted, the silicone band can ensure complete closure of an eyelid; if levator muscle function is intact, complete and frequent blinking is also achieved. By using this technique, a paralyzed lower eyelid is usually restored to its normal position. However, postoperative ptosis of the upper eyelid is expected. The known complications of this technique include erosion of the silicone band through the soft tissues and extrusion; in addition, the material eventually becomes fatigued, and the procedure needs to be repeated.

Gold Weight Implantation.   A gold weight can also be used to reanimate a paralyzed upper eyelid. These weights are available commercially, and the appropriate weight is chosen in the office by taping a gold weight to the paralyzed eyelid and assessing lid closure when the patient is in a sitting position. Under local anesthesia, the natural eyelid crease is first marked and incised. Using blunt dissection, a pocket is then created between the orbicularis muscle and the tarsal plate in the central portion of the upper eyelid (Fig. 5). An implant of appropriate weight is inserted into this space and is anchored with permanent sutures. The eyelid height and closure are assessed at this time by having the patient open and close the eyelid. When the desired result is achieved, the skin incision is closed. Although the incidence of extrusion, migration, or infection of the gold implant is extremely low, there is a cosmetic drawback because in some patients with pale and thin skin, the implant can be noticeable. Furthermore, blinking is not as complete or as natural as that achieved by the silicone band or palpebral spring.

Palpebral Spring Insertion.   To achieve the maximal effect of reanimation, the use of a palpebral spring may be combined with a levator-strengthening procedure. The palpebral spring is fashioned from an orthodontic, stainless steel wire. It is prefabricated preoperatively by the surgeon into a V-shape to conform to the natural contour of the upper lid and the periorbital region of the patient (Fig. 6). The patient's natural eyelid crease is marked, anesthetized, and incised. Laterally and superiorly, the dissection is carried out to the orbital rim. The apex of the implant is anchored laterally to the orbital rim with Dacron mesh and permanent

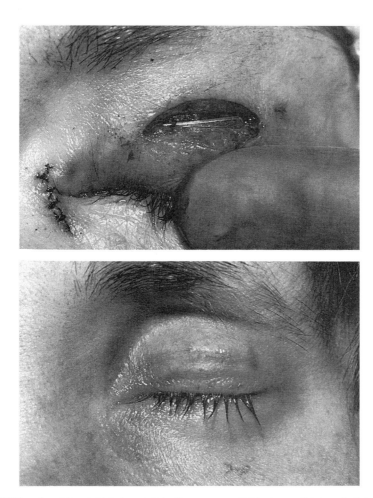

FIGURE 5.   A gold weight is inserted in the upper eyelid between the tarsal plate and the orbicularis muscle. It is anchored with a permanent suture. The lower photograph shows a patient 2 weeks after insertion of a gold weight. The patient has thin skin and very little orbital fat, so the gold weight is noticeable.

sutures. The upper arm of the implant, conforming to the contour of the lateral portion of the superior orbital rim, is anchored to this area with permanent sutures. The lower arm, conforming to the contour of the upper eyelid, is inserted between the orbicularis muscle and the tarsal plate. In most cases, Dacron mesh is used to aid in anchoring the implant at its apices. Tension in the spring is adjusted intra-operatively to achieve the desired blinking and closure, after which the skin incision is closed in the usual manner. The functional and cosmetic results of the palpebral spring are excellent; lid closure is complete, and the frequency and completeness of the blink approaches that of normal. However, the procedure is technically more difficult and is fairly time-consuming. In addition, occasional erosion through the soft tissue, infection, dislodging, and fatigue of the spring have been noted.

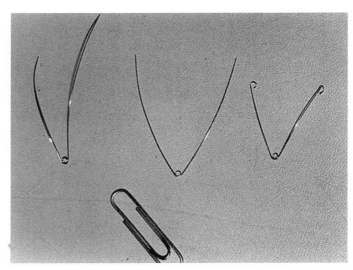

FIGURE 6.   Stainless steel wire is used to make a V-shaped spring to be implanted in the eyelid. A small paper clip is used for comparison of size.

TRAUMA TO THE ADNEXA

Clarity of vision and comfort of the eye are maintained mainly by the lacrimal apparatus, which consists of three portions: the secretory, distributional, and excretory systems. The secretory system includes the lacrimal gland, oil glands, and mucin glands; together, they produce the three-layered precorneal tear film. The distributional portion includes the eyelid and its blinking mechanism. The excretory system includes the puncta, canaliculi, and nasolacrimal duct. The afferent nerve supply is the fifth cranial nerve, and the efferent arm is the seventh cranial nerve.[24] When the secretory portion of the lacrimal system is injured, a dry eye and discomfort will result. Treatment in such a case typically consists of constant lubrication by means of artificial tears and ointment. In addition, the drainage system can be occluded by punctal plugs or by surgical techniques. When the eyelid is injured, proper blinking and closure may be affected (*see* earlier discussion). When the excretory portion of the lacrimal system is injured, excessive tearing may result, which can result in discomfort and which may be embarrassing to the patient.

Treatment of such a problem is usually surgical, as the drainage system needs to be probed and irrigated, and the proper diagnosis made. Depending on the exact nature of the injury and the location and extent of the obstruction, silicone intubation of the canalicular system may be performed, or a dacryocystorhinostomy, with or without insertion of a Pyrex tube, may be necessary (Fig. 7).[25,53] The success rate of these various procedures is generally quite high. Recently, lasers have been used for some of these procedures, and early reports show very promising results.

Ptosis as a result of trauma can usually be corrected surgically (Fig. 8). It is advisable, however, to wait for the initial edema to subside in the acute stage. In the case of a nerve injury, a 6-month waiting period before surgery is the rule. Severe ptosis can deprive the patient of normal, single, binocular vision and depth perception, in addition to being a cosmetic blemish. A partial ptosis may be

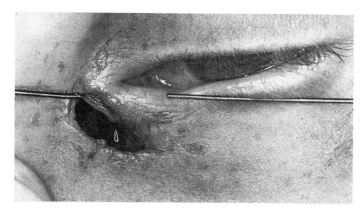

FIGURE 7. A laceration in the medial canthal area that involves the canalicular system. At times, silicone intubation of the canalicular system can restore function of the drainage system. Frequently, a dacryocystorhinostomy with the insertion of a Pyrex tube is necessary.

corrected via an external approach for levator resection or a levator tuck; severe ptosis may be corrected with a frontalis muscle sling, using either fascialata or a silicone band.[5] However, the correction of ptosis must be weighed against the possibility of creating a situation in which exposure keratitis can develop. Careful assessment of the patient's Bell's phenomenon, levator function, and orbicularis function is important.

BLOW-OUT FRACTURES OF THE ORBIT

Orbital fractures are generally the result of blunt trauma to the orbital region. Motor vehicle accidents are the most common cause of such injuries, although a blunt object, such as a fist, baseball, or even tennis ball can cause an orbital fracture. Clinical signs of an orbital fracture include periorbital edema, ecchymosis,

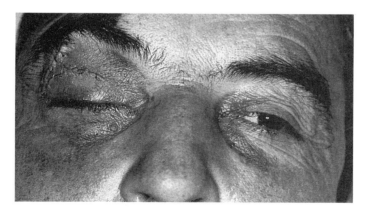

FIGURE 8. This patient has complete ptosis as a result of the initial trauma and lacks normal binocular vision and depth perception. Surgical repair of this ptosis must be weighed against the possibility of his developing exposure keratitis.

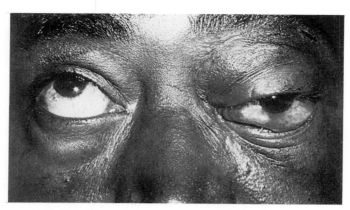

FIGURE 9.   Typical clinical picture of a patient suffering from a blow-out fracture of the orbit. The left eye is proptotic, chemotic, and unable to move freely in upward gaze.

conjunctival chemosis, subconjunctival hemorrhage, crepitance in the periorbital soft tissue, epistaxis, tearing, photophobia, enophthalmos, exophthalmos, and hypoesthesia along the infraorbital nerve distribution (Fig. 9).[48] The extent of damage to the periorbital soft tissue, bony confines, and the ocular structures is highly variable. At the one extreme, a patient may have many of the clinical signs but without serious injury of the globe itself, and thus have no visual sequelae. At the other extreme, the optic nerve may be injured, with resultant severe loss of visual function but no other significant clinical signs. In between, there are varying degrees of injury to the visual system, and the sensory system, the motor system, or both may be involved. To properly assess the extent of the injury and to render appropriate treatment and anticipate and prevent possible complications, an ophthalmologist should be involved in the care of these patients from the very first.

Examination.   A complete ocular examination is essential, and visual acuity should be carefully checked and recorded; the presence or absence of afferent pupillary defect should be assessed. Whenever a decrease in vision is present, an explanation should be diligently sought. For example, the cornea may be abraded, the lens may be dislocated, iritis may be present, or the retina may be contused or detached. A thorough examination with a slitlamp and funduscope is essential in the identification of these causes. Exophthalmometry is used to determine if endophthalmos or exophthalmos is present.

When diplopia or ocular motility limitation is present, its cause should be investigated. There are many possible causes for these conditions, including contused muscles, an entrapped muscle, damage of the nerve supply to the muscle, or restriction secondary to edema or pain.[11] The muscle most commonly affected is the inferior rectus, although the medial or the superior rectus muscle may be affected. In cases of diplopia or motility limitation, it is necessary to perform serial motility examinations over the next 7 to 10 days. Local application of a cold compress, oral steroid administration, or both may hasten the resolution of edema and pain. If improvement in motility is seen within a few days, the cause of the motility limitation is likely to be either orbital edema or contusion to the extraocular muscles. However, if no improvement is seen and the serial measurements stabilize, it is likely that the muscle is entrapped or that a nerve is damaged. In

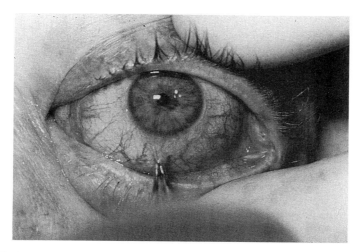

FIGURE 10. Forced duction test. With appropriate anesthesia, the inferior rectus muscle insertion is grasped with a forceps. The globe is moved gently superiorly and inferiorly.

these cases, a forced duction test is most helpful. The inferior fornix is first anesthetized by inserting a cotton pledget soaked in 4% cocaine. A toothed forceps is used to grasp the insertion of the inferior rectus muscle. By gently rotating the globe superiorly, the examiner can almost always determine the cause of the motility limitation (Fig. 10). In the case of muscle paralysis, the globe can be rotated easily, whereas in the case of an entrapped muscle, some resistance will be felt. In general, if diplopia is noted only in extreme upgaze or lateral gaze, and if there is no other clinical indication, conservative management may be the choice. Aggressive surgical intervention often makes the diplopia even worse; that is, the patient often develops diplopia in primary or down gaze. Diplopia in the extreme gazes may be unnoticeable or avoided by turning of the head; diplopia in primary gaze or in down gaze, however, is extremely debilitating and is often difficult to correct.

Surgical Treatment. The indications for surgical intervention in a blow-out fracture of the orbit are (1) entrapment of extraocular muscles, (2) diplopia in primary or down-gaze, or (3) enophthalmos of greater than 3 mm.[54] Several surgical approaches can be used. In general, ophthalmologists prefer the conjunctival or the subciliary approach, although some do prefer the intraoral approach. The first two approaches afford the surgeon direct visualization of the orbital contents and do not entail working through a contaminated region. Following the incision of the conjunctiva or the skin, dissection is carried down to the periorbita at the inferior orbital rim. The periorbita is then dissected and reflected, providing a clear view of the orbital contents and orbital floor. Incarcerated tissue is freed at this time, and an implant or autograft of appropriate size can be placed. The purpose of these implants is to restore orbital volume as well as to cover the fracture site. With the intraoral approach, the soft tissue over the maxilla is dissected and retracted. When the anterior wall of the maxilla is removed, the surgeon has a clear view of the orbital floor from below. Repair of the fracture is accomplished in most cases by packing the antrum.[8,14,48,54]

Surgical intervention for a blow-out fracture of the orbit does not always result in complete resolution of the problem. Some of the more commonly seen complications include residual enophthalmos, residual diplopia, ectropion, and lacrimal dysfunction. Although late enophthalmos is difficult to correct, problems such as lacrimal dysfunction or ectropion can be corrected with further surgery. Small amounts of residual diplopia can be managed satisfactorily with prisms in most cases, and some patients learn to turn their head in the appropriate direction to eliminate the annoying diplopia. Strabismus surgery is necessary for patients with large deviations and for those who do not benefit sufficiently from prisms.

Midfacial Trauma. Patients suffering from midfacial trauma often have ocular involvement and should be evaluated and treated by an ophthalmologist to minimize visual complications. Midfacial traumas include fractures of the frontal sinus, nasoethmoidal complex, pygomatic complex, and maxilla. For most patients with midfacial fractures, definitive reconstructive surgery is deferred until initial edema of the soft tissue has subsided. Children, however, should have surgery much sooner, and a precise reduction of the fractures must be achieved because bone healing and molding take place very rapidly in the young.[1,12,42,52]

If the posterior table of the frontal sinus is fractured, it should be repaired by a neurosurgeon. If the anterior table alone is involved, the sinus mucosa and the frontoethmoidal duct should be carefully inspected before repairing the bony defect. It is important that no sinus mucosa is incarcerated in the fracture site and that an adequate sinus drainage system is established in order to prevent the development of a mucocele. Repair of an anterior table fracture can be accomplished via the existing laceration, through a suprabrow incision, or by means of a coronal flap.[26,43]

In repairing a nasoethmoidal fracture, care should be taken to ensure that the medial canthal tendons are properly reattached if they have been disinserted; in many cases, transnasal wiring of the tendons will be necessary. The nasal lacrimal drainage system should be carefully identified and retracted to preclude further damage during surgery. To repair a nasoethmoidal fracture, a coronal flap, open-sky approach, or a modified dacryocystorhinostomy incision can be used.[10,40]

Zygomatic fractures are the most commonly encountered fractures in midfacial trauma. These fractures are difficult to classify, and depending on the location and the nature of the fracture, many different techniques can be used for their reduction. A simple depressed fracture of the zygomatic arch can be repaired via a Gillies' approach. This calls for a small incision over the temporal area, through which an elevator is inserted in the appropriate anatomic plane to reach the depressed arch. The fracture can then be reduced manually. A displaced or rotated tripod fracture can be reduced with a Gillies' technique through a percutaneous approach, via the intraoral route, or by means of a coronal flap. In many instances, the orbital floor or walls are fractured when the zygomatic complex is injured; when indicated, orbital fractures can be repaired at the same time.[15,21,55]

Fractures of the maxilla can be reduced most readily via a Caldwell-Luc technique but may also be approached intranasally or via the existing wound. In cases in which the maxillary antrum needs to be packed, care should be taken so that no undue pressure is exerted on the orbital contents and to ensure that an adequate antral window is created.[15,31]

Fixation Methods. To achieve the best result both functionally and cosmetically, facial fractures should be accurately reduced and fixated and the soft tissues meticulously repaired. Surgical stainless steel wires are used to approximate the bony fragments, but three-dimensional stabilization is often difficult to achieve. The use of metallic miniplates and screws, however, affords a rigid three-dimensional fixation of the bony structures and promotes rapid primary healing.[22,30] Indeed, we find this technique to be most beneficial to the patient, as it yields excellent results and causes very few complications. Hardware, fabricated of various rare metals and of various designs, is available commercially.

For many patients with eyelid or orbital trauma, the cosmetic defect is their greatest concern. Scars in the facial or periorbital area can be revised by various techniques, such as Z-plasty, multiple Z-plasty, local flaps, or free grafts.[14,20,23,44] Many of these patients have ectropion or entropion of the eyelid, which can be corrected surgically. In some patients, traumatic ptosis of the upper lid may be present. Ptosis noted at the initial examination may be secondary to periorbital edema and often improves spontaneously when the edema subsides. However, if ptosis persists for more than 6 months, despite resolution of edema, surgical correction may be necessary. In most of these trauma cases, dehiscence or disinsertion of the levator aponeurosis is seen.

RETINAL DETACHMENT

Retinal detachment is a separation between outer retinal pigment epithelium and the inner sensory retina. Such a separation occurs when there is traction on the inner sensory layer or when an opening, such as a hole, a break, or a tear, permits accumulation of fluid between the two layers. Retinal breaks result usually from vitreous traction on the sensory retina secondary to retinal degeneration or following penetrating or blunt trauma to the eye. In general, retinal detachment occurs more frequently in men than in women, in eyes with a degenerative myopia, in the aged, and following cataract surgery.[16,17] Trauma accounts for approximately 15% of the total retinal detachments; these traumatic detachments are usually late sequelae of the original injury, with about 80% occurring within 2 years of the initial incident and the remaining 20% occurring at the moment of injury or shortly thereafter. The most common type of retinal break seen in young patients with trauma to the eye is a dialysis, which consists of a disinsertion of the retina at the ora serrata, anteriorly. This is seen most commonly in the superior nasal quadrant of the eye. A giant tear of the retina refers to a tear of the retina that affects more than one quadrant.[9,45]

Retinal edema occurs often after a direct blow to the eye. In such cases, vision is reduced, and the prognosis for central acuity is guarded. Late pigmentary macular changes, a macular cyst, or a macular hole may develop. With a severe enough contusion to the globe, choroidal rupture may occur; initially, this may be obscured by a large intraocular hemorrhage. Neovascularization in the area of rupture may also develop, which can lead eventually to transudation, hemorrhage, and macular detachment.[19,50]

The patient with a retinal detachment usually experiences flashes of light, which result from vitreous traction on the retina, or a sudden shower of black dots in the peripheral visual field, which results from vitreous hemorrhage at the point of a retinal break. The diagnosis of retinal detachment is made on the funduscopic findings of the retina (Fig. 11). First the pupils are dilated pharmacologically, and both eyes are examined for comparison. The best way to make a diagnosis of retinal detachment and locate the holes and tears is to perform the technique of indirect ophthalmoscopy. Ophthalmologists use special head gear, magnifying

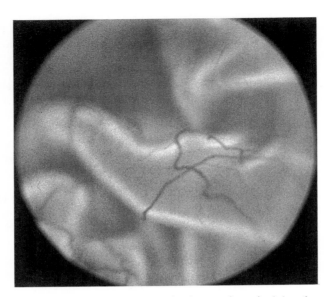

FIGURE 11. A typical funduscopic picture of a retinal detachment.

lens, and light source to perform this examination. Indirect ophthalmoscopy combined with scleral depression enables the examiner to study the entire retina from the optic disc to the ora serrata.

The treatment of traumatic retinal detachment is surgical. Once the diagnosis is established, immediate treatment is indicated to prevent macular involvement, if this has not yet detached. In order to reattach the retina, the holes or breaks have to be closed first, and the subretinal fluid must be drained. Retinal holes are closed by creating adhesion between the edge of the hole and the retinal pigment epithelium by means of either cryosurgery or diathermy.[6,36] Drainage of the subretinal fluid is achieved by perforating the choroid through the sclera, although the subretinal fluid usually reabsorbs when the retinal hole is sealed. Once the holes are identified and closed, various techniques are used to buckle the sclera and the choroid to keep the retina in good contact with the retinal pigment epithelium. Selection of a particular procedure depends on the type of hole and the number of quadrants of retina involved. A radially placed implant is usually sufficient to close a single horseshoe-shaped hole, whereas an encircling band around the circumference of the eye may be required to seal multiple holes in multiple quadrants. In addition, silicone oil or air injected into the vitreous cavity may help to keep the retina attached. In penetrating injuries of the globe, early vitrectomy is also indicated.[7,13,18,33–35]

ENUCLEATION AND EVISCERATION

Only rarely is enucleation performed as a primary procedure following trauma, but it may be done, for example, in patients with a severe gunshot wound to the eye and in whom the globe is ruptured beyond repair.

The patient who undergoes enucleation will typically experience four predictable phases of psychiatric adjustment: denial, depression or anger, acceptance, and rehabilitation. The loss of an eye is especially devastating because the patient not only experiences a significant sensory deprivation but also must adjust to an altered body image concerning the most cosmetically crucial part of the body. Enucleation is often necessary in the treatment of an intraocular malignancy, but these patients have time to prepare for this eventuality. Losing an eye to trauma is sudden and unexpected, and these patients are ill-prepared for the adjustments required of them. In general, unless the globe is shattered beyond repair, enucleation is not performed as a primary procedure in trauma cases.

The usual practice is to repair the globe as much as possible, even though the physician realizes that recovery of vision is beyond any hope. Following the initial repair, the physician then discusses with the patient and the patient's family the clinical findings, making them understand that there is no hope of regaining vision, thereby preparing them for the inevitable enucleation. Once the patient realizes the situation after a few days and is able to accept this fact, it will be easier for the patient to undergo enucleation.

Enucleation is performed also in patients with a blind eye that is painful or cosmetically objectionable. In rare instances, this procedure is performed to remove a traumatized eye that still retains some vision, in order to preclude the development of sympathetic ophthalmia in the remaining eye.[39,51] Sympathetic ophthalmia is the most dreaded complication of ocular trauma affecting the noninjured eye from weeks to many years following the initial injury. It is thought to be of autoimmune origin. When the injury involves prolapse of the uveal tissues, and if the injured eye is not removed in a timely fashion, a severe inflammatory response is incited via an unknown mechanism in the uninvolved good eye, which may eventually be totally destroyed.

Enucleation is performed under general anesthesia. A 360° peritomy is performed, the conjunctiva and Tenon's capsule are dissected, and the extraocular muscles are identified, tagged with sutures, and disinserted. The optic nerve is severed, and the eyeball is then removed.[44] Many different types of implants and surgical techniques have been described to achieve the best cosmetic results. The goals are to restore orbital volume and to maintain the best possible motility for the prosthetic eye. For more than a century, ophthalmologists have been trying to devise an ideal implant that would achieve these goals. Recently, an integrated hydroxyapatite orbital implant has shown promise.[41]

Known complications resulting from enucleation include ptosis, depressed superior sulcus, enophthalmus, sagging of the lower eyelid, entropion, extropion, extrusion, and migration of the implant.[53-55] Enucleation, therefore, should not be looked on as simply the removal of an eye; rather, it is part of a rehabilitation program for the patient, and requires a strong patient-physician relationship. Following surgery, the patient needs to be referred to an ocularist and to be fitted with the appropriate prosthetic eye (Fig. 12).

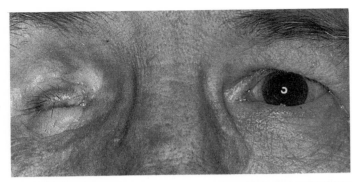

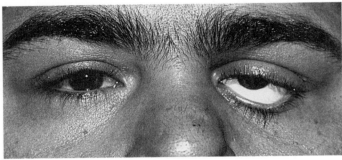

FIGURE 12.   *Top*, An enucleation that was performed poorly, leaving the patient with a severely contracted socket. This problem can be corrected surgically. *Lower*, This patient has a poorly fitted prosthesis in the left socket following an enucleation. The opthalmologist and ocularist need to work closely together with the patient to achieve the best result.

REFERENCES

1. Anderson RL, Panje WR, Gross CE: Optic nerve blindness following blunt forehead trauma. Ophthalmology 89:445–455, 1982.
2. Arion HG: Dynamic closure of the lids in paralysis of the orbicularis muscle. Int Surg 57:48–50, 1972.
3. Baker DC, Conley J: Reanimation of facial paralysis. In English GM (ed): Otolaryngology. Philadelphia, JB Lippincott, 1982.
4. Barclay TL, Roberts AC: Restoration of movement to the upper eyelid in facial palsy. Br J Plast Surg 22:257–261. 1969.
5. Beard C: Ptosis, 3rd ed. St. Louis, CV Mosby, 1981, pp 66–174.
6. Campochiaro PA, Kaden IH, Vidaurri-Leal J, et al: Cryotherapy enhances intravitreal dispersion of viable retinal pigment epithelial cells. Arch Ophthalmol 103:434–436, 1985.
7. Chang S, Reppucci V, Zimmerman NJ, et al: Perfluorocarbon liquids in the management of traumatic retinal detachments. Ophthalmology 96:785–792, 1989.
8. Converse JM, Smith B: On the treatment of blowout fractures of the orbit. Plast Reconstr Surg 62:100–104, 1978.
9. Cox MS, Schepens CL, Freeman HM: Retinal detachment due to ocular contusion. Arch Ophthalmol 76:678–685, 1966.
10. Cruse CW, Blevins PK, Luce EA: Naso-ethmoid-orbital fractures. J Trauma 20:551–556, 1980.
11. Fujino T, Makino K: Entrapment mechanism and ocular injury in orbital blowout fracture. Plast Reconstr Surg 65:571–576, 1980.
12. Giovinazzo VJ: The ocular sequelae of blunt trauma. Adv Ophthalmic Plast Reconstr Surg 6:107–114, 1987.
13. Glaser BM: Treatment of giant retinal tears combined with proliferative vitreoretinopathy. Ophthalmology 93:1193–1197, 1986.

14. Glover AG: Eyelid burns. In Singleton BJ, Hersh PS, Kenyon KR (eds): Eye Trauma. St. Louis, Mosby YearBook, 1991, pp 315–322.
15. Gruss JS, Van Wyck L, Phillips JH, Antonyshyn O: The importance of the zygomatic arch in complex midfacial fracture repair and correction of posttraumatic orbitozygomatic deformities. Plast Reconstr Surg 85:878–890, 1990.
16. Hagler WS: Retinal dialysis: A statistical and genetic study to determine pathogenic factors. Trans Am Ophthalmol Soc 78:686–733, 1980.
17. Haimann MH, Burton TC, Brown CK: Epidemiology of retinal detachment. Arch Ophthalmol 100:289–292, 1982.
18. Han DP, Mieler WF, Abrams GW, et al: Vitrectomy for traumatic retinal incarceration. Arch Ophthalmol 106:640–645, 1988.
19. Hart CD, Raistrick R: Indirect choroidal tears and late onset serosanguinous maculopathies. Graefes Arch Clin Exp Ophthalmol 218:206–210, 1982.
20. Hartford CE: Methods of reducing burn scar deformity. In Stark RB (ed): Plastic Surgery of the Head and Neck, vol 1. New York, Churchill Livingstone, 1987, pp 282–285.
21. Jackson IT: Classification and treatment of orbitozygomatic and orbitoethomoid fractures: The place of bone grafting and plate fixation. Clin Plast Surg 16:77–91, 1989.
22. Jackson IT, Somers PC, Kjar JG: The use of Champy miniplates for osteosynthesis in craniofacial deformities and trauma. Plast Reconstr Surg 77:729–736, 1986.
23. Jelks GW, Smith BC: Reconstruction of the eyelids and associated structures. In McCarthy JG (ed): Plastic Surgery. Philadelphia, WB Saunders, 1990, pp 1671–1784.
24. Jones LT, Wobig JL: Neuro-Physiology. Birmingham, UK, Aesculapius Publishing Company, 1976, p 74.
25. Jones LT, Wobig JL: Surgery of Eyelids and Lacrimal System. Birmingham, UK, Aesculapius Publishing Company, 1976, pp 194–230.
26. Larrabee WF Jr, Travis LW, Tabb HG: Frontal sinus fractures—Their suppurative complications and surgical management. Laryngoscope 90:1810–1813, 1980.
27. Lessa S, Carreirao S: Use of an encircling silicone rubber string for the correction of lagophthalmos. Plast Reconstr Surg 61:719–723, 1978.
28. Levine RE: Management of the eye after acoustic tumor surgery. In House WF, Luetje CM (eds): Acoustic Tumors, Management, vol 2. Baltimore, University Park Press, 1979, p 105.
29. Liu D: Gold weight lid load as a secondary procedure. Plast Reconstr Surg 87:854–858, 1991.
30. Luhr HC: Stabile fixation von Oberkiefer-Mittelgesichtsfrakturen durch Mini-Kompression platten. Dtsch Zahnaerztl Z 34:851, 1979.
31. Manson PN, Crawley WA, Yaremchuk MJ, et al: Midface fractures: Advantages of immediate extended open reduction and bone grafting. Plast Reconstr Surg 76:1–10, 1985.
32. Marrone AW: Thermal eyelid burns. In Hornblass A, Hanio CT (eds): Oculoplastic, Orbital and Reconstructive Surgery, vol 1, Eyelids. Baltimore, Williams & Wilkins, 1988, pp 433–437.
33. McCuen BW II, Hida T, Sheta SM: Transvitreal cyanoacrylate retinopexy in the management of complicated retinal detachment. Am J Ophthalmol 104:127–132, 1987.
34. Meredith TA, Gordon PA: Pars plana vitrectomy for severe penetrating injury with posterior segment involvement. Am J Ophthalmol 103:549–554, 1987.
35. Michels RG: Vitrectomy methods in penetrating ocular trauma. Ophthalmology 87:629–645, 1980.
36. Michels RG, Rice TA, Blankenship G: Surgical techniques for selected giant retinal tears. Retina 3:139–153, 1983.
37. Morel-Fatio D, Lalardrie JP: Palliative surgical treatment of facial paralysis. The palpebral spring. Plast Reconstr Surg 33:446–456, 1964.
38. Newell FW: Ophthalmology: Principles and Concept, 6th ed. St. Louis, CV Mosby, 1986.
39. Nunery WR, Hetzler KJ: Improved prosthetic motility following enucleation. Ophthalmology 90:1110–1115, 1983.
40. Paskert JP, Manson PN, Iliff NT: Nasoethmoidal and orbital fractures. Clin Plast Surg 15:209–223, 1988.
41. Perry AC: Advances in enucleation. Ophthalmol Clin North Am 4:173–182, 1991.
42. Petro J, Tooze FM, Bales CR, Baker G: Ocular injuries associated with periorbital fractures. J Trauma 19:730–733, 1979.
43. Remmler D, Boles R: Intracranial complications of frontal sinusitis. Laryngoscope 90:1814–1824, 1980.
44. Robson MC, Zachary LS, et al: Repair of traumatic cutaneous injuries involving the skin and soft tissue. In Georgiade NG, et al (eds): Essentials of Plastic, Maxillofacial, and Reconstructive Surgery. Baltimore, Williams & Wilkins, 1987, pp 117–122.
45. Ross WH: Traumatic retinal dialyses. Arch Ophthalmol 99:1371–1374, 1981.

46. Samii M: Facial nerve grafting in acoustic neurinoma. In Terzis JK (ed): Microreconstruction of Nerve Injuries. Philadelphia, WB Saunders Company, 1987, pp 651–660.
47. Smellie GD: Restoration of the blinking reflex in facial palsy by a simple lid-load operation. Br J Plast Surg 19:279–283, 1966.
48. Smith B, Regan WF Jr: Blow-out fracture of the orbit: Mechanism and correction of internal orbital fracture. Am J Ophthalmol 44:733–739, 1957.
49. Smith JW: Advances in facial nerve repair. Surg Clin North Am 52:1287–1306, 1972.
50. Smith RE, Kelley JS, Harbin TS: Late macular complications of choroidal ruptures. Am J Ophthalmol 77:650–658, 1974.
51. Spivey BE: Enucleation: A remaining challenge. Aust J Ophthalmol 8:69–74, 1980.
52. Steidler NE, Cook RM, Reade PC: Incidence and management of major middle third facial fractures at the Royal Melbourne Hospital: A retrospective study. Int J Oral Surg 9:92–98, 1980.
53. Veirs ER: Malleable rods for immediate repair of the traumatically severed lacrimal canaliculus. Trans Am Acad Ophthalmol Otolaryngol 66:263–264, 1962.
54. Wilkins RB, Havins WE: Current treatment of blow-out fractures. Ophthalmology 89:464–466, 1982.
55. Winstanley RP: The management of fractures of the zygoma. Int J Oral Surg 10(suppl 1):235–240, 1981.

JOHN L. SHEN, MD

PERIPHERAL NERVE INJURY FOLLOWING TRAUMATIC BRAIN INJURY

From the
Adult Brain Injury Service
Rancho Los Amigos Medical
  Center
Downey, California

Correspondence to:
John L. Shen, MD
Adult Brain Injury Service
Rancho Los Amigos Medical
  Center
7601 E. Imperial Highway
800 Annex
Downey, CA 90242

It is well established that cognitive deficits are the most common and serious sequelae following a traumatic brain injury (TBI). However, concomitant peripheral nerve injuries (PNIs) can coexist in this population, especially in patients with moderate to severe brain and polymusculoskeletal trauma.[36,87,111] Stone and Keenan[111] found the prevalence of PNI in adults with severe TBI to be 34%. Cosgrove et al.[19] reported a conservatively low 10% in their population. This disparity may be secondary to differences among patients studied (acute versus chronic, mild versus severe) or the criteria in selecting patients for diagnostic evaluation. Philip and Philip[87] screened 157 children with TBI, of whom 7% had a concomitant PNI. Garland and Bailey[36] reported that of 254 consecutive patients admitted to the Head Trauma Service at Rancho Los Amigos Medical Center, 11% were identified as having 10 previously undiagnosed fractures or dislocations and 29 undetected PNIs. Another study found that the incidence of traumatic peripheral nerve lesions of the upper limb was twice that in the lower limb (5% and 2.7%, respectively).[45] Goodall[44] cited, in order of decreasing frequency, that the radial, ulnar, peroneal, median, and sciatic nerves were most vulnerable. PNI is commonly associated with long-bone fractures,[51] but other risk factors include improper limb positioning, ill-fitting casts, nerve complications after surgery, and spasticity.

Heterotopic ossification (HO) has been associated with TBI and PNI. The etiology of HO formation has not yet been elucidated (*see* the later chapter by Garland).[124] Patients with spinal cord injury and severe TBI frequently develop ectopic bone growth. Garland and Keenan[37] reported that 11% of 496 adults with TBI developed significant HO, with the hip as the most commonly involved joint. Nerve entrapment as a complication of HO formation may occur.[9] Varghese and coworkers[116] reported case findings of ulnar nerve compression as a complication of HO formation. Brooke et al.[9] published similar findings and recommended computed tomographic scanning to help localize the site of compression.

DIAGNOSIS

Nerve conduction studies and electromyography (EMG) are useful adjuncts to confirm or dispute the clinical diagnosis. Fibrillation potentials and positive sharp waves are considered the hallmark of injury to the lower motor neuron, neuromuscular junction, or muscle fiber.[7] However, recent articles suggest that certain upper motor neuron disorders, including stroke and spinal cord injury, may demonstrate abnormal spontaneous potentials in paralytic extremities, probably secondary to trans-synaptic degeneration of motor neurons.[3,10] In this circumstance, nerve conduction velocities of the involved extremity are typically normal.[10,43]

A flail extremity in a trauma victim usually indicates a plexus injury until proven otherwise, particularly if associated with a shoulder or pelvic fracture.[37] However, mild weakness that is masked by central paresis in a limb can be overlooked. The presence of motor weakness, sensory loss, skin changes, asymmetrical hyporeflexia, atrophy, and fasiculations in an appropriate distribution are signs that should lead one to suspect a peripheral nerve lesion. Typically, the TBI patient is in a confused or unresponsive state, which tends to make the detection of a PNI more difficult.[117] Therefore, a high index of suspicion is necessary to identify peripheral nerve lesions in this population. The early documentation of a nerve injury allows the patient to receive appropriate early rehabilitation while awaiting nerve regeneration.

ULNAR NERVE

Ulnar nerve entrapments occur most commonly in the region of the elbow.[12,13] Three possible sites of compression are the retroepicondylar groove, the humero-ulnar aponeurotic arcade, and distal to the two heads of the flexor carpi ulnaris.[14] Other, less common areas of involvement may include the hand,[78,83] wrist,[29,128] and axilla. Two general types of ulnar nerve lesions at the elbow have been described[33]: neuropathy in relation to the medial epicondylar groove associated with a history of elbow fracture or dislocation (tardy ulnar palsy), and entrapment distal to the two heads of the flexor carpi ulnaris and normally not associated with clinical or roentgenographic evidence of joint deformity (cubital tunnel syndrome).[13,77]

The majority of patients complain of numbness, hypesthesia, or both on the volar surface of the ulnar half of the palm. Sometimes, numbness is detected in the laterodorsal aspect of the hand (dorsal ulnar cutaneous nerve), which may indicate a lesion proximal to the wrist. Weakness may manifest in the abductor digiti minimi, flexor digitorum profundus to the fourth and fifth digits, flexor carpi ulnaris, and the first dorsal interosseous. When the adductor pollicis and flexor pollicis brevis weaken, the metacarpophalangeal joints of the thumb will lose its stability, producing a vicarious movement known as Froment's sign.[47] In severe and long-standing cases, atrophy of the intrinsic muscles leads to a claw hand deformity.

After TBI, focal entrapment of the ulnar nerve is relatively common at the elbow.[111] Factors that predispose to injury at this level include elbow trauma, elbow flexor spasticity, periarticular HO, decreased mobility, and prolonged recovery period.[54] Keenan et al.[54] reported that the incidence of late ulnar neuropathy occurred in 2.5% of 25 patients. All of the patients they studied had residual spasticity and nerve entrapment within the neurologically impaired upper extremity. It has been reported that 26% of HO formation occurs around the elbow in brain-injured patients.[37] If the elbow is traumatized, risk for HO in that region is even higher.[23,38,48] Garland and Keenan[37] reported that 90% of patients with elbow dislocations or fractures develop periarticular HO. We have witnessed a large number of our TBI patients who have developed ulnar neuropathies related to HO entrapping the nerve along with persistent elbow flexion (Fig. 1). If HO is suspected, plain radiographs and a bone scan can delineate the maturity of bone-forming activity. Kincaid[56] believes that the number of fascicles are reduced in the elbow area and hence may make the nerve even more susceptible to compression.

Comatose patients are prone to developing compartment syndromes,[100] which may be another source of ulnar neuropathy. Furthermore, improper positioning of the upper limb is detrimental to the ulnar nerve secondary to a pressure neuritis.[37] Brain-injured patients are very often positioned with their elbows flexed, resting on a hard surface. This position exacerbates an ulnar nerve compression.

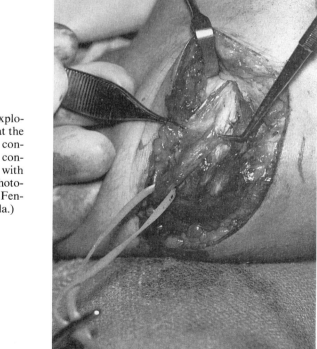

FIGURE 1. Surgical exploration of the ulnar nerve at the elbow. The ulnar nerve is constricted, hyperemic, and congested and is associated with heterotopic ossification (Photograph courtesy of Colin Fennell, MD, Calgary, Canada.)

Electrodiagnosis can aid in localizing the entrapment. Motor nerve conduction slowing across the elbow is a clue that compression may be localized to the elbow.[13,75,77] Recently, Campbell and associates[14] recommended that short-segment incremental studies can identify compression levels more accurately than the standard inching technique. Evaluation of the compound motor action potential amplitude is also necessary. Miller[77] concluded that if decrement of the evoked action potential amplitude above the elbow as compared with below the elbow exceeds 10%, it is considered abnormal.

The **choice of treatment** appears to depend on the nature of the entrapment and the surgeon's preference. For entrapments without HO formation, initially splinting the elbow in extension at nighttime is recommended. In patients with HO, surgery is generally the first approach because of the inflammatory HO formation and difficulty in positioning the joint in extension. Under anesthesia, the patient's ankylosed joint can be manipulated manually to determine whether a soft tissue contracture exists. Surgical choices include simple decompression, anterior transposition, or medial epicondylectomy. A decompression procedure is preferred in subacute cases, tardy ulnar palsies without deformities, and idiopathic cases.[16] If HO is present at the cubital tunnel, an anterior subcutaneous transposition is recommended.[37] Medial epicondylectomy or submuscular transposition may enhance the formation of HO postoperatively and is therefore contraindicated.

MEDIAN NERVE

Carpal tunnel syndrome is caused by the compression of the median nerve at the wrist. Carpal tunnel syndrome implies an underlying disorder, and many etiologies have been identified.[22,112] The symptoms may include weakness, pain, paresthesia, and numbness in the median nerve distribution. Weakness may become a debilitating factor impairing a patient's activities of daily living skills. Some patients may exhibit a positive Tinel's sign, Phalen's sign, or a tethered median nerve stress test[59] (pain radiating to the proximal volar forearm when the index finger is hyperextended).

Patients with chronic disabilities, including those with spinal cord injuries,[41] postpoliomyelitis,[118,121] traumatic myelopathies, and stroke, are at risk for median mononeuropathy at the wrist. Patients who use mobility devices may develop carpal tunnel syndrome, involving almost always the side of frequent hand usage. Gellman and associates[41] speculated that excessive and repetitive forceful extension of the wrist that occurs during transfer or propelling of a wheelchair will cause a rise in pressure within the carpal canal, predisposing the nerve to injury. Interestingly, Haas et al.[46] had reported seven patients who developed symptoms and signs of carpal tunnel syndrome after being involved in motor vehicle accidents.

A common feature after severe TBI is a spastic flexion deformity of the upper extremity. Patients typically exhibit elbow, wrist, and finger flexion spasticity with shoulder adduction (Fig. 2). Wrist flexion spasticity may cause prolonged mechanical compression of the median nerve.[109] In 1981, Gelberman et al.[40] described a technique to measure the intracarpal canal pressures of able-bodied patients with electrodiagnostically proven carpal tunnel syndrome. The mean pressures during forced wrist flexion and extension were 94 and 110 mm Hg, respectively. They proposed that increased pressure could be one of several factors for the causation of carpal tunnel syndrome. This is in contrast to a study by Orcutt et al.[82] who described 10 brain-injured patients who had developed carpal tunnel syndromes from prolonged spastic posturing in flexion of the wrists and fingers. Carpal tunnel

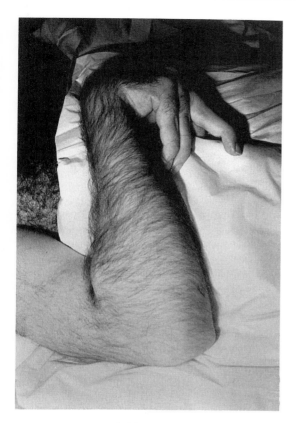

FIGURE 2. Right upper extremity demonstrating spasticity with hyperflexion of the elbow, wrist, and fingers, causing compression of the median nerve at the wrist and ulnar nerve at the elbow. (Photograph courtesy of Lance Stone, DO, San Diego, CA.)

pressures averaged 11 mm Hg in the resting position. They established that increased intracanal pressures did not contribute to the development of carpal tunnel syndrome. Marin and associates[70] demonstrated that hyperflexion of the wrist for 5 minutes in control subjects and in patients with carpal tunnel syndrome caused a significant increase in distal sensory latency during nerve conduction study. We speculate that the combination of spastic flexion deformities of the wrist and fingers, which tethered the median nerve against the transverse carpal ligament and the tight flexor sublimus tendons, put the nerve at risk for carpal tunnel syndrome.

Nerve conduction studies are useful adjuncts to the diagnosis of carpal tunnel syndrome in TBI, especially where a history is unreliable or unobtainable. Several articles have been published describing different methods of detection.[17,25,55,69,85,90,114,127]

Conservative treatment of spastic hand deformities in patients with carpal tunnel syndrome may include motor-point blocks with 5% phenol to the forearm muscle flexors, followed by serial casting or splinting. If that fails, a carpal tunnel release with wrist and finger flexor tendon lengthening is advocated.[82]

RADIAL NERVE

The radial nerve can be compromised by either a humeral fracture, compression,[34] or a traction injury. Most traumatic radial nerve injuries are secondary to midshaft humeral fractures, especially those spiral in type.[49,99] A fracture in the lower third of the humerus can also present with a radial neuropathy,[44] which results when the proximal bony fragment displaces radially and the distal portion proximally, compressing the radial nerve. It has been proposed that the radial nerve travels close to the inferior lip of the spiral groove.[49,68] As the nerve approaches the lateral supracondylar ridge, it pierces the lateral intermuscular septum. Holstein and Lewis[49] believe that the nerve is relatively immobile at this point and is easily injured with fractures of the humerus.

In the confused TBI patient with spasticity, closed reduction of the fracture places the radial nerve at risk because of an inability to maintain adequate reduction. Therefore, open reduction and internal fixation are recommended.[37] The radial nerve can also sustain a traction injury without fracturing the humerus.[119]

The treatment of a wrist drop is mostly supportive, since the majority recover spontaneously. The primary goal is to prevent the development of joint contractures. Barton[5] recommended a passive splint made of plaster holding the wrist and metacarpophalangeal joints in extension. Later, the splint can be bi-valved anteriorly and posteriorly for nighttime use. A dynamic splint which permits active flexion of all the joints and passively returns them to the extended position will reduce the risk for joint immobilization. Electrical stimulation of the denervated muscles has not been found to be effective.[5] A transected radial nerve can be microsurgically repaired along with tendon transfers, producing a fair recovery.[32]

POSTERIOR INTEROSSEOUS NERVE

The posterior interosseous nerve is the motor branch of the radial nerve, and as it enters the supinator muscle, it adheres tightly around the radial head. Traction or compression[28] caused by injuries of the forearm may injure the posterior interosseous nerve. Spontaneous recovery can be expected in 60% of the patients within the first 8 weeks after injury. Therefore, routine exploration of the nerve is not indicated.[105] In forearm fractures following TBI, anterior elbow HO or synostosis of the intermuscular membrane may form, causing nerve compression. Fracture of the ulnar with dislocation of the radial head (Monteggia fracture) has also been associated with posterior interosseous nerve palsy.[65,104,105]

Clinically, patients demonstrate weakness in wrist extension with a radial drift, finger extension at the level of the metacarpophalangeal joint, and thumb extension and thumb abduction.[20] Radial deviation of the wrist is due to the strong unopposed extensor carpi radialis longus and brevis with paralysis of the extensor carpi ulnaris. Patients may complain of pain in the elbow region, which is aggravated by forced supination or resisted wrist dorsiflexion.[15] The diagnosis is confirmed with needle EMG studies.

BRACHIAL PLEXOPATHY

Brachial plexus injury is of great significance in view of the associated severe residual morbidity. The sequelae involve a combination of physical and psychological disabilities. All too often, patients recover enough insight to discern their profound deficit, only to become grossly absorbed with a sense of anger and frustration. Therefore, it is important that the physician screen for this type of malady with a high index of suspicion, because it is often missed. Garland and Bailey[36] stressed that if a TBI patient presents with a shoulder girdle fracture and a flail upper extremity, brachial plexopathy must be ruled out, especially if the patient was operating a motorcycle. Not surprisingly, Rosson[95] described that the

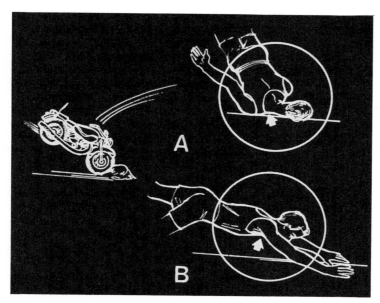

FIGURE 3. *A,* Forceful lateral flexion of the head away from the shoulder, producing a C5–C6 root, upper trunk brachial plexopathy, or both. *B,* Hyperabduction of the arm, causing a C8–T1 root, lower trunk plexus lesion, or both. (Photograph courtesy of Lance Stone, DO, San Diego, CA.)

majority of patients with brachial plexus lesions after motorcycle accidents were young males (less than 20 years old), had less than 1 year of driving experience, and were not adequately trained. A displaced fracture of the midclavicle[23] after a fall[96] or motorcycle accident[36] may also injure the brachial plexus. Football players are at risk for upper trunk plexopathy.[24,93] Fracture and dislocation of the cervical spine should also alert one to a possible plexopathy.[72]

Motor vehicle accidents expose individuals to rapid and unprotected impacts (Fig. 3). When the neck is stretched laterally with the arm drawn inward, it often produces a upper trunk or C5-6 root injury (Erb's paralysis). The result is a functional hand with a nonfunctional shoulder. Conversely, when the arm is hyperabducted, the lower trunk or C8–T1 root is stretched or torn (Klumpke's paralysis).[113] This would produce a clinical picture of someone who has proximal selective control but lacks fine hand movements.

By far, traction to the brachial plexus is the most common mechanism of injury. This is usually due to distractions of the head from the shoulder.[63,98,107] Traction forces usually disrupt the continuity at the root level because the neurofibrils are quite thin in this area.[62] Because the sensory cell bodies are located in the dorsal root ganglion, an avulsion injury (preganglionic) will degenerate the motor axons but preserve the integrity of the sensory axons. Hence, preganglionic lesions carry a poor prognosis for recovery because microsurgical intervention at this level is not likely to produce an improvement.

In contrast, injuries distal to the dorsal root ganglion (postganglionic) carry a better prognosis for recovery. The possibility of spontaneous recovery is greater if certain neurostructures are maintained despite some axonal loss.[62] In addition, surgical reanastomoses have better outcomes.

Certain factors may contribute to the overall prognosis, however. In 1981, Rorabeck and Harris[94] reported that isolated upper trunk injuries carry the best prognosis. Lesions of the lower trunk did not respond well to reinnervation. Leffert and Seddon,[63] however, noted that infraclavicular lesions had a better outcome than supraclavicular lesions. Also, pain that persists for more than 6 months, a combined cord and root lesions, and the presence of a Horner's sign typically carry poor prognosis.[94]

Nerve conduction testing will elucidate the nature of the lesion. Sensory nerve action potential (SNAP) will be normal in preganglionic lesions because the dorsal root ganglion is still intact with its axon.[122,125] On the other hand, postganglionic lesions will have abnormal SNAP[55] and absent voluntary motor units in the corresponding myotome.[122] Compound muscle action potentials will demonstrate maximal changes approximately 7 days after injury.[125] Comparing the values on the involved extremity to the contralateral side is necessary. Needle EMG testing of the paraspinal and limb muscles 3 weeks after the insult could aid in localizing the lesion within the plexus.

For entire brachial plexus injury, the arm should be supported by a sling; this may circumvent the development of pain secondary to chronic shoulder subluxation. Active-assisted range-of-motion exercises of the arm are encouraged. The skin should be routinely inspected because of the increased likelihood of sustaining environmental assaults. During the time of nerve regeneration, the patient should be evaluated for activities of daily living, social, and vocational pursuits. Finally, a custom-made orthosis would be appropriate for those who have achieved and demonstrated maximum cognitive recovery to warrant its effective usage.

SUPRASCAPULAR NERVE

The suprascapular nerve is a branch of the upper trunk, which is the union of C5 and C6 roots. Traumatic injury to this nerve can be secondary to a fall on the shoulder, fracture of the scapular notch, anterior shoulder dislocation, or repetitive strain of the upper extremity.[57] Traction is the usual mechanism of injury, probably secondary to scapular protraction, shoulder abduction, or hypermobility of the neck.[108] The majority of patients complain of generalized pain in the proximal shoulder. Because the suprascapular nerve has no cutaneous sensory distribution, this pain cannot be not localized.[74] Lee and Khunadorn[61] found that a lesion of the suprascapular nerve is not associated with pain in the hemiplegic shoulder. Patients may have weakness, with shoulder abduction and external rotation. Diagnosis can be confirmed by needle EMG studies and by stimulating at Erb's point, recording over the supraspinatus or infraspinatus muslce.[57] Frequently, this PNI is not detected until noticeable atrophy of the supraspinatus and infraspinatus has occurred.

AXILLARY NERVE

Axillary nerve palsy associated with anterior shoulder dislocation is well known.[67,74] Liveson[67] points out that the specific mechanism of injury will help to clarify the pattern of nerve damage. As in most PNI, stretching with traction of the nerve is involved. For example, a shoulder dislocation following a fall on an outstretched arm may result in isolated axillary nerve palsy. In severe cases, the posterior cord may be involved. The prognosis for recovery is considered good[6] and is managed with therapy and arm support until spontaneous recovery occurs.

FACIAL NERVE

It is not uncommon for TBI patients to have temporal bone fractures and associated peripheral facial nerve palsy. A detailed description of the facial nerve anatomy is beyond the scope of this chapter.[53,89]

The facial nerve may be injured by penetrating[31] or nonpenetrating trauma.[123] The nerve can be injured within the fallopian canal (i.e., in the perigeniculate and labyrinthine portion of the nerve)[73, 129] associated with fractures of the petrous bone. Facial nerve injury secondary to lacerations, stabbing, and gunshot wounds to the face are usually detected weeks after the initial insult because of the localized swelling that may mask its presentation. Duncan[31] and colleagues reported that 60% of the gunshot victims to the head have sustained facial nerve damage.

Fractures of the temporal bone can be classified either as longitudinal or transverse. About 90% of all temporal bone fractures are longitudinal in type. These fractures originate in the temporal squama, proceed through the mastoid process, and terminate in the middle ear.[88] Facial nerve palsy occurs in approximately 20% of longitudinal fractures.[31] Prognosis for facial nerve recovery is considered to be good.

In contrast, transverse fractures run perpendicular to the longitudinal axis of the petrous portion of the temporal bone. The nerve usually sustains injury in the tympanic and geniculate segment. Prognosis for recovery for patients with transverse fracture is less favorable than for those with longitudinal fractures.

Clinically, patients may exhibit various signs, including weakness of the ipsilateral forehead muscles and nasolabial fold, miosis, loss of corneal sensation and taste papillae, and ptosis of the ipsilateral eyelid. Depending on the site of the lesion, dysgeusia, hyperacusis, retroauricular pain, reduced salivary flow, and decreased tear production may also occur. Chronic lesions may produce "crocodile tears," a phenomenon whereby salivary fibers aberrantly regenerate to the pterygopalatine ganglion.

Electrodiagnostic testing may help with decision making about whether to explore versus observe. In the case of a peripheral facial palsy, electroneuronography provides the most reliable information for prognostication if performed on the fifth day.[30] The amplitude of the direct motor nerve evoked response is probably the most useful in determining prognosis as compared to the latency.[42] A maximum stimulation test is also considered to be useful.[35] Needle EMG assesses the viability of surviving and degenerating motor fibers. Finally, abnormal growth of regenerating axons may give rise to hemifacial spasms,[71] myokymia,[115] or both.

The debate about the treatment of facial nerve injuries is far from resolved.[2,18] For some surgeons, the general rule is to explore those with immediate facial paralysis and conservatively wait with those with delayed paralysis. McKennan and Chole[73] advocate that traumatic, delayed-onset paralysis does not necessitate surgical decompression under any routine circumstances. Adegbite et al.[1] found no statistically significant difference in recovery of function between patients with an immediate as opposed to a delayed onset of seventh nerve palsy. They advocated a conservative approach and recommended surgical treatment in patients with complete facial palsy persisting for 12 to 18 months postinjury. However, as Adkins and Osguthorpe point out,[2] this depends on the cause, site of trauma, mechanism of injury, residual auditory function, and electrical studies. When complete facial nerve disruption has occurred, a microsurgical reanimation procedure, e.g., a cranial nerve XII to VII crossover, is highly effective. Even with this guideline, there is still a great controversy and debate as to the most judicious method of treatment.[18]

FEMORAL NERVE

Femoral nerve neuropathy is well described in the literature, occurring commonly as a complication of operative procedures.[91] Other causes include stretch injuries associated with vigorous athletic exercises and hemorrhage secondary to anticoagulation. Compression of the femoral nerve's epineurium secondary to a blunt trauma without hematoma formation has been reported.[21]

The lateral femoral cutaneous nerve, a purely sensory nerve derived from the L2 and L3 nerve roots, innervates the anterolateral aspect of the proximal thigh. The nerve enters the lower extremity by passing through the lateral tip of the inguinal ligament. At this point, the nerve can become entrapped, producing the condition called meralgia paresthetica.[60] Several authors claim trauma as a cause. However, in our experience, we have witnessed that obesity may lead to entrapment of the nerve. Some TBI patients become sedentary and lack the initiative to exercise after their hospital discharge. An obese and protuberant abdomen may partially explain why the lateral femoral cutaneous nerve becomes compressed.

Electrodiagnostic studies help with the diagnosis. A side-to-side comparison of the SNAP amplitude is more useful for diagnosis than are sensory nerve conduction velocity and somatosensory evoked potential latency.[60] One must exclude a proximal femoral nerve injury or L4 radiculopathy, which may present similarly to a meralgia paresthetica.[84] Conservative treatment includes nonsteroidal anti-inflammatory medications, weight reduction, and heel lifts.[79] Surgery is advocated for refractory cases.[79]

SCIATIC NERVE

Injuries to the sciatic nerve are rare, but when they do occur they are often traumatic in nature. Fractures and dislocations of the hip, injections into the gluteal muscles, and hip surgery account for most of the causes. Sciatic nerve compression by HO has also been described as a complication after a femoral fracture.[27,92] Typically, the common peroneal division of the sciatic nerve is more vulnerable than its tibial component. Needle EMG testing of the short head of the biceps femoris pinpoints a suspected lesion that is proximal to the knee.

PERONEAL NERVE

The TBI patient may develop a peroneal nerve palsy secondary to a femoral fracture,[36,103] an ill-fitting cast about the fibular head,[103,120] a compartment syndrome,[100,106] ankle sprain,[64] and improper positioning during surgery.[126] The nerve is commonly compressed at the fibular head because of its superficial location. For example, an externally rotated leg, as seen in a comatose individual, places pressure over the nerve (Fig. 4). Proximal tibial and fibular joint disruption with adduction of the knee also produce a common peroneal neuropathy. Traction injuries are responsible for a small number of cases.[36]

Clinically, the patient exhibits a foot drop. The Achilles reflex and inverters of the foot are normally preserved.[79] A spastic lower extremity with an absent Babinski reflex may suggest a deep peroneal nerve injury. Abnormal sensory changes present over the dorsum of the foot and the web space between the first and second toes.

Nerve conduction studies of the peroneal nerve are accessible,[103] but as Wilbourn[126] points out, it is difficult to localize the precise site of the lesion. Kanakamedala and Hong[52] have described a method of short-segment stimulation across the fibular head, which could be a sensitive technique for mild compression.

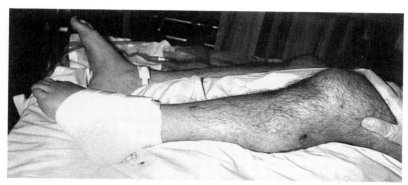

FIGURE 4. Left foot drop secondary to compression at the fibular head. Note the pressure ulcer and swelling over the proximal fibula. (Photograph courtesy of Lance Stone, DO, San Diego, CA.)

The compound muscle potential conducted to the tibialis anterior is required because it provides prognostic information for recovery of a foot drop.[126] Neurapraxic fibers, manifested as a partial conduction block over a short nerve segment, signify that viability of the axons is maintained and correlates with good functional recovery.[11] Needle EMG of the lower lumbosacral paraspinal muscles will help with differentiating L5–S1 radiculopathy from common peroneal mononeuropathy.

A patient with a foot drop can be fitted with a bivalved anteroposterior splint set in neutral position while the patient is in bed. And for those who ambulate a dorsiflexion-assisted/ankle-foot orthosis will help with foot clearance during swing. An equinus contracture should be managed with serial casting and then converted into an anteroposterior splint. Tendo-Achilles lengthening is recommended for cases refractory to conservative treatment.

OBTURATOR NERVE

The adductor muscles of the thigh are innervated by the obturator nerve. The sensory fibers supply the medial thigh and hip and knee joints. An isolated lesion to this nerve is rare. The majority of cases are associated with pelvic fractures, intraabdominal surgery,[8,86] hip arthroplasty,[102] and labor of childbirth. Femoral nerve conduction studies and needle EMG of the adductor muscles are essential to differentiate this disorder from a lumbar radiculopathy.

LUMBOSACRAL PLEXOPATHY

Lumbosacral plexopathy is an uncommon phenomenon after TBI. When it does occur in this population, it represents only a small percentage of the total injuries.[19] Stevens[109] believes that the proximal muscles of the hip and the bony pelvic ring protect the plexus. Injuries tend to occur distal to the spinal ganglion, and avulsion of the lumbosacral roots[101] is normally not encountered. Furthermore, nerve injuries are more likely to develop in double vertical pelvic fractures,[50] with displacement of the pelvic ring.[109]

Automobile accidents represent the leading cause of lumbosacral plexus injury. Traction injury, with stretching of the neural elements, is the major mechanism of insult. The lumbosacral trunk, superior gluteal, and obturator nerves are frequently injured.[50] This disorder is associated with a poor prognosis.

TARSAL TUNNEL SYNDROME

As the tibial nerve travels around the medial malleolus, it may become entrapped under the flexor retinaculum, compressing the distal branches of the medial plantar, lateral plantar, and calcaneal nerves. This has been coined the tarsal tunnel syndrome. Interestingly, Augustijn and Vanneste[4] recently described tarsal tunnel syndrome developing in patients with lesions that were proximal to the ankle. This syndrome is rare and has been associated with many entities. However, in the TBI population, tarsal tunnel syndrome could commonly be associated with ankle sprain, distal tibial or ankle fracture, or calcaneal eversion secondary to an abnormal displacement of the forefoot.[26]

Individuals afflicted with tarsal tunnel syndrome usually complain of burning, numbness, or paresthesia in the foot and toes, sometimes radiating up the leg.[58,81] However, in the confused TBI patient, he or she will likely generalize the problem to the entire foot. During a physical examination, the ability to differentiate a concomitant peripheral sensory neuropathy from an actual tarsal tunnel syndrome may be difficult. Orthodromic stimulation of the medial and lateral plantar nerves, as proposed by Saeed and Gatens,[97] offers one method to distinguish between these diseases. The sural (sensory) nerve should also be tested for evidence of a peripheral neuropathy. Surgical decompression of the flexor retinaculum is the procedure of choice for refractory cases. Recently, Oh and associates[80] reported that nerve conduction studies and clinical symptoms improved in all three patients who had undergone decompression 14 months to 3.5 years ago.

CONCLUSIONS

The majority of peripheral nerve injuries in TBI patients can be related to their initial trauma, improper limb positioning, postoperative complications, or iatrogenic causes. Clinicians must be vigilant in screening for these injuries because neuropathies may have subtle presentations. It is not uncommon that the majority of peripheral nerve injuries are detected while the patient is undergoing acute rehabilitation. This underscores the point that physiatrists and other rehabilitation specialists are in a position to contribute to the early diagnosis of peripheral nerve injury and offer definitive treatment that could lead to better recovery.

REFERENCES

1. Adegbite AB, Khan ML, Tan L: Predicting recovery of nerve function following injury from a basilar skull fracture. J Neurosurg 75:759–762, 1991.
2. Adkins WY, Osguthorpe JD: Management of trauma of the facial nerve. Otolaryngol Clin North Am 24:587–611, 1991.
3. Aisen ML, Brown W, Rubin M: Electrophysiologic changes in lumbar spinal cord after cervical cord injury. Neurology 42:623–626, 1992.
4. Augustijn P, Vanneste J: The tarsal tunnel syndrome after a proximal lesion. J Neurol Neurosurg Psychiatry 55:65–67, 1992.
5. Barton NJ: Radial nerve lesions. Hand 5:200–208, 1973.
6. Berry H, Bril V: Axillary nerve palsy following blunt trauma to the shoulder region: A clinical and electrophysiological review. J Neurol Neurosurg Psychiatry 45:1027–1032, 1982.
7. Bhala RP: Electromyographic evidence of lower motor neuron involvement in hemiplegia. Arch Phys Med Rehabil 50:632–637, 1969.
8. Bischoff C, Schoenle PW: Obturator nerve injuries during intra-abdominal surgery. Clin Neurol Neurosurg 93:73–76, 1991.
9. Brooke MM, Heard DL, de Lateur BJ, et al: Heterotopic ossification and peripheral nerve entrapment: Early diagnosis and excision. Arch Phys Med Rehabil 72:425–429, 1991.
10. Brown W, Snow R: Denervation in hemiplegic muscles. Stroke 21:1700–1704, 1990.

11. Brown WF, Watson BV: Quantification of axon loss and conduction block in peroneal nerve palsies. Muscle Nerve 14:237–244, 1991.
12. Campbell WW, Pridgeon RM, Riaz G, et al: Variations in anatomy of the ulnar nerve at the cubital tunnel: Pitfalls in the diagnosis of ulnar neuropathy at the elbow. Muscle Nerve 14:733–738, 1991.
13. Campbell WW, Pridgeon RM, Sahni SK: Entrapment neuropathy of the ulnar nerve at its point of exit from the flexor carpi ulnaris muscle. Muscle Nerve 11:467–470, 1988.
14. Campbell WW, Pridgeon RM, Sahni KS: Short segment incremental studies in the evaluation of ulnar neuropathy at the elbow. Muscle Nerve 15:1050–1054, 1992.
15. Carfi J, Dong MM: Posterior interosseus syndrome revisited. Muscle Nerve 8:499–502, 1985.
16. Chan RC, Paine KW, Varughese G: Ulnar neuropathy at the elbow: Comparison of simple decompression and anterior transposition. Neurosurgery 7:545–550, 1980.
17. Cioni R, Passero S, Paradiso C, et al: Diagnostic specificity of sensory and motor nerve conduction variables in early detection of carpal tunnel syndrome. J Neurol 236:208–213, 1989.
18. Coker NJ: Management of traumatic injuries to the facial nerve. Otolaryngol Clin North Am 24:215–227, 1991.
19. Cosgrove JL, Vargo M, Reidy ME: A prospective study of peripheral nerve lesions occurring in traumatic brain-injured patients. Am J Phys Med Rehabil 68:15–17, 1989.
20. Cravens G, Kline DG: Posterior interosseus nerve palsies. Neurosurgery 27:397–402, 1990.
21. D'Amelio LF, Musser DJ, Rhodes M: Bilateral femoral nerve neuropathy following blunt trauma. J Neurosurg 73:630–632, 1990.
22. Dawson DM, Hallett M, Millender LH: Entrapment Neuropathies. Boston, Little, Brown & Company, 1990.
23. Della SD, Narakas A, Bonnard C: Late lesions of the brachial plexus after fracture of the clavicle. Ann Chir Main Memb Super 10:531–540, 1991.
24. Di Benedetto M, Markey K: Electrodiagnostic localization of traumatic upper trunk brachial plexopathy. Arch Phys Med Rehabil 65:15–17, 1984.
25. Di Benedetto M, Mitz M, Klingbeil GE, et al: New criteria for sensory nerve conduction especially useful in diagnosing carpal tunnel syndrome. Arch Phys Med Rehabil 67:586–589, 1986.
26. DeLisa JA, Saeed MA: The tarsal tunnel syndrome. Muscle Nerve 6:664–670, 1983.
27. Derian PS, Bibighaus AJ: Sciatic nerve entrapment by ectopic bone after posterior fracture-dislocation of the hip. South Med J 67:209–210, 1974.
28. Derkash RS, Niebauer JJ: Entrapment of the posterior interosseus nerve by a fibrous band in the dorsal edge of the supinator muscle and erosion of a groove in the proximal radius. J Hand Surg 6A:524–526, 1981.
29. Dodds GA, Hale D, Jackson WT: Incidence of anatomic variants in Guyon's canal. J Hand Surg 15A:352–355, 1990.
30. Dumitru D, Nicholas EW, Porter LD: Electrophysiologic evaluation of the facial nerve in Bell's palsy. Am J Phys Med Rehabil 67:137–144, 1988.
31. Duncan NO, Coker NJ, Jenkins HA, et al: Gunshot injuries of the temporal bone. Otolaryngol Head Neck Surg 94:47–55, 1986.
32. Edwards P, Kurth L: Postoperative radial nerve paralysis caused by fracture callus. J Orthop Trauma 6:234–235, 1992.
33. Electrodiagnosis of ulnar neuropathies. Lancet ii:25–26, 1987.
34. Fernandez E, Pallini R, Talamonti G: Sleep palsy (Saturday-night palsy) of the deep radial nerve. J Neurosurg 66:460–461, 1987.
35. Fisch U: Surgery for Bell's palsy. Arch Otolaryngol 107:1–11, 1981.
36. Garland DE, Bailey S: Undetected injuries in head-injured adults. Clin Orthop 155:162–165, 1981.
37. Garland DE, Keenan MA: Orthopedic strategies in the management of the adult head-injured patient. Phys Ther 63:2004–2009, 1983.
38. Garland DE, O'Hollaren RM: Fractures and dislocations about the elbow in the head-injured adult. Clin Orthop 168:38–41, 1982.
39. Garland DE, Ruzza BE, Waters RL: Forceful joint manipulation in head-injured adults with heterotopic ossification. Clin Orthop 169:133–138, 1982.
40. Gelberman RH, Hergenroeder PT, Hargens AR, et al: The carpal tunnel syndrome. A study of carpal canal pressures. J Bone Joint Surg 63A:380–383, 1981.
41. Gellman H, Chandler DR, Petrasek J, et al: Carpal tunnel syndrome in paraplegic patients. J Bone Joint Surg 70A:517–519, 1988.
42. Gilchrist JM: AAEM case report #26: Seventh cranial neuropathy. Muscle Nerve 16:447–452, 1993.

43. Goldkamp O: Electromyography and nerve conduction studies in 116 patients with hemiplegia. Arch Phys Med Rehabil 48:59–63, 1967.
44. Goodall RJ: Nerve injuries in fresh fractures. Tex Med 52:93–95, 1956.
45. Groswasser Z, Cohen M, Blankstein E: Polytrauma associated with traumatic brain injury: Incidence, nature and impact on rehabilitation outcome. Brain Inj 4:161–166, 1990.
46. Haas DC, Nord SG, Bome MP: Carpal tunnel syndrome following automobile accidents. Arch Phys Med Rehabil 62:204–206, 1981.
47. Haymaker W, Woodhall B: Peripheral Nerve Injuries: Principles of Diagnosis, 2nd ed. Philadelphia, WB Saunders, 1959.
48. Hoffer M, Brody G, Ferlic F: Excision of heterotopic ossification about elbows in patients with thermal injury. J Trauma 18:667–670, 1978.
49. Holstein A, Lewis GB: Fractures of the humerus with radial-nerve paralysis. J Bone Joint Surg 45A:1382–1388, 1963.
50. Huittinen VM: Lumbosacral nerve injury in fracture of the pelvis: A postmortem radiographic and pathoanatomical study. Acta Chir Scand Suppl 429:3–43, 1972.
51. Huittinen VM, Slätis P: Nerve injuries in double vertical pelvic fractures. Acta Chir Scand 138:571–575, 1972.
52. Kanakamedala RV, Hong CZ: Peroneal nerve entrapment at the knee localized by short segment stimulation. Am J Phys Med Rehabil 68:116–122, 1989.
53. Karnes WE: Diseases of the seventh cranial nerve. In Dyck PJ, Thomas PK, Lambert EH, et al (eds): Peripheral Neuropathy. Philadelphia, WB Saunders, 1984, pp 1266–1299.
54. Keenan MA, Kauffman DL, Garland DE, et al: Late ulnar neuropathy in the brain-injured adult. J Hand Surg 13A:120–124, 1988.
55. Kimura J: Electrodiagnosis in Diseases of Nerve and Muscle: Principles and Practice, 2nd ed. Philadelphia, FA Davis, 1989.
56. Kincaid JC: AAEE minimograph #31: The electrodiagnosis of ulnar neuropathy at the elbow. Muscle Nerve 11:1005–1015, 1988.
57. Kiss G, Komar J: Suprascapular nerve compression at the supraglenoid notch. Muscle Nerve 13:556–557, 1990.
58. Kuritz HM, Sokoloff TH: Tarsal tunnel syndrome. J Am Podiatr Med Assoc 65:825–840, 1975.
59. LeBan MM, MacKenzie JR, Zemenick GA: Anatomic observations in carpal tunnel syndrome as they relate to the tethered median nerve stress test. Arch Phys Med Rehabil 70:44–46, 1989.
60. Lagueny A, Deliac MM, Deliac P, et al: Diagnostic and prognostic value of electrophysiologic tests in meralgia paresthetica. Muscle Nerve 14:51–56, 1991.
61. Lee KH, Khunadorn F: Painful shoulder in hemiplegic patients: Study of the suprascapular nerve. Arch Phys Med Rehabil 67:818–820, 1986.
62. Leffert RD: Brachial plexus injuries. New Engl J Med 291:1059–1067, 1974.
63. Leffert RD, Seddon H: Infraclavicular brachial plexus injuries. J Bone Joint Surg Br 47B:9–22, 1965.
64. Lemont H: Perineural fibrosis of the superficial peroneal nerve complicating ankle sprain: A case report [letter]. Foot Ankle 11:414, 1991.
65. Lichter RL, Jacobsen T: Tardy palsy of the posterior interosseus nerve with a Monteggia fracture. J Bone Joint Surg 57A:124–125, 1975.
66. Lister GD, Belsole RB, Kleinert HE: The radial tunnel syndrome. J Hand Surg 4A:52–59, 1979.
67. Liveson JA: Nerve lesions associated with shoulder dislocation: An electrodiagnostic study of 11 cases. J Neurol Neurosurg Psychiatry 47:742–744, 1984.
68. Lotem M, Fried A, Levy M, et al: Radial palsy following muscular effort. J Bone Joint Surg 53B:500–506, 1971.
69. MacDonell RAL, Schwartz MS, Swash M: Carpal tunnel syndrome: Which finger should be tested? An analysis of sensory conduction in digital branches of the median nerve. Muscle Nerve 13:601–606, 1990.
70. Marin EL, Vernick S, Friedmann LW: Carpal tunnel syndrome: Median nerve stress test. Arch Phys Med Rehabil 64:206–208, 1983.
71. Martinelli P, Giuliani S, Ippoliti M: Hemifacial spasm due to peripheral injury of facial nerve: A nuclear syndrome? Move Disord 7:181–184, 1992.
72. McGowin JF, Schlitt M, McCloskey JJ: Brachial plexus injuries associated with cervical spine fractures. J Spinal Disord 2:104–108, 1989.
73. McKennan KX, Chole RA: Facial paralysis in temporal bone trauma. Am J Otol 13:167–172, 1992.
74. Mendoza FX, Main K: Peripheral nerve injuries of the shoulder in the athlete. Clin Sports Med 9:331–342, 1990.

75. Miller RG: The cubital tunnel syndrome: Diagnosis and precise localization. Ann Neurol 6:56–59, 1979.
76. Miller RG: Ulnar nerve lesions. In Brown WF, Bolton CF (eds): Clinical Electromyography. Stoneham, MA, Butterworth, 1987, pp 97–117.
77. Miller RG: AAEM case report #1: Ulnar neuropathy at the elbow. Muscle Nerve 14:97–101, 1991.
78. Murphy TP, Parkhill WS: Fracture-dislocation of the base of the fifth metacarpal with an ulnar motor nerve lesion: Case report. J Trauma 30:1585–1587, 1990.
79. Nakano KK: The entrapment neuropathies. Muscle Nerve 1:264–279, 1978.
80. Oh SJ, Arnold TW, Park KH, Kim DE: Electrophysiological improvement following decompression surgery in tarsal tunnel syndrome. Muscle Nerve 14:407–410, 1991.
81. Oh SJ, Sarala PK, Kuba T, Elmore RS: Tarsal tunnel syndrome: Electrophysiologic study. Ann Neurol 5:327–330, 1979.
82. Orcutt SA, Kramer WG, Howard MW, et al: Carpal tunnel syndrome secondary to wrist and finger flexor spasticity. J Hand Surg 15A:940–944, 1990.
83. Pastacaldi P, Rossi B, Sartucci F, et al: Compression of the deep palmar branch of the ulnar nerve: Clinical and electromyographic findings after a new method of decompression. Hand 15:106–109, 1983.
84. Pease WS: Entrapment neuropathies. Phys Med Rehabil: State Art Rev 3:741–756, 1989.
85. Pease WS, Cannell CD, Johnson EW: Median to radial latency difference test in mild carpal tunnel syndrome. Muscle Nerve 12:905–909, 1989.
86. Pellegrino MJ, Johnson EW: Bilateral obturator nerve injuries during urologic surgery. Arch Phys Med Rehabil 69:46–47, 1988.
87. Philip PA, Philip M: Peripheral nerve injuries in children with traumatic brain injury. Brain Inj 6:53–58, 1992.
88. Potter JM, Braakman R: Injury to the facial nerve. Handbk Clin Neurol 24:105–117, 1976.
89. Proctor B: The anatomy of the facial nerve. Otolaryngol Clin North Am 24:479–504, 1991.
90. Redmond MD, Rivner MH: False positive electrodiagnostic tests in carpal tunnel syndrome. Muscle Nerve 11:511–517, 1988.
91. Reinstein L, Alevizatos AC, Twardzik FG, et al: Femoral nerve dysfunction after retroperitoneal hemorrhage: Pathophysiology revealed by computerized tomography. Arch Phys Med Rehabil 65:37–40, 1984.
92. Reinstein L, Eckholdt JW: Sciatic nerve compression by preexisting heterotopic ossification during general anesthesia in the dorsal lithotomy position. Arch Phys Med Rehabil 64:65–68, 1983.
93. Robertson WC, Eichman PL, Clancy WG: Upper trunk brachial plexopathy in football players. JAMA 241:1480–1482, 1979.
94. Rorabeck CH, Harris WR: Factors affecting the prognosis of brachial plexus injuries. J Bone Joint Surg Br 63B:404–407, 1981.
95. Rosson JW: Closed traction lesion of the brachial plexus—An epidemic among young motorcyclists. Injury 19:4–6, 1988.
96. Rumball KM, DaSilva VF, Preston DN, et al: Brachial plexus injury after clavicular fracture: Case report and literature review. Can J Surg 34:264–266, 1991.
97. Saeed MA, Gatens PF: Compound nerve action potentials of the medial and lateral plantar nerves through the tarsal tunnel. Arch Phys Med Rehabil 63:304–307, 1982.
98. Schwartzman RJ: Brachial plexus traction injuries. Hand Clin 7:547–556, 1991.
99. Shaw JL, Sakellarides H: Radial-nerve paralysis associated with fractures of the humerus. A review of forty-five cases. J Bone Joint Surg 49A:899–902, 1967.
100. Shields RW, Root KE, Wilbourn AJ: Compartment syndromes and compression neuropathies in coma. Neurology 36:1370–1374, 1986.
101. Sidhu JS, Dhillon MK: Lumbosacral plexus avulsion with pelvic fractures. Injury 22:156–158, 1991.
102. Siliski JM, Scott RD: Obturator-nerve palsy resulting from intrapelvic extrusion of cement during total hip replacement. J Bone Joint Surg 67A:1225–1228, 1985.
103. Smith T, Trojaborg W: Clinical and electrophysiological recovery from peroneal palsy. Acta Neurol Scand 74:328–335, 1986.
104. Spar I: A neurologic complication following Monteggia fracture. Clin Orthop 122:207–209, 1977.
105. Spinner M, Freundlich BD, Teicher J: Posterior interosseous nerve palsy as a complication of Monteggia fractures in children. Clin Orthop 58:141–145, 1968.
106. Sridhara CR, Izzo KL: Terminal sensory branches of the superficial peroneal nerve: An entrapment syndrome. Arch Phys Med Rehabil 66:789–791, 1985.

107. Stanwood JE, Kraft GH: Diagnosis and management of brachial plexus injuries. Arch Phys Med Rehabil 52:52–60, 1971.
108. Steinman I: Painless infraspinatus atrophy due to suprascapular nerve entrapment. Arch Phys Med Rehabil 69:641–643, 1988.
109. Stevens JC: Lumbosacral plexus lesions. In Dyck PJ, Thomas PK, Lambert EH, Bunge R (eds): Peripheral Neuropathy. Philadelphia, WB Saunders, 1984, pp 1425–1434.
110. Stevens JC: AAEE minimonograph #26: The electrodiagnosis of carpal tunnel syndrome. Muscle Nerve 10:99–113, 1987.
111. Stone L, Keenan MA: Peripheral nerve injuries in the adult with traumatic brain injury. Clin Orthop 233:136–144, 1988.
112. Szabo RM: Carpal tunnel syndrome–general. In Gelberman RH (ed): Operative Nerve Repair and Reconstruction. Philadelphia, JB Lippincott, 1991, pp 869–888.
113. Tracy JF, Brannon EW: Management of brachial-plexus injuries (traction type). J Bone Joint Surg 40A:1031–1042, 1958.
114. Uncini A, Lange DJ, Solomon M, et al: Ring finger testing in carpal tunnel syndrome: A comparative study of diagnostic utility. Muscle Nerve 12:735–741, 1989.
115. Valls-Sole J, Tolosa ES, Pujol M: Myokymic discharges and enhanced facial nerve reflex responses after recovery from idiopathic facial palsy. Muscle Nerve 15:37–42, 1992.
116. Varghese G, William K, Desmet A, Redford JB: Nonarticular complication of heterotopic ossification: A clinical review. Arch Phys Med Rehabil 72:1009–1013, 1991.
117. Wainapel SF, Rao PU, Schepsis AA: Ulnar nerve compression by heterotopic ossification in a head-injured patient. Arch Phys Med Rehabil 66:512–514, 1985.
118. Waring WP, Werner RA: Clinical management of carpal tunnel syndrome in patients with long term sequelae of poliomyelitis. J Hand Surg 14A:865–869, 1989.
119. Weiss AP, Idler RS: Radial nerve rupture after a traction injury: A case report. J Hand Surg 17:69–70, 1992.
120. Weiss AP, Schneck RC, Sponseller PD, et al: Peroneal palsy after early cast application for femoral fractures in children. J Pediatr Orthop 12:25–28, 1992.
121. Werner R, Waring W, Davidoff G: Risk factors for median mononeuropathy of the wrist in postpoliomyelitis patients. Arch Phys Med Rehabil 70:464–467, 1989.
122. Wertsch JJ: Polyradiculopathy and plexopathy. Phys Med Rehabil Clin North Am 1:101–119, 1990.
123. Williams MJ: Blunt trauma leading to facial nerve paralysis. J Emerg Med 9:27–28, 1991.
124. Wharton GW: Heterotopic ossification. Clin Orthop 112:142–149, 1975.
125. Wilbourn AJ: Electrodiagnosis of plexopathies. Neurol Clin 3:511–529, 1985.
126. Wilbourn AJ: AAEE case report #12: Common peroneal mononeuropathy at the fibular head. Muscle Nerve 9:825–836, 1986.
127. Wongsam PE, Johnson EW, Weinerman JD: Carpal tunnel syndrome: Use of palmar stimulation of sensory fibers. Arch Phys Med Rehabil 64:16–19, 1983.
128. Wu JS, Morris JD, Hogan GR: Ulnar neuropathy at the wrist: Case report and review of literature. Arch Phys Med Rehabil 66:785–788, 1985.
129. Ylikoski J: Facial palsy after temporal bone fracture: (Light and electron microscopic findings in two cases). J Laryngol 102:298–303, 1988.

MARK F. LEW, MD
CHERYL H. WATERS, MD, FRCPC

POST-TRAUMATIC MOVEMENT DISORDERS

From the
Division of Movement Disorders
Department of Neurology
University of Southern California
School of Medicine
Los Angeles, California

Correspondence to:
Mark F. Lew, MD
Division of Movement Disorders
Department of Neurology
University of Southern California
School of Medicine
1510 San Pablo, #615
Los Angeles, CA 90033

Cerebrospinal trauma may produce hyperkinetic or akinetic movement disorders. Delay between the injury and appearance of clinical symptoms often obscures a definitive cause-and-effect relationship. This review discusses reported cases in which trauma led to an excess of movement—dyskinesia—or a paucity of movement—parkinsonism.

Accidents are now the fourth most common cause of death at all ages and the leading cause below age 40.[46] Although severe head injuries account for almost 75% of accidental deaths, many are nonfatal. From these are derived the most common types of head injury inciting subsequent movement disorders: concussion, contusion, diffuse axonal injury, and hemorrhage.

Concussion

Concussion is defined as a temporary, reversible neurologic deficiency caused by trauma resulting in immediate, temporary loss of consciousness.[18] Generally, both retrograde and post-traumatic amnesia follow, with the duration of amnesia being directly correlated to the severity of brain injury. The amnesia resolves in less than 24 hours, or more serious brain damage exists.

Contusion

A cortical contusion is a bruise of the brain's surface and is characteristic of a mechanical injury. Coup contusions are evident at the site of cranial impact, whereas contrecoup contusions occur opposite the location of cranial impact. Contusions are likely to be found in the inferior temporal and frontal areas, as the brain surface moves over the irregular boney prominence normally found in these skull regions.

Diffuse Axonal Injury

Diffuse axonal injury most frequently occurs as a consequence of blunt injuries to the brain. Clinically, patients lose consciousness soon after the initial insult and have a prolonged comatose or persistent vegetative state. Shear forces and angular rotation of the head, with damage to cerebral white matter, brain stem, and the corpus callosum, are felt to cause diffuse axonal injury.[23,38]

Hemorrhage

Epidural hematomas are due to bleeding between the calvarium and the dura mater. Characteristically, they are caused by a blow to the head with subsequent temporal bone fracture and laceration of the middle meningeal artery. A rapidly progressive clinical course ensues, culminating in death or coma if surgical decompression is delayed.

Subdural hematoma develops if blood accumulates in the subdural space because of rupture of the bridging veins. Subdural hematoma is clinically less fulminant than epidural hematoma. Clots are most frequently found in the temporoparietal region.

PARKINSON'S DISEASE/PARKINSONISM

Idiopathic Parkinson's disease is a disorder caused by the degeneration of the neuromelanin-containing neurons predominantly located in the substantia nigra (pars compacta). These neurons characteristically contain Lewy bodies, or intracytoplasmic eosinophilic inclusions. Clinically, the tetrad of resting tremor, cogwheel rigidity, akinesia, and loss of postural reflexes predominate.

Secondary parkinsonism may be caused by:
1. toxins, e.g., 1,2,3,6-tetrahydro-1-methyl-4-phenylpyridine and manganese;
2. infectious agents, e.g., human immunodeficiency virus and other encephalitides;
3. medications, e.g., neuroleptics;
4. metabolic disorders, e.g., Wilson's disease; or
5. trauma.

A wealth of literature exists suggesting that brain trauma may cause Parkinson's disease. In 1817, James Parkinson, in his landmark *Essay on the Shaking Palsy,*[39] hypothesized that a medullary injury might be the anatomic locus of this ailment. Charcot, the famous French neurologist, later offered that emotional trauma or exposure to the cold or damp environment could cause Parkinson's disease.[19] Reports of parkinsonism after closed-head trauma in World War I[15] as well as the striking epidemic of parkinsonism following von Economo's encephalitis established a central insult as the likely cause of Parkinson's disease.

Patrick and Levy[40] found 22 of 146 cases (15%) of Parkinson's disease to be related to trauma. However, the incidence of trauma in the control population was not specified. In his 1934 review of 86 cases of paralysis agitans and trauma, Grimberg[20] felt that only two of these cases were true post-traumatic parkinsonism. A necessary condition for this diagnosis, in his estimation, was direct head trauma forceful enough to cause definitive brain damage. Schwab and England[43] suggested that only head injury severe enough to lead to midbrain hemorrhage could cause parkinsonism. These patients generally present with a host of neurologic sequelae aside from parkinsonism, including pyramidal and cerebellar dysfunction.

Although there are many reports of post-traumatic parkinsonism, few include post-mortem pathologic evaluation. Bruetsch and De Armond[7] reported on a 60-year-old laborer who fell from a height of 8 feet, landing on his hips and shoulders and striking his occiput. There was no loss of consciousness. "Stiffness" and "muscular rigidity" occurred within days. A formal neurologic exam 8 months later was remarkable for parkinsonian features. Autopsy revealed a fracture of the inner table of the occiput and petrous bones. There was depigmentation of the substantia nigra and petechial hemorrhage in the striatum and midbrain, findings consistent with trauma. No Lewy bodies were found. In another case, presented by Nayernouri[36] in 1985, a 37-year-old man became profoundly parkinsonian several weeks after blunt head trauma. Computed tomographic (CT) scanning, although initially unremarkable, revealed bilateral, low-density lesions in the substantia nigra when the scan was repeated.

Traumatic encephalopathy due to diffuse brain injury in boxers has been well documented over the years. The "punch-drunk" state was first described in 1928 by Martland.[33] Dementia pugilistica and the punch drunk of boxers can present with signs of diminished facial expression, slurred speech, bradykinesia, dementia, and a resting tremor.[10,34] The severity of this form of post-traumatic parkinsonism has clearly been shown to correlate with the duration of one's career and the number of contests fought.[45] This brain damage is thought to be due to a cumulative effect of continued blows to the head over time, and symptoms can continue to surface even years after a career is over. Neuropathologic correlates to parkinsonism in this population include depigmentation and neuronal loss of the substantia nigra, with cortical and brainstem petechial hemorrhages. No Lewy bodies were seen.[9]

Thus, severe head trauma can cause parkinsonian features as part of a more involved neurologic syndrome. Mesencephalic damage is often evident on pathologic evaluation or imaging studies.[7,36] Because midbrain injury is usually lethal, post-traumatic parkinsonism is quite rare. Whether trauma can permanently aggravate existing Parkinson's disease or potentiate preclinical Parkinson's disease remains to be determined. Better controlled clinical studies are needed to clarify the relationship between Parkinson's disease and trauma.

PARKINSON-PLUS SYNDROMES

Post-traumatic progressive supranuclear palsy is another akinetic-rigid syndrome that presents with Parkinson-like features, often with a prominent vertical gaze palsy but without tremor. Post-traumatic progressive supranuclear palsy is an extremely rare occurrence. Two cases were reported by Koller et al.[28] in otherwise previously healthy patients who sustained significant falls. Both developed clinical stigmata of progressive supranuclear palsy, including diminished vertical extraocular movements, bradykinesia, increased tone, and gait imbalance. CT scan results of the brain on one patient were entirely normal. The other showed diffuse brainstem atrophy.

CHOREA AND BALLISMUS

Chorea refers to involuntary, irregular, purposeless, rapid, unsustained movements that flow from one body part to another. Prototypical choreic movements are seen in Huntington's chorea. Random choreic movements can be partially suppressed and can be incorporated into a repertoire of purposeful movements called parakinesia.[17] Chorea is frequently combined with sinuous, slow, writhing movements called athetosis. *Ballism* is considered very large amplitude, exaggerated choreic movements. Because these movements are very rapid, they are often flinging and flailing in nature. Both chorea and ballism have been ascribed to lesions of the contralateral subthalamic nucleus, striatum, and thalamic nuclei.[27]

Chandra et al.[8] reported on a case of a 28-year-old who fell from a three-story building at age 9, sustaining severe left hemispheric damage. Sequelae included right-sided spastic hemiparesis and choreoathetoid movements of the right arm. CT scanning showed a left-sided brain hypodensity with a dilated left ventricle. These involuntary movements responded to valproic acid therapy, in spite of the absence of electroencephalographic correlates.

Drake et al. described 3 cases of closed-head injury in men aged 18 to 30 who developed paroxysmal choreoathetosis 4 to 6 weeks after impact.[12] CT scan results in this group were normal. Electroencephalograms showed no evidence of cortical seizure focus in each case. Etiology was thought to be secondary to subcortical Duret hemorrhages.

Subdural hematoma and hemorrhagic infarct have also been suggested to cause post-traumatic chorea and ballism. The first case reported in the literature involved a 12-year-old boy who developed diffuse chorea 2 weeks after receiving chemotherapy.[4] CT scanning revealed a large left-sided subdural hematoma with left-to-right shift of midline structures. On neurosurgical evacuation, abnormal involuntary movements ceased. Although this case is not post-traumatic, there are a number of cases in the literature, as described below. Kotogal et al.[29] reported on an elderly man who suffered multiple falls and developed confusion with continuous bilateral upper-extremity choreoathetoid movements. CT scanning confirmed bilateral subdural hematoma, with compression of the lateral ventricles. Subcortical dysfunction secondary to compression was the likely cause of chorea.

Lodder and Baard[30] reported on a case of a 75-year-old woman with diabetes who developed bilateral ballism, more predominantly in the upper extremities, after suffering mild head trauma. CT scanning showed bilateral hemorrhagic infarction of the caudate and putamen. Symptoms spontaneously resolved in several weeks in conjunction with full resorption of hemorrhagic lesions on follow-up CT scanning.

The previous references indicate that chorea and ballism due to trauma may be paroxysmal or persistent. Although more likely to follow extensive brain damage, post-traumatic chorea and ballism remain relatively rare entities.

DYSTONIA

Dystonia refers to twisting movements that are sustained and repetitive. They can be brief and shock-like, as in myoclonic dystonia, or prolonged, lasting for minutes to hours, called dystonic postures. When a single body part is affected, this condition has been named focal dystonia, i.e., spasmodic torticollis or nuchal dystonia. If two or more contiguous body regions are involved, this is called segmental dystonia. Hemidystonia refers to unilateral body involvement.

Reports of focal dystonia following head trauma are sparse. Drake details the case of a 19-year-old who sustained severe closed-head injury in a car accident.[11] After suffering prolonged intracranial hypertension and 6 weeks of coma, he developed paroxysmal laterocollis with rotation to the left. CT scanning showed only atrophy with mild enlargement of the ventricles. Electroencephalography revealed no evidence of related seizure activity. Another case of focal dystonia was reported by Messimy et al.[35] concerning an otherwise well 30-year-old man who sustained a nonconcussive right-sided head injury in a car accident. Four years later, he developed left arm dystonia. CT scanning showed calcification of the contralateral caudate nucleus.

Many reports document an association between head trauma and hemidystonia. Marsden et al.[32] noted that 3 of 28 cases were related to trauma, whereas Pettigrew and Jankovic[41] found 3 of 22 patients to have post-traumatic hemidystonia. Brett et al.[6] described the case of a 5-year-old girl pedestrian involved in a traffic accident. She grazed the right side of her face but did not lose consciousness. Over the next 24 months, she developed progressive right hemidystonia. CT scanning revealed a low-density area in the left putamen. Andrew et al. reported on the case of an 8-year-old boy who was involved in a traffic accident and 1 day later had left-sided involuntary movements.[3] By age 24, he had developed a combination of left-hemibody myoclonic jerks, orofacial dystonia, hemiballism, and torsion dystonia. CT scanning showed a right caudate and putamen hypodensity. Stereotactic thalamotomy reduced the involuntary movements.

Maki et al. described four children who had mild head trauma that led to similar basal ganglia infarcts and hemidystonia or hemiparesis within minutes to hours afterwards.[31] Shearing or rotational forces from the trauma rupturing the perforating middle cerebral artery branches is the likely mechanism involved.

TICS

Tics can be separated into two categories: abnormal movements (motor tics), and abnormal sounds (phonic tics). When the two are combined, the designation of Gilles de la Tourette syndrome is often applied. Simple motor tics are abrupt isolated movements, such as eye blinking, shoulder shrug, or nose twitching, involving only one group of muscles. Complex motor tics consist of coordinated movements resembling normal motor acts or gestures that are inappropriately intense and timed.[17] They may be purposeful, like touching the nose, touching other people, throwing, or hitting. Nonpurposeful tics include head shaking and trunk bending. Simple phonic tics would be throat clearing and sniffing, whereas barking and verbalizations are considered complex phonic tics.

There are only four cases of trauma-related tic disorders in the current literature. The first report was by Erickson and Persson in 1969, about a 3-year-old boy who suffered a depressed right temporal nonconcussive skull fracture after being knocked down by a motorcycle.[14] He soon developed eye, face, and shoulder tics. By age 12, he developed tongue and cheek biting, along with phonic tics, including loud, bellowing noises. Episodes responded at times to diazepam, phenytoin, and barbiturates. Fahn described an 18-year-old man who lost consciousness for several minutes after being hit in the face by a steel girder and knocked against a wall.[16] Two or 3 months later, he developed simple facial tics. Several years later, he had a large repertoire of complex motor tics and some vocal tics. Clonazepam helped intermittently.

Koller et al. reported on a case of simple motor tics following closed-head trauma.[28] Singer et al. presented the case of a 27-year-old man who lost consciousness after closed-head injury while a passenger in a van involved in an accident.[44] Several weeks later, he developed motor tics, including eye blinking and facial tics.

TREMOR

Tremor is an involuntary movement characterized by rhythmic oscillations of a body part. Tremor can be resting or movement related. Tremors with movement are additionally subdivided into (1) postural or static tremor, (2) with movement from point to point or intention or kinetic tremor, and (3) target-specific tremor.[21] Tremor following less severe head trauma is generally asymptomatic postural or kinetic in nature. There can be associated head, trunk, or leg involvement. A cerebellar or rubral tremor occurs with more severe injury to the midbrain or cerebellar outflow tracts. This tremor affects the trunk and the more proximal limb portions, usually worsens with target-directed movement, and often includes dysmetria.

Biary et al. described seven patients who sustained less severe head trauma and developed tremor weeks after injury.[5] In each case CT scanning and electroencephalographic results were normal. β-blockers, anticonvulsants, and clonazepam did not help much. Ellison reported on two children who developed debilitating action tremor following severe head injury.[13] Both responded dramatically to propranalol. Obeso and Norbone[37] related a case of disabling post-traumatic postural tremor in a 13-year-old girl after loss of consciousness for 1 week. She responded to combination valproic acid and propranalol. Glutethimide helped decrease post-traumatic tremor in one patient.[1]

Andrew et al.[2] reported on eight young patients who underwent stereotactic thalamotomy to treat kinetic or postural tremor after severe head injury. All eight had dramatic improvement of their tremor and function of the involved limb. A midbrain lesion was felt to be the anatomic locus involved in these subjects.

MYOCLONUS

Myoclonus is a sudden brief jerk caused by either muscle contraction (positive myoclonus) or brief lapses of muscle contraction in active postural muscles (negative myoclonus or asterixis).[17] Myoclonus cannot be voluntarily controlled. Whole body myoclonus is called generalized myoclonus. Multifocal myoclonus affects many body parts randomly, whereas focal or segmental myoclonus is confined to a particular body region. Myoclonus may be present at rest, in a particular posture, with movement, i.e., action myoclonus, or it may be stimulus sensitive, i.e., reflex myoclonus.

Hallet et al. described a 21-year-old woman who sustained severe head injury, remaining unconscious for several days.[22] There was no documented hypoxia. Soon after, she had generalized myoclonus with voluntary movement. Some 20 years later, she developed facial and bulbar myoclonus and consequent difficulty eating. Cortical reflex myoclonus was then diagnosed. A case of post-traumatic segmental myoclonus was detailed by Jankovic and Pardo[25] in a study of 37 patients. This patient had facial and platysma muscle involvement.

Palatal or branchial myoclonus has rarely been reported following head injury. Riley and Brock described the case of an alcoholic who sustained multiple head traumas with resultant palatal myoclonus.[42] Jacobson and Gorman reported on a case of oculopalatal myoclonus in an infantry man after he received multiple shrapnel wounds to the head and neck.[24] Keane has described two cases of galloping tongue, which is a rhythmic, involuntary tongue movement after severe head and neck trauma.[26]

In summary, most if not all movement disorders have occurred after significant head injury. Further studies of post-traumatic movement disorders may help illuminate the mechanism of human motor control.

REFERENCES

1. Aisen M, Holzer M, Rosen M, et al: Glutethimide treatment of disabling action tremor in patients with multiple sclerosis and traumatic brain injury. Arch Neurol 48:513–515, 1991.
2. Andrew J, Fowler CJ, Harrison MJG: Tremor after head injury and its treatment by stereotaxic surgery. J Neurol Neurosurg Psychiatry 45:815–819, 1982.
3. Andrew J, Fowler C, Harrison MJ: Hemidystonia due to focal basal ganglia lesion after head injury and improved by stereotaxic thalamotomy. J Neurol Neurosurg 45:276–282, 1982.
4. Bean SC, Ladisch S: Chorea associated with subdural hematoma in a child with leukemia. J Pediatr 90:255–259, 1977.
5. Biary N, Cleeves L, Findley L, Koller W: Post traumatic tremor. Neurology 39:103–106, 1989.
6. Brett BM, Hoare RD, Sheehy MP, Marsden CD: Progressive hemidystonia due to focal basal ganglia lesion after mild head trauma. J Neurol Neurosurg Psychiatry 44:442–460, 1981.
7. Bruetsch WL, De Armond M: The parkinsonism syndrome due to trauma. A clinico-anatomical study of a case. J Nerv Ment Dis 81:531–543, 1935.
8. Chandra V, Spunt AL, Rosinowitz MS: Treatment of post traumatic choreoathetosis following head injury. Ann Neurol 2:447–448, 1977.
9. Corsellis J, Bruton C, Freeman-Browne D: The aftermath of boxing. Psychol Med 3:270–303, 1989.
10. Critchley M: Medical aspects of boxing, particularly from a neurological standpoint. BMJ 1:357, 1957.
11. Drake ME: Spasmodic torticollis after closed head injury. J Natl Med Assoc 79:561–563, 1987.
12. Drake ME, Jackson RD, Miller CA: Paroxysmal choreoathetosis after head injury. J Neurol Neurosurg Psychiatry 49:837–843, 1986.
13. Ellison PH: Propranolol for severe post head injury action tremor. Neurology 28:197–199, 1978.
14. Erikson B, Persson T: Gilles de la Tourettes syndrome. Two cases with organic brain injury. Br J Psychiatry 115:351–353, 1969.
15. Factor S, Sanchez-Ramos J, Weiner WJ: Trauma as an etiology of Parkinsonism: A historical review of the concept. Mov Disord 3:30–37, 1988.
16. Fahn S: A case of post traumatic tic syndrome. In Friedhoff AJ, Chase TNP (eds): Gilles de La Tourette Syndrome. Advances in Neurology, vol 35. New York, Raven Press, 1982, pp 349–350.
17. Fahn S, Marsden D, Jankovic J: A Comprehensive Review of Movement Disorders for the Clinical Practitioner. Aspen, CO, August 1991 course syllabus, p 284.
18. Genarelli TA: Cerebral concussion and diffuse brain injuries. In Cooper PR (ed): Head Injury. Baltimore, Williams & Wilkins, 1982, p 83.
19. Goetz CG: Charcot on Parkinson's disease. Mov Disord 1:27–32, 1986.
20. Grimberg L: Paralysis agitans and trauma. J Nerv Ment Dis 79:14–42, 1934.
21. Hallet M: Classification and treatment of tremor. JAMA 226:1115–1117, 1991.
22. Hallett D, Chadwick D, Marsden CD: Cortical reflex myoclonus. Neurology 29:1107–1125, 1979.
23. Holbourn AHS: Mechanics of head injuries. Lancet ii:438, 1943.
24. Jacobson MB, Gorman WF: Palatal myoclonus and primary nystagmus following trauma. J Neurol Neurosurg Psychiatry 62:796–801, 1949.
25. Jankovic J, Pardo R: Segmental myoclonus: Clinical and pharmacological study. Arch Neurol 43:1025–1033, 1986.
26. Keane JR: Galloping tongue: Post-traumatic, episodic rhythmic movements. Neurology 34:251–252, 1984.
27. Koller WC, Nauseida PA, Weiner WJ, Klawans HL: The pharmacology of ballismus. Clin Neuropharmacol 4:157–174, 1979.
28. Koller W, Wong G, Lang A: Post traumatic movement disorders: A review. Mov Disord 4:20–36, 1989.
29. Kotagal S, Shuter E, Horenstein S: Chorea as a manifestation of bilateral subdural hematoma in the elderly man. Arch Neurol 38:195–201, 1981.
30. Lodder J, Baard WC: Paraballismus caused by bilateral hemorrhagic infarction in the basal ganglia. Neurology 31:484–486, 1981.
31. Maki Y, Akimoto H, Enomoto T: Injuries of basal ganglia following trauma in children. Childs Brain 7:113–123, 1980.
32. Marsden CD, Obeso JA, Zaran JJ, Lang AE: The anatomical basis of hemidystonia. Brain 108:463–483, 1980.
33. Martland HS: Punch drunk. JAMA 91:1103–1107, 1928.
34. Mawdsley C, Ferguson FR: Neurological disease in boxers. Lancet ii:795–801, 1963.
35. Messimy R, Diebler C, Metzger J: Dystonie de torsion de membre superieur gauche probablement a un traumatisme cranien. Rev Neurol (Paris) 133:199–206, 1977.

36. Nayernouri T: Post traumatic parkinsonism. Surg Neurol 24:263–264, 1985.
37. Obeso JA, Norbone J: Post-traumatic tremor and myoclonic jerking. J Neurol Neurosurg Psychiatry 46:488, 1983.
38. Oppenheimer DR: Microscopic lesions in the brain following head injury. J Neurol Neurosurg Psychiatry 31:299, 1968.
39. Parkinson J: Essay on the Shaking Palsy. London, Whittingham and Rowland, For Sherwood, Neely and Jones, 1817.
40. Patrick HV, Levy PM: Parkinson's disease: A clinical study of one hundred and forty-six cases. Arch Neurol Psychiatry 7:711–720, 1922.
41. Pettigrew LC, Jankovic J: Hemidystonia: A report of 22 patients and review of the literature. J Neurol Neurosurg Psychiatry 48:650–657, 1985.
42. Riley HA, Brock S: Rhythmic myoclonus. Arch Neurol Psychiat 29:276, 1933.
43. Schwab RS, England AC: Parkinsonism due to various specific causes. In Vinken PJ, Bruyn GW (eds): Handbook of Clinical Neurology, vol 6, 1st ed. Amsterdam, North Holland Publishing Co., 1968, pp 230–233.
44. Singer C, Sanchez-Ramos J, Weiner WJ: A case of post traumatic tic disorder. Mov Disord 4:342–344, 1989.
45. Stiller JW, Weinberger DR: Boxing and chronic brain damage. Psychiatr Clin North Am 8:339–356, 1985.
46. US Department of Health, Education, Welfare: National Center for Health Statistics. Hyattsville, MD, Vital Statistics of the United States, 1975, 1979.

LANCE R. STONE, DO
DANIEL Y. SHIN, MD

MANAGEMENT OF HYPERTONICITY USING CHEMICAL DENERVATION FOLLOWING TRAUMATIC BRAIN INJURY

From the
Center for Brain Injury
   Rehabilitation (LRS)
San Diego Rehabilitation Institute
San Diego, California;
Department of Physical Medicine
   and Rehabilitation (LRS, DYS)
University of California at Irvine
   School of Medicine
Irvine, California;
Department of Neurology (LRS,
   DYS)
University of Southern California
   School of Medicine
Los Angeles, California;
   and
Electrodiagnostics Laboratory
   (DYS)
Rancho Los Amigos Medical
   Center
Downey, California

Correspondence to:
Lance R. Stone, DO
San Diego Rehabilitation Institute
6645 Alvarado Road
San Diego, California 92120

Clinicians treating traumatic brain injury (TBI) patients should be familiar with the technical considerations of nerve blocks for management of hypertonicity. More importantly, an understanding of which TBI patients are at risk for this complication and their prognosis for recovery needs to be established prior to treatment. This chapter attempts first to identify which patient group is likely to develop hypertonicity, then discusses the differential diagnosis of abnormal movement. The history of phenol as a therapeutic agent and specific clinical indications are presented in the second section. Finally, botulinum toxin A is introduced as the newest and most selective treatment for hypertonicity in the chapter's concluding section.

CLASSIFICATION OF TRAUMATIC BRAIN INJURY

Nonpenetrating TBI can be classified into two groups, *focal* or *diffuse*, based on the pathology.[5,8,54] Focal injury can be further subdivided into focal cortical contusion,[23] subcortical hemorrhages,[2] and infarcts within a distinct arterial territory.[1,43,62,87] Diffuse pathologic injury results from shear strains, known as diffuse axonal injury,[3,40] or is related to hypoxic-ischemic events following cardiovascular,[63,93,100] respiratory,[21,93] or increased intracranial pressure complications.[92,96] The late sequelae of these injuries frequently cause disturbances of cognition, behavior, executive functioning, and personality.[11,16,78,103] During the early stages of recovery, TBI patients are typically in rehabilitation hospitals where abnormal motor function and hypertonicity may predominate and complicate their therapy.[15,39,88]

FOCAL INJURIES

Focal cortical contusions usually occur at the frontal and temporal poles[55] and generally do not directly affect the more posteriorly represented primary and unimodal sensory and motor cortex. An exception may be a laceration or contusion directly involving the motor cortex underlying the point of contact from, for example, an assault with a blunt object. Subcortical hemorrhages due to rupture of small perforating arterial branches, such as the lenticulostriate or anterior choroidal, supplying the basal ganglia and internal capsule can produce motor disorders. These lesions infrequently occur, in approximately 3% of all nonpenetrating injuries, and are therefore of lesser clinical consequence.[2,65] Infarction resulting from compromise of a particular artery may arise through brain swelling, producing neurologic deficits related to functions within its distribution.

Cerebral infarction within the territory of the posterior cerebral artery often associated with transtentorial herniation is by far the most common.[43,45] The clinical syndrome of posterior cerebral artery territory infarction varies according to the site of occlusion and the availability of collaterals. Incomplete or partial posterior cerebral artery syndromes are the rule. Occlusion of the posterior cerebral artery can potentially produce a greater spectrum of deficits than occlusion of any other artery because both the upper brainstem, which is densely organized with important structures, and the inferior parts of the temporal and medial parts of the occipital lobe lay within its domain. Another type of infarction resulting from herniation causes elongation and finally rupture of the paramedian perforating arteries of the midbrain tegmentum (Duret hemorrhages). Rosenblum[108] proposes that vascular lesions of the midbrain and rostral pons are frequent in fatal cases of head trauma and that such lesions are probably an immediate consequence of trauma rather than delayed herniation. Nevertheless, the outcome of Duret hemorrhages involving brainstem structures render recovery almost impossible. If these patients survive, they may remain in a persistent vegetative state[67,109] and are unlikely to be treated in acute rehabilitation settings.

DIFFUSE INJURIES

Diffuse axonal injury (DAI) results from shear and tensile strain damage to axons. The distribution of DAI is distinctive, following a gradient occurring from the cortical-subcortical junction toward the midbrain, with greater concentrations of axonal perturbation deeper within the hemispheres associated with more severe rotational acceleration forces.[40,108] There is a tendency to involve the corpus callosum and dorsolateral midbrain in the severest injuries.[3] Microscopic examination of DAI reveals scattered axon retraction balls in the white matter and demyelination in areas where the axons converge into tracts, e.g., the cerebral peduncles.[3] DAI may cause temporary, reversible axoplasmic swelling or complete and irreversible axonal disruption.[32] DAI has the greatest capacity to damage corticospinal pathways at many levels, including the cerebral cortex, subcortical white matter, internal capsule, and brainstem. In the subcortical white matter, the corticospinal fibers are intermingled with corticorubrospinal, corticoreticulospinal, corticovestibulospinal, corticotectospinal, and ascending thalamocortical fibers. Thus, shearing strains may simultaneously affect both corticospinal and extrapyramidal motor systems.

Hypoxic-ischemic injury may be superimposed on a DAI and manifest itself in various syndromes.[43,87,91,108] Diffuse and boundary-zone hypoxic-ischemic injury are the two forms that are of the most clinical importance. Diffuse hypoxic-ischemic injury is usually a delayed complication of increased intracranial pressure or cardiorespiratory arrest. Selective neuronal necrosis occurs that may be global or confined to the third, fifth, and sixth lamina of the cerebral cortex (pseudolaminar necrosis), Purkinje cells of the cerebellum, and pyramidal cells in Somner's sector of the hippocampus.[91] DAI may cause deafferentation by axotomy, whereas diffuse hypoxic-ischemic brain injury tends to cause widespread death of neurons. The abnormal control of voluntary movement and muscle tone observed after diffuse hypoxic-ischemic injury may be difficult to distinguish clinically from DAI.

Boundary-zone hypoxic-ischemic injury is usually due to a transient episode of perfusion failure.[1,43,91] This failure tends to produce hypoxic damage that is concentrated between territories of the major cerebral arteries, so-called watershed zones. Boundary-zone hypoxic-ischemic injury involves unimodal and heteromodal cortex and produces disorders of language, visual recognition, visual motor integration, and visual scanning, with sparing of the primary motor cortex.[5] Severe hypotension may result in infarcts in the basal ganglia, which under normal circumstances is nourished by small penetrating arteries and lacks a collateral supply.

In summary, DAI and diffuse hypoxic-ischemic injury are theoretically the two major pathologic processes that are most likely to produce motor dysfunction and hypertonicity following nonpenetrating TBI. There are estimated to be between 50,000 to 70,000 severe TBI survivors per year.[75] Overall, DAI is distinguished in about one-third of severe brain injuries.[44] This is probably an underestimation because the features of DAI may be subtle and masked by other forms of brain injury. The presence of diffuse hypoxic damage is difficult to estimate. During acute rehabilitation, clinicians are likely to encounter motor dysfunction and hypertonicity as a complication of diffuse hypoxic-ischemic injury and DAI.[39,88] Without appropriate treatment, disabling musculotendinous contractures and abnormal, dyssynergic patterns of movement occur, further complicating the patient's recovery and outcome.

DISORDERS OF MOVEMENT

Dysfunction of active and passive movement following TBI can be a manifestation of abnormalities of muscle tone, i.e., rigidity, spasticity, athetosis, dystonia, paratonia, flaccidity or disturbances of sensorimotor integration, optic ataxia, or constructional apraxia. Additionally, a reduction in intention, i.e., abulia, decreased initiation and attention, hemineglect, and hemiakinesia can all impair normal movement. Finally, resistance to movement may represent collagen transformation within the normal viscoelastic property of muscle and connective tissue elements.[56] Evaluation using nerve blocks consisting of lidocaine, phenol, or botulinum A toxin (Botox) cannot influence disturbances of intention or sensorimotor integration, but their effect on muscle tone may help to clarify the underlying resistance to movement.

DISORDERS OF TONE

Rigidity, spasticity, and dystonia are the three forms of abnormal muscle tone observed following a TBI that may contribute to the development of musculotendinous contracture and restricted purposeful function. In severe DAI, all three forms may be present in the same patient in separate limbs, requiring careful clinical observation and analysis by the examiner prior to embarking on treatment to normalize tone and voluntary movement.

Clinical *spasticity* is that form of hypertonicity marked by increased involuntary contractile resistance of muscle to passive range of motion. The resistance is proportionate to the velocity of movement secondary to hyperexcitability of the stretch reflex.[76]

Rigid muscles are continuously or intermittently firm and tense. The increased restraint on passive movement that characterizes rigidity is not proceeded by an initial free interval and has an even or uniform quality throughout the range of movement of the limb. Rigidity is present in all muscle groups, both flexor and extensor, but it tends to be more prominent in those that maintain a flexed posture.[4]

Dystonia, as defined by the Scientific Advisory Board of the Dystonic Medical Research Foundation, is a syndrome of sustained muscle contraction, frequently causing twisting and repetitive movements or abnormal postures.[34] Dystonias have been classified into four types: focal, segmental, multifocal, and generalized. In the authors' experience, dystonia best characterizes the abnormal tone that requires chemical denervation following TBI.

EARLY VERSUS LATE HYPERTONICITY

Hypertonicity is usually greatest during the period of spontaneous neurologic recovery typically occurring within the first 6 months following injury. It is an important treatment principle that any permanent neurosurgical or orthopedic surgical procedures intended to control hypertonicity should be avoided during this recovery phase. Phenol[39] and botulinum toxin type A[60] are ideal therapeutic agents because of their reversible mechanism of action. Lidocaine has both a therapeutic and diagnostic role in managing early- and late-appearing hypertonic disorders.[68] In early stages, it can be useful in predicting the response to phenol or botulinum toxin type A and can also be applied prior to serial or inhibitory casting. In the late stages of recovery, lidocaine can assist the clinician in predicting the functional outcome of a musculotendinous release, muscle transfer, or muscle lengthening. The appropriate management for hypertonicity presenting between 6 and 18 months following injury can be vexing as whether to recommend surgical versus continuing nonsurgical treatment.

In this circumstance, prognostic factors including the patient's age,[53] selective motor control,[39] length of coma,[53,54] post-traumatic amnesia,[54] superimposed secondary complications, e.g., hypoxia or infarction,[54] depth of lesion on magnetic resonance imaging[80] and level of care on discharge are evaluated.[68] The majority of patients complete their neurologic recovery by 18 to 24 months. Younger patients have the greatest potential for continuing improvement because of the inherent plasticity of their nervous system. Functional improvement after 2 years is usually the result of surgery, adaptive equipment, assistive devices, and environmental compensations.

GENERALIZED VERSUS FOCAL HYPERTONICITY

After the prognosis for motor return and stage of recovery has been established, the clinician evaluates whether the hypertonicity is generalized or focal. Generalized hypertonicity will not be responsive to local nerve or motor-point blocks. Multiple contributing overactive muscle groups, both superficial and deep, make neurolysis and neuromuscular blockade impractical and technically unfeasible. In distinction, focal hypertonic muscles lend themselves well to this technique. The treatment for both early and late generalized hypertonicity that is complicated by the emergence of contractures or skin breakdown will be first pharmacologic (dantrolene sodium)[131] then surgical lengthening or selective posterior rhizotomy.[64] Intrathecal implantable infusion pumps may assume a future role in this circumstance but have not been adequately researched in the TBI population.[64,102,135] Occasionally, focal nerve blocks may be of benefit in generalized hypertonicity. For example, obturator and musculocutaneous nerve blocks may enhance perineal care and elbow hygiene, respectively.[68]

CAUSE-SPECIFIC VERSUS SYMPTOMATIC THERAPY

Prior to chemical denervation, the approach to hypertonicity can be divided into two strategies: treatment directed at a reversible cause contributing to the condition, and therapy that alleviates symptoms but does not influence the pathogenesis of the injury.

Hydrocephalus provides an example of a cause-specific etiology. The incidence of post-traumatic ventricular dilatation has been reported to be between 30.5[46] and 72%.[79] Severe disturbance of gait, motor performance, and hypertonicity have been observed, which may improve with shunting.[119,123] If residual symptoms persist following shunting, then symptomatic treatment, such as nerve blocks, should be considered. Chronic subdural hematomas and hygromas, depending on their location and mass affect, may produce fluctuating abnormalities of tone, including hemiparesis. The treatment is surgical evacuation unless the subdural is small and exerting little mass effect. Drug-induced movement disorders are probably the more common cause-specific complication observed. Those due to anticonvulsants may be treated by discontinuing or reducing the dosage of the anticonvulsant.[24] Extrapyramidal symptoms, including rigidity and acute dystonic reactions secondary to neuroleptic drugs or other dopamine receptor antagonists, such as metoclopramide, may respond to parenteral administration of anticholinergics or antihistamines.[29,59,99]

The great majority of patients with symptomatic hypertonic disorders require localized nerve blocks or neuromuscular blockade designed to depress the final common pathway during CNS reorganization and recovery. The remainder of this chapter discusses hypertonicity management that uses local pharmacologic therapeutic treatment with phenol, lidociane, and botulinum toxin type A. Their historical uses, mechanisms of action, specific indications, and technical applications will be described.

PHENOL NEUROLYSIS

History

Carbolic acid, more familiarly known as phenol, is a remarkably toxic agent that, despite its potential to destroy tissue, has found therapeutic uses in rehabilitation. The clinical success of phenol benefits from its destructive protein-denaturing effect. Historically, its application can be grouped into the treatment of four general conditions. beginning with antiseptic use followed by peripheral vascular disease, pain control, and more recently, spasticity management.

Phenol was first established as a medicinal agent by Lister for antiseptic purposes in 1867.[81] Both subcutaneous[133] and intrathecal[126] injections of phenol were employed in the treatment of tetanus caused by the anaerobic, spore-forming rods, *Clostridium tetani*. The exotoxin tetanospasmin was denatured by phenol in vitro, which led to treatment of the disease. Phenol has few current legitimate uses as an antiseptic today because of the more effective and less toxic substances now available. Some additional clinical conditions that have benefited from phenol take advantage of its neurolytic effect. Both Doppler,[28] in 1925, and Binet,[10] in 1933, applied 7% aqueous phenol to exposed blood vessels for the treatment of peripheral vascular insufficiency. The vasodilation was presumed to result from the destruction of autonomic perivascular fibers. More recently, authors have reported on chemical paravertebral sympathectomy using phenol for peripheral vascular disease. Reid[106] described a technique of injecting phenol to induce a lumbar sympathectomy. Subsequently, Hughes-Davies and Rechman[57] have published on their experience of 124 injections. Although intermittent claudication was not altered, improved superficial blood flow, temperature, and healing of pregangrenous skin changes and resting pain were major benefits.

Putnam and Hampton[104] carried out one of the earliest uses of phenol neurolysis for the relief of pain in a series of gasserian ganglion injections. With the introduction of carbamazepine, microvascular decompression, and high-frequency nerve stimulators capable of producing easily controlled lesions, the use of chemical neurolysis for the treatment of trigeminal neuralgia became obsolete.[4,127]

Nevertheless, phenol continued to be used as a neurolytic agent for the treatment of pain. Maher[89] first introduced the injection technique of intrathecal phenol neurolysis for intractable cancer pain. Phenol has gained widespread acceptance and enhanced application since its use reported by Maher. Alterations in technique, variations in concentrations, and constituents of the various solutions for pain are well documented but are beyond the scope of this review.

In 1959, Kelly and Gautier-Smith[69] and Nathan[97] simultaneously reported on the intrathecal injection of phenol in glycerine on anterior nerve roots, causing a flaccid paralysis and relieving spasticity caused by upper motor neuron lesions. Since then, phenol neurolysis has emerged in the treatment of spasticity. Following Kelly and Gautier-Smith and Nathan's success with intrathecal phenol, the experience with phenol can be categorized into central and peripheral uses.

Various techniques, concentrations, and carriers have been reported in the use of intrathecal phenol to effect a chemical rhizolysis in spastic paraplegia.[7,73,82,83,101,117,118,133] It was reported that the majority of patients treated benefited, but more recent reports are less conclusive. Phenol has several undesirable characteristics, including transient relief of symptoms and indiscriminate and nonselective nerve damage. Intrathecal phenol may reduce bladder function in patients who still maintain a spinal reflex and may destroy sensation, rendering the skin more prone to injury.[82,97,101,133] In addition, there is the potential of producing severe degenerative and reactive changes, such as arachnoiditis, meningitis, vascular thrombosis, and demyelination.[121,133] Subsequent surgical therapy is thus rendered more difficult. Intrathecal phenol has not been advocated for hypertonicity management following TBI. Its popularity for use in paraplegia has waned in favor of more selective and less destructive procedures, including implantable intrathecal pumps,[64,102,135] selective microrhizotomies, medication, tendon lengthening and release, and peripheral uses of phenol.[68,133]

Intravenous Use

The peripheral use of phenol for spasticity began shortly after its use in the subarachnoid space. Cooper et al.[20] reported on the only and perhaps most unusual series of patients treated for the relief of spasticity by perfusioning a limb with a 0.36% phenol dextran solution for 15 minutes. They treated 12 patients and were able to reduce spasticity in nine limbs.

Paravertebral Use

In an effort to avoid the complications of intrathecal blocks and to yield a more selective effect on spastic hip and knee flexors in paraplegics, Meelhuysen et al.[90] performed paravertebral lumbar somatic blocks. With the patient positioned, they located the nerve just after its emergence from the intravertebral foramen with a Teflon-coated needle and a nerve stimulator. The phenol was reconstituted in water to either a 5% or 3% concentration, depending on the completeness of the spinal cord injury. Hip flexor spasticity was treated by injecting into L2, 3, 4, and knee flexor spasticity, by L5–S1 nerve block. Of the 31 blocks, 21 yielded some relaxation, with electromyographic evidence of denervation. Overall lumbar and sacral paravertebral nerve blocks are technically more cumbersome than intrathecal procedures but have the advantage of high selectivity.

Koyama et al.[74] conducted direct major and minor psoas intramuscular phenol blocks under ultrasonic monitoring in an attempt to reduce x-ray exposure and minimize the risk of organ and vascular injury. No significant complications occurred, and hip range of motion improved in all patients. Extensive anatomic knowledge and skill in echographic procedures is required before attempting the procedure. Blocking of a single nerve root results in loss of spasticity in several different muscles or muscle groups. Paravertebral blocks can spread more widely than planned, creating undesired results. It can also cause an unacceptable sensory impairment and deafferentation pain syndrome due to blocking of a mixed nerve.

The effort to become more selective with phenol and better manage upper extremity spasticity led to the peripheral nerve approach. These procedures can be grouped into closed (percutaneous) and open (intraneural) injections. The use of dilute phenol, 2% and 3% in water, had been first reported in 1969 by Khalili et al.[72] in a large series, to provide temporary relief of spasticity. This series covered 293 blocks and 120 patients and resulted in 10 months of improvement and a 10% complication rate of deafferentation pain.

Katz et al.,[66] Fusfeld,[36] Glass et al.,[41] Brattstrom et al.,[13] and Copp and Keenan[22] all subsequently reported varying duration of effectiveness and deafferentation pain as a complication that ranged from 3 to 10%. Multiple explanations for this variation in results include the concentration of phenol and the type of solvent used, the length of contact time with a nerve, differences in technique of application, localization and selection of block site, and lack of standardization of reporting results.

In peripheral nerves with a major sensory contribution, Mooney et al.[94] attempted to avoid post-block deafferentation pain and sensory loss by performing surgical open intraneural motor branch injections. This technique was further refined by Braun et al.,[14] who used 5% phenol in a glycerin solution. The primary application has been for injection of motor branches of the posterior tibial and musculocutaneous nerves. The desired response or effect may be more prolonged, and deafferentation pain may be avoided; however, the technique is more difficult, is time consuming, and requires surgery.

Intramuscular Use

In contrast to percutaneous peripheral neurolysis, "motor-point" neurolysis can diminish hypertonicity in individual muscles while avoiding deafferentation pain or sensory loss. Tardieu and Hariga[128] are two investigators credited for introducing this injection approach using dilute alcohol. Cain and Liebgold[17] subsequently demonstrated a technique of using dilute solutions of phenol. Halpern and Meelhuysen observed Cain and Liebgold then went on to report a large series of patients.[49] Successful relaxation of hypertonia was achieved concurrently with improvement of function in 114 of 122 muscles injected in 39 patients. The effects persisted up to 6 months or longer. Cain et al.[17] and Khalili and Benton[70] both reported their results the same year. The results were variable, as were the concentrations and volumes of phenol injected. This technique continues to be popular, and reports of different applications injecting various muscles have demonstrated good results.[12,42,52,68,74]

Chemistry

Phenol is a benzene ring with a hydroxyl group substituting for a hydrogen ion. Phenol consists of colorless crystals with a somewhat aromatic odor. It is soluble in water at room temperature in a ratio of 1:15. Phenol is not available as a ready-to-use pharmaceutical preparation but must be reconstituted from an analytical-grade phenol. Phenol is highly soluble in glycerin and diffuses from it slowly, an advantage in open injections that prevents spread; it also allows for highly localized tissue fixation. When phenol is to be mixed with glycerin, great care must be taken that both phenol and glycerin are free of water, or the necrotizing effect of the phenol-glycerin mixture will be much greater than anticipated.

Concentration

Phenol has been used as a neurolytic agent in various solutions and concentrations. Its current application in the TBI patient is open motor branch neurolysis, percutaneous nerve injection, and motor-point injection. For open motor branch neurolysis, a 3% phenol in glycerin preparation was used by Roper[107] and in 1982, by Garland et al.,[38] and this continues to be an effective concentration. Motor-point blocks have been performed with concentrations ranging from 3 to 7%.[12,17,22,42,49,52,68,70,74,133] Khalili and Betts[71] reported on peripheral nerve injections in a series of 193 muscles and 120 patients using 2% and 3% aqueous phenol. Spasticity improved for an average of 198 days. Katz et al.[66] published on a series of 56 injections in 22 patients. Their results were less impressive: 50% reduction of spasticity, with duration of effect greater than 1 month in only 16%. Brattstrom et al.[13] reported on 90 blocks in 57 patients using 2 to 3% solutions. The average duration of effect was 18 months. Coop and Keenan in 1972[22] used 3 to 5% aqueous phenol but did not report on duration of effect.

Pathophysiology

Phenol has been demonstrated to have an immediate local anesthetic effect and, when acting as such, has a selective effect, as do other anesthetics.[98] Local anesthetics appear to block the influx of sodium ions through ionic pores, thereby preventing depolarization. Effectiveness is determined by surface area-to-volume ratio of nerve and agent concentration. Consequently, thinner gamma fibers, which have greater relative surface area, are most easily paralyzed, whereas alpha fibers are less susceptible to the effects of local anesthetic agents. This explanation is particularly applicable to electrophysiologic results recorded shortly after phenol injection in spinal rootlets of cats, which showed a selective effect on small-diameter fibers.[58,98]

Schaumburger et al.,[114] in their acute electrophysiologic and histologic experiments, observed an initial fall in amplitude of the slower myelinated (delta) and nonmyelinated (C potentials) that very slightly antedated the fall of the rapidly conducting alpha fibers. The faster potentials then began to decline at approximately the same rate, resulting in no evidence of a significant differential effect.

Histologic studies showed no selective fiber effect, findings that dispute acute electrophysiologic studies suggesting that phenol has a persistent differential blockade effect, as described in cat spinal roots. Stewart and Lourie,[124] in 1963, observed nonselective degeneration in cat rootlets; as the concentration and duration of application were increased, nerve damage increased *pari passu.*

Phenol causes protein coagulation and necrosis. Its affinity in vitro for minced aorta was shown to be greater than that of brain neurophospholipid. This is consistent with the concept that phenol affects protein and with the fact that many of the complications of phenol are due to its damaging effects on perineural vascular elements. The neurolytic action of phenol and subsequent wallerian degeneration and regeneration account for the reversible tissue effect of phenol.

According to Sunderland,[125] the rate of functional regeneration of peripheral nerve is in the order of 1.5 ± 0.1 mm/d following crush injuries. This time sequence explains the eventual return of hypertonicity in most patients. There are patients in whom relief is permanent, resulting from vascular thrombosis and nerve infarction. For regeneration of fibers to occur, the cell body must survive and the endoneural tube and Schwann cells must remain viable. Permanent relief of hypertonicity thus may be clinical evidence of anterior horn cell death, dorsal root ganglion, or Schwann cell loss, varying according to the site of injection of the phenol.[42,98,114,124,133] Another etiology may be the shrinkage of the neurolemmal sheath following wallerian degeneration and the development of endoneural fibrosis, obstructing axonal regrowth, or loss of normal endplates in the prolonged delay of reinnervation.[35]

Complications

Nerve blocks for the provision of denervation, like any other invasive procedure, carry risk inherent to the procedure. To help minimize these complications, nerve blocks should be performed by clinicians knowledgeable not only in the technique but also in coping with potential local and systemic adverse effects.

LOCAL

Transient local muscle discomfort and soreness related to the trauma of injection is universally present to some degree. The chief complaint noted by Halpern and Meelhuysen[49] was the presence of discomfort or pain of mild intensity in the area of injection lasting about 2 days following motor-point neurolysis. This was observed mainly in the children injected with a 7% solution. Analgesics were not required, but activity was inhibited during this period. No pain followed injections with 3% solutions. This is representative of most intramuscular phenol studies, which report local pain, swelling and discomfort, requiring ice, elevation, acetaminophen, and nonsteroidal anti-inflammatory drugs.[12,17,37,52,70,133] In studies in which mixed motor and sensory nerves were injected percutaneously at the peripheral or paravertebral level, painful paresthesias have been reported at between 3 and 10%.[22,42,71,72,133] This may be transient or last up to 3 months. In an effort to avoid deafferentation pain, the open surgical technique of identifying the motor branches was developed.[14,42,94,107,133] Garland et al.[38] reported on 16 open tibial nerve blocks; 1 patient complained of dysesthesia of the foot, which gradually resolved without interfering with therapy. Minimal tenderness and swelling at the surgical site was transient in most patients.

Sensory loss can also occur with injection of mixed nerves. Typically, this sensory loss is not complete and has negligible consequences in mixed nerves with small sensory representations. Injection of mixed nerves with a sensory supply involving the hand or weight-bearing surfaces should be avoided.

Injection into a viscera is a serious complication related to improper technique and may potentially be seen with obturator nerve injection (bladder) and subscapularis, pectoral (pneumothorax) motor-point blocks. Their occurrence has not been reported in the literature.

A subcutaneous injection may cause extensive skin necrosis. Phenol has great penetrability into tissues. The skin may turn red and eventually sloughs, leaving the cutaneous surfaces stained a light brown. If phenol has been applied locally to skin, it can be removed effectively with 50% alcohol, glycerin, vegetable oils, or even water.[33] The clinician is cautioned not to inject too superficially under the skin. Infection is a rare complication because phenol is an antiseptic agent, and therefore, it is not necessary to prepare the skin.

Although not described in the literature, multiple motor-point blocks in the forearm may precipitate edema and result in a compartment syndrome. Neither Garland et al.[37] nor Halpern and Meelhuysen[49] mentioned the volume of phenol injected at one sitting. It has been our practice to limit volume to 10 mL. Caution should be used in patients who are on anticoagulants. To minimize risk, anticoagulated patients stop taking warfarin sodium 1 to 2 days before the procedure. Loss of useful muscle function must always be considered prior to performing a block. When weakness does occur, it usually represents the unmasking of paresis, underlying an increase in tone that was useful to the patient. In a situation where there is a possibility that a reduction of hypertonicity may have undesirable functional consequences, one should always try a diagnostic anesthetic block before injecting phenol. This can be helpful in predicting the outcome of a phenol nerve block. We strongly emphasize that nerve blocks be performed only following a careful consideration of the functional pathokinesiologic consequences of changes in the dynamic balance of the musculoskeletal system.

More serious local complications, such as venous thrombosis, although rare, may occur.[86] Greater caution should be exercised when injecting the paravertebral area because of the possibility of intrathecal injection or spinal cord infarction.[9,90]

SYSTEMIC

Phenol is effectively metabolized by liver enzymes. It can reach the circulation from all sites of administration, even when applied to intact skin. The principal pathways are conjugation to the glucuronides and oxidation to quinol compounds or to carbon dioxide and water, and excretion as various conjugates via the kidney.[33] The toxic dose of phenol in adults is estimated to be between 8 and 15 g or about 0.75 and 1.5 g/body weight.[42,49,133] Deichman and Keplinger[26] cite death after the ingestion of as little as 1 g in an adult. An accidental intravascular injection of phenol may cause systemic, nonlethal toxic effects. In general, these include cardiovascular and central nervous system depression and collapse.

Morrison et al.[95] studied the incidence of cardiac dysrhythmias in children receiving dilute phenol (5% in water) for neurolysis at the motor-point insertion. Cardiac dysrhythmias occurred in 3 of 16 patients (19%). No correlation could be made between the dosage and blood concentrations of phenol and the incidence of dysrhythmias in this study population. The long duration (33 ± 8 minutes) of phenol administration may have been a factor in the lower-than-expected incidence of dysrhythmias in the pediatric series, in contrast to the experience reported in the plastic surgery literature, in which rapid absorption following chemical face peels and possible greater plasma concentrations might have been contributing factors. Safe doses, duration of administration or absorption of phenol, and the threshold blood concentration, in which dysrhythmias may become more pronounced, have not been established. Administered systemically by accident phenol stimulates the CNS and causes muscle tremors and eventually, convulsions.[33,42,133] Stimulation is followed by depression, and death results from respiratory failure.

Circulation is also remarkably depressed by phenol, and blood pressure falls secondary to central vasomotor depression and toxic reaction on the myocardium and small blood vessels. In this circumstance, treatment is entirely supportive. Prevention of a systemic reaction includes careful technique and use of a lure-lock control syringe because it facilitates aspiration and other maneuvers with one hand. Our prevailing practice is to limit the maximum dose in one setting to 20 mL of a 5% solution (1 g). Goggles should be used by the physician to prevent any eye exposure by dislodgement of the syringe from the needle and consequent spraying of phenol. The patient's eyes should also be protected. It is ideal to perform the blocks in a setting where the equipment and drugs are readily available to treat any complications. This would include a tray containing epinephrine and a laryngoscope. It is not necessary to routinely place a Hep-Lock or cardiac monitor on the patient. This recommendation does not apply to children, who will require anesthesia with halothane nitrite oxide in a day-surgery setting.[95]

In conclusion, adverse side effects following phenol nerve block are extremely rare when the procedure is performed by an experienced physician. However, there are a few potential complications such that informed consent should be required in patients or guardians for those who do not have the capacity to understand the risk.

CLINICAL APPLICATION

Chemical neurolysis has evolved from a novel neurolytic procedure to basic management of abnormal muscle tone interfering with the rehabilitation of patients following a TBI. Nerve blocks can be categorized into two types: diagnostic and therapeutic. Diagnostic nerve blocks use local short-acting anesthetics, whereas therapeutic nerve blocks generally employ toxins like phenol and botulinum toxin type A. The following discussion will be limited to therapeutic nerve blocks, although it should be understood that diagnostic nerve blocks may need to be performed initially to appreciate the consequence of a more long-lasting neurolytic block.

Indications

In general, the benefits of using chemical denervation following TBI are to avoid the CNS effects of antispasmodic medications, avoid irreversible surgical effects, and direct treatment to specific hypertonic muscle groups.

Common clinical situations necessitating chemical neurolysis are the following:
1. impending soft tissue contracture formation resulting in a loss of motion despite aggressive physical or occupational therapy and serial casting, range-of-motion exercises, and use of physical modalities;

2. functionally disabling conditions, such as hip extensor hypertonicity interfering with seating;
3. hip adductor hypertonicity, causing a scissoring gait; or ankle clonus, interfering with transfers, gait, and bracing;
4. to facilitate perineal hygiene by diminishing hip adductor hypertonicity;
5. shoulder adductor hypertonicity control for axillary care and finger flexor tone control for hand hygiene.

For some patients, nerve blocks can be used to prevent a pressure-induced neuropathy. This has been observed in hyperflexed joints, for example, causing ulnar nerve compression at the elbow or median nerve entrapment at the wrist, with severe wrist flexor tone. Another common indication would be to prevent skin breakdown by reducing hip flexor tone to achieve better positioning and pressure relief of a sacral ulcer. Hip adductor tone reduction can decrease the risk of skin breakdown at the medial aspect of the knee.

Preparation

In preparing for a nerve block, one should be equipped with the following: a constant-current stimulator, a surface-probing electrode, a large surface anode, and Teflon-coated 22-gauge sterile hypodermic needles from 37 to 75 mm in length with exposed tips. The needles will act as a cathode. Exploring with the needle, a motor nerve can be localized at the site where the least current is required to elicit a muscle contraction. For the neurolytic block, a 5% aqueous solution of crystalline phenol is used. For the anesthetic or diagnostic blocks, either 1% lidocaine or 0.25% bupivacaine hydrochloride is used.

Principles

In performing a neurolytic block, the following principles should be considered:

- Consistent patterns of hypertonicity should be identified over time.
- If multiple blocks are required in the limb, proximal muscles should be managed prior to approaching distal muscles. For example, if the patient has both hip and knee flexor hypertonicity, blocking the knee flexor may aggravate the hip flexor hypertonicity because of unopposed hip flexor tone. By controlling the hip flexors first, knee flexors may become relaxed by breaking flexor synergy patterns. By the same token, elimination of hip adductor spasticity frequently results in the reduction of knee extensor and ankle equinus.
- Hypertonicity usually affects a group of muscles that serve a specific function. The next consideration, therefore, is to identify the common myotomes when multiple muscle group tone is present. Muscles supplied by different nerves may share the same myotomal innervation. For example, hip flexor and adductors share the second through fourth lumbar myotomes. Thus, second and third lumbar paraspinal blocks can abolish both hip flexor and adductor tone simultaneously.
- If a mixed nerve with a significant number of cutaneous nerve fibers is blocked, there is a risk of developing painful paresthesia. All efforts should be made to avoid injecting phenol directly into mixed nerves, which have high cortical sensory representation. For nerves with high sensory components, motor-point blocks or open phenol blocks are preferred.

In the following sections, the use of peripheral nerve blocks as diagnostic and therapeutic procedures in the rehabilitation management of TBI patients is presented. The technique and anatomic approach for accurate localization are

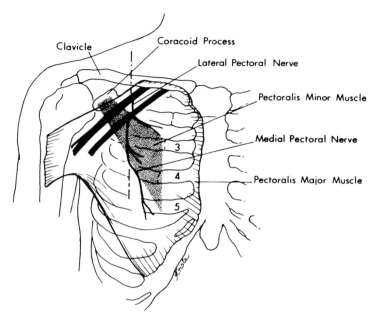

FIGURE 1. **Medial and lateral pectoral nerve** (anterior chest view). The medial and lateral pectoral nerves originate from the medial and lateral cord of the brachial plexus, respectively, at the midclavicular line.

described and illustrated. The emphasis is placed upon the most common clinical indications. Given a proper understanding of anatomy, virtually any nerve or its motor branches can be blocked if the clinical evaluation identifies it as contributing to a disabling deformity.

NERVE BLOCKS FOR UPPER EXTREMITY DEFORMITIES

Shoulder Adductors

MEDIAL AND LATERAL PECTORAL NERVES

Shoulder adduction deformity may result from hypertonia involving the pectoralis major and minor muscles. The clavicular head of pectoralis major is innervated by the lateral cord of the brachial plexus. The lateral pectoral nerve becomes superficial at the intersection of the line formed by the upper margin of the pectoralis minor and a perpendicular line dropped from the midpoint of the clavicle. It is useful to demarcate the triangular borders of the pectoralis minor from its origin at the coracoid process to its insertion at the third through fifth costosternal junction. (Fig. 1)

The medial pectoral nerve originates from the C8 and T1 spinal nerves through the medial cord of the brachial plexus and innervates the sternal muscles. The medial pectoral nerve can be located by using a surface stimulator at the intersection of the lower border of the pectoralis minor and a perpendicular line drawn from a midclavicular point. Special care should be taken to avoid entering the pleural cavity.

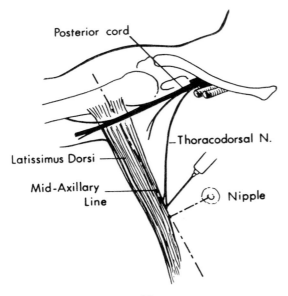

FIGURE 2. **Thoracodorsal nerve** (anterior chest view). The thoracodorsal nerve originates from the posterior cord of the brachial plexus.

THORACODORSAL NERVE

One of the strongest adductors of the shoulder is the latissimus dorsi muscle, which is innervated by the thoracodorsal nerve arising from the posterior cord either posteriorly or anteriorly (Fig. 2). It is easier to approach this nerve anteriorly, as the latissimus dorsi muscle can be easily separated from the lateral chest wall because the nerve passes between these two structures. Special care needs to be taken with the thoracodorsal nerve, as it travels with the same-named artery. To localize this nerve, a perpendicular line is drawn from the midaxillary point. With a surface electrode, this nerve is easily located on the midaxillary line 1.5 inches above the nipple line between the latissimus dorsi and chest wall. The nerve may be approached more precisely with the use of a Teflon-coated needle. Strong shoulder adduction should be seen with a current <2 mA.

LOWER SUBSCAPULAR NERVE

In addition to the pectoralis major and latissimus dorsi muscles, the teres major muscle is another source of shoulder adductor deformity. Teres major is innervated by the lower subscapular nerve (Fig. 3), which originates from the C5 and C6 spinal nerves through the posterior cord of the brachial plexus (Fig. 4). The lower subscapular nerve enters teres major as it travels downward parallel to the thoracodorsal nerve at its lateral position. The nerve is localized midway between the acromion and the inferior angle of the scapula along its lateral border. After the nerve is localized with the surface stimulator, a Teflon-coated needle is inserted toward the midportion of teres major parallel to the chest wall to localize the nerve.

Elbow Flexors

Elbow flexor synergy may result from hypertonia involving the muscle groups innervated by the musculocutaneous nerve or from abnormal tone in the brachioradialis, which is innervated by the radial nerve. The combination of these two muscle groups is common.

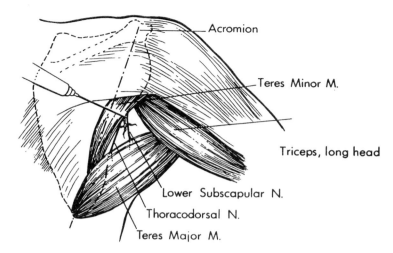

FIGURE 3. **Lower subscapular nerve** (posterior shoulder view, the scapula is shown in dotted lines) is visualized in its relation to thoracodorsal nerve and teres major.

RADIAL NERVE

Hypertonicity involving the brachioradialis can be managed either by percutaneous motor-point blocks using phenol or by a motor branch neurolysis through an open surgical approach. The radial nerve may be easily located by palpating the nerve in the radial groove of the humerus. Temporary block at this location, using a local anesthetic agent, is a useful technique in facilitating serial casting or in determining the degree of contracture formation.

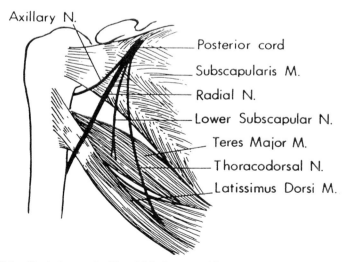

FIGURE 4. **Posterior cord of brachial plexus** and its branches, the axillary, radial, lower subscapular, and thoracodorsal nerves (posterior shoulder view, the scapula is removed).

Musculocutaneous Nerve

The musculocutaneous nerve originates from the lateral cord of the brachial plexus at a slightly higher level than the origin of the median nerve. The musculocutaneous nerve runs obliquely downward and laterally to supply the coracobrachialis muscle and then down to the biceps and brachialis.

In the axillary approach, the needle is inserted below the tendon of the pectoralis major close to its insertion into the humerus, and anterior to the axillary artery. The needle is advanced parallel to the arm and directed toward the coracoid process. The tip of the needle will first lie in proximity to the median nerve, as evidenced by a contraction of the wrist and finger flexors. When the needle is advanced approximately 1 cm further, its tip will be near the musculocutaneous nerve, and a visible contraction of the biceps will be observed. The needle should remain anterior to the lateral plane of the axillary artery. This position can be assured by pressing down on the axillary artery with the index finger.

Another approach can be made by inserting a needle perpendicularly into the coracobrachialis muscle substance immediately posterior to the pectoralis major tendon. With the arm in an abducted position, the axillary artery is palpated posteriorly, and the artery should be compressed using the palpating fingertip to avoid an accidental injection into the axillary artery. The musculocutaneous nerve is encountered at a depth of less than 2 cm within the coracobrachialis muscle. The nerve is anterior and lateral to the axillary neurovascular sheath at this location (Fig. 5).

Wrist and Finger Flexors

To treat finger and wrist flexor deformities, median or ulnar nerve blocks can be performed. Usually, these nerve blocks are performed diagnostically by using lidocaine to determine the flexibility of the flexor tendons. Nerve blocks are also used to facilitate serial casting for the treatment of closed-fist deformities with wrist flexion hypertonicity.

Median Nerve

The median nerve (Fig. 6) lies medial to the brachial artery beneath the bicipital aponeurosis at the elbow. It leaves the antecubital fossa by dipping between the two heads of the pronator teres to supply most of the muscles in the anterior compartment of the forearm. Branches to the pronator teres usually originate while the nerve is still in the antecubital fossa. The median nerve may be approached in the antecubital fossa. However, due to its proximity to the brachial artery in the antecubital fossa, it is preferable to approach the median nerve at a lower level.

Usually, the needle is inserted 1 inch below and 1 inch anterior to the medial epicondyle and advanced horizontally until a visible response to stimulation is noted in the corresponding muscles.

Ulnar Nerve

Diagnostic ulnar nerve blocks are commonly performed at the wrist in Guyon's canal to determine the presence of intrinsic hypertonicity. Occasionally, ulnar nerve blocks can be done using local anesthetics above the elbow to relieve wrist and long-finger flexor tone on the ulnar side. This block can be performed in conjunction with median nerve blocks prior to serial casting.

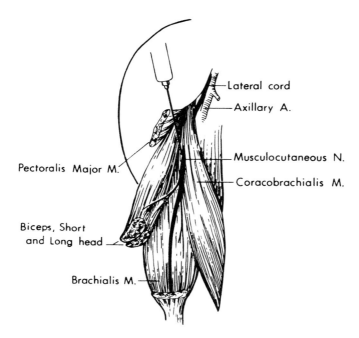

FIGURE 5. **Musculocutaneous nerve.** The nerve is shown behind the pectoralis major tendon and in the substance of coracobrachialis muscle.

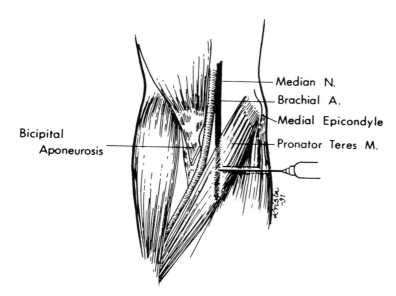

FIGURE 6. **Median nerve.** The nerve is localized in the distal to the antecubital fossa, away from the brachial artery.

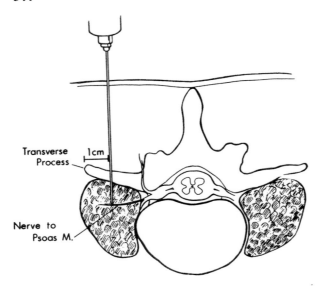

FIGURE 7. Direct spinal nerve branches to the psoas major at the third and fourth intertransverse space (coronal section at the upper margin of the fourth lumbar spine).

Both median and ulnar nerve blocks using phenol are undesirable because of the risk of painful paresthesia. In this case, motor-point blocks to the long-finger and wrist flexors in the forearm are more desirable. Multiple injections to different parts of the motor point may be required.

NERVE BLOCKS FOR LOWER EXTREMITY DEFORMITIES

Hip Flexors

The main hip flexor is the iliopsoas muscle, which consists of the psoas major and the iliacus muscle. Both psoas major and the iliacus muscle are innervated by branches from the femoral nerve. The psoas major also receives direct branches from the second and the third lumbar spinal nerves. These direct branches can be approached at the fourth and fifth intertransverse space (Fig. 7). L2 and L3 spinal nerves innervating the psoas muscle are most commonly found at the site close to the tip and anterior to the transverse process (Fig. 8). In the third and fourth lumbar intertransverse space, the spinal nerves to the femoral and obturator nerves are frequently encountered. The L2 and L3 nerve fibers contributing to the femoral nerve pass posterolateral to the spinal nerves innervating the psoas muscle. The fibers supplying the obturator nerve, however, are located posteromedial to the spinal nerves entering into the psoas major muscle (Fig. 9).

Therefore, if a contraction of the quadriceps muscle is seen while the branches to the psoas major muscle are approached, the needle should be withdrawn and redirected anteromedially. If the patient has hip flexion and adductor hypertonicity, this can be controlled at the L4–L5 intertransverse space by blocking the L2–L3 spinal nerves.

Hip Adductors

Obturator nerve block is one of the most commonly performed nerve blocks in the lower extremities (Fig. 10). The obturator nerve originates in the substance

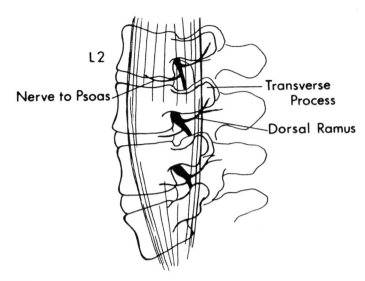

FIGURE 8. **Anterior rami** of the direct spinal nerve branches to the psoas major (lateral view).

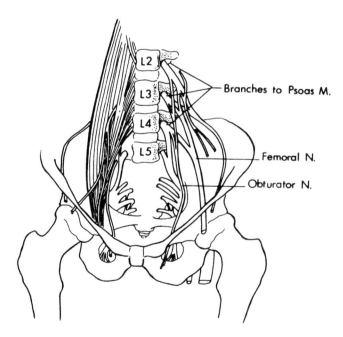

FIGURE 9. **Lumbar plexus** branches to psoas major, and its relation to the femoral nerve (posterolateral) and to the obturator nerve (posteromedial) at the third and fourth lumbar spaces.

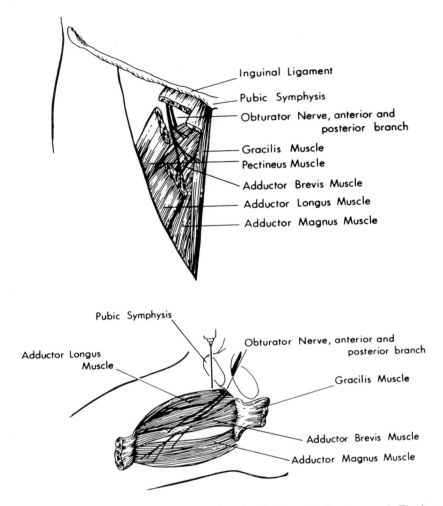

FIGURE 10. The **obturator nerve.** Anterior view is shown in the top panel. The lower panel shows the sagittal section of the right pelvis and the upper thigh across the obturator foramen, showing the anterior and the posterior branches of the obturator nerve.

of the psoas major muscle from the L2–L4 spinal nerves. It leaves the pelvis through the obturator canal, where it divides into the anterior and posterior branches, supplying all adductors of the hip. The two branches of the obturator nerve lie almost at the same sagittal plane, with the posterior branch at a deeper plane than the anterior branch (Fig. 10, lower panel). Both branches can be approached by inserting a needle vertically between the adductor longus and the pectineus muscle, 2 to 3 cm distal to the inguinal ligament.

Hip Extensors
Severe hip extensor hypertonicity rarely may interfere with sitting. The inferior gluteal nerve, which innervates the most powerful hip extensor, the gluteus

maximus, arises from the posterior divisions of the lumbosacral plexus. This nerve receives fibers from the fifth lumbar and the first and second sacral spinal nerves. The nerve then parallels the sciatic nerve beneath the lower border of the piriformis muscle and turns sharply posterolateral to the sacrotuberous ligament to enter the gluteus maximus.

The gluteus maximus originates from the posterior surface of the sacrum and inserts into the gluteal tuberosity of the femur. To localize the nerve, a needle is inserted in the center of the quadrilateral borders of the muscle. A strong contraction is obtained with a needle insertion depth of less than 3 cm. If any contraction is seen in the hamstring muscles, the needle should be withdrawn to avoid an accidental injection into the sciatic nerve.

Knee Extensors

Knee extensor hypertonicity may be useful for the patient's transfers and standing. However, severe knee extensor hypertonicity in the nonambulatory patient may interfere with sitting. In this circumstance, abnormal quadriceps tone can be controlled by blocking the femoral nerve. The nerve is localized by using a surface stimulator positioned in the groin, lateral to the femoral artery. To obtain good relaxation of the quadriceps muscle following the block, a proximal approach to the nerve is desirable because the femoral nerve divides into a number of terminal branches shortly below the inguinal ligament.

Knee Flexors

Lidocaine injection is the most common use of a sciatic nerve block, prior to casting a spastic knee flexion contracture. To localize the sciatic nerve, a line is drawn between the upper aspect of the greater tuberosity of the femur and the posterior superior iliac spine. This line should coincide with the upper border of the piriformis muscle and also the upper border of the sciatic notch. A perpendicular and bisecting line is then drawn. A point 3 cm distal on the perpendicular line represents the injection point. A second verification of the injection point may be made by projecting a line from the greater trochanter of the femur to a point one to two cm below the sacral cornua. The bisecting line crossing perpendicularly at three cm below the first line also represents the point overlying the sciatic nerve as it exits the pelvis. As the needle is advanced, the gluteus maximus muscle contraction will be noticed first. With further advancement of the needle, a stronger hamstring muscle contraction will be noticed as the gluteus muscle contraction ceases.

Ankle Plantar Flexors

A posterior tibial nerve block (Fig. 11) is indicated in spastic equinovarus deformity of the foot that is resistant to conservative therapy. Commonly, posterior tibial nerve block is performed by using a local anesthetic to facilitate a serial casting program applied in the management of spastic equinovarus deformity of the ankle. There is a high incidence of painful paresthesia after percutaneous phenol block of this nerve. Therefore, selective motor branch blocks through an open approach is recommended if the patient requires long-term control of tone or has recurrent contracture following multiple serial casting.

The tibial nerve can be approached for a block either at the apex of the popliteal fossa or at the popliteal crease. At the apex, the nerve is easy to locate because it is superficially located between the medial and lateral hamstrings.

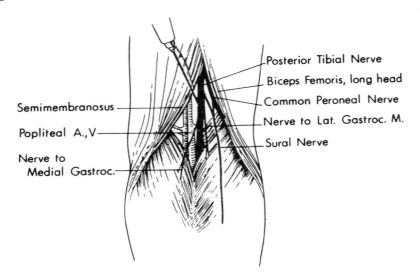

FIGURE 11. **Posterior tibial nerve** (posterior view of the right leg at the popliteal crease). The needle is located on the tibial nerve, distal to the origin of the sural nerve.

Injecting the nerve proximally guarantees blockage of the branches to the gastrocnemius, which usually exits from the main trunk high in the fossa. Unfortunately, a block at this level is also proximal to the origin to the sural nerve and is more likely to be complicated by paresthesia if phenol is used. Another drawback in blocking the nerve at the apex of the fossa is the close proximity of the peroneal nerve, which may be affected by the block.

At the popliteal crease, the nerve may be approached by inserting the needle one fingerwidth lateral to the midpoint and directing it anteriorly. The advantage of this approach at the popliteal crease is that the injection point is away from the peroneal nerve and distal to the point of origin of the sural nerve. But at this level, the fibers to the gastrocnemius may escape the block.

BOTULINUM TOXIN NEUROMUSCULAR BLOCKADE

History

Despite the recognition of botulism over 200 years ago, a cause-and-effect relationship between the toxin released by the bacterium *Clostridium botulinum* and this severe illness was not established until 1897.[129] Research has identified seven serologically distinct neurotoxins; only types A, B, and E have been linked to cases of fatal food poisoning in humans.[50] Type A is the only one that can be crystallized and is widely available for clinical use in the United States. Type F is being studied at some centers for those patients who develop antibodies to type A.

The initial description of therapeutic application using local injections of botulinum toxin type A was for the treatment of strabismus as an alternative to surgical correction.[115] The therapeutic goal was to preferentially block extraocular muscle neuromuscular junctions, causing subsequent muscle weakness in an effort to enhance convergence. Various putative therapeutic agents, including α-bungarotoxin, had been considered prior to botulinum toxin type A, but each had undesired side effects, including lack of selectivity, short duration of action, and substantial antigenicity. The FDA has approved the use of botulinum toxin type A for the treatment of strabismus and blepharospasm associated with dystonia, including benign essential blepharospasm or facial nerve disorders, in patients 12 years of age or above. The therapeutic scope of conditions treated with botulinum toxin type A has expanded to include dystonic and nondystonic involuntary movements, including spasms accompanying stroke, demyelinating disease, and tremor.

A position paper published by the American Academy of Neurology Therapeutics and Technology Assessment Subcommittee[6] concludes that botulinum toxin type A is accepted as a safe and efficacious modality for the treatment of cervical dystonia (torticollis), adductor laryngeal dystonia (spasmodic dysphonia), oromandibular dystonia, and hemifacial spasm. Neuromuscular blockade with botulinum toxin type A may also be promising in patients with other forms of focal dystonia, including writer's cramp and hyperkinetic movement disorders, such as tics and segmental myoclonus. Motor dysfunction due to abnormally increased muscle tone, such as spasticity, may be ameliorated by botulinum toxin type A. The effects of botulinum toxin type A on spasticity in children with cerebral palsy are also being studied. Injections of botulinum toxin type A into spastic external urethral sphincter muscles have been found to improve bladder function of patients with spinal cord injury and detrusor sphincter dyssynergia.[30,31] In one small study, local injections of botulinum toxin type A into the puborectalis muscle were effective in treating anismus in intractable constipation.[48]

Pharmacology of Botulinum Toxin

There are seven immunologically distinct but structurally similar toxins: A, B, C_1, D, E, F, and G.[50] When isolated from bacterial cultures, the toxins are naturally complexed with nontoxic proteins and hemagglutinin.[120] Type A is the only toxin that has a dimer containing hemagglutinin, and this characteristic allows it to be crystallized. When injected locally into skeletal muscles, the nontoxic proteins do not enhance the toxicity of the neurotoxin and may even interfere slightly. However, when ingested, the nontoxic proteins may enhance toxicity greatly, possibly by protecting the neurotoxin from proteolytic enzymes of the gut. The neurotoxin component of the complex has a molecular mass of approximately 150,000.[120]

The toxin is synthesized as a single chain and in this form the toxin molecule has relatively little paralytic action. The single-chain toxin molecule can be cleaved by certain proteolytic enzymes to yield a dichain molecule in a process called "nicking." The two chains have different molecular weight, consisting of a heavy chain (100,000 daltons) linked by a disulfide bond to a light chain (50,000 daltons). In this form, the toxin exerts its effect at the neuromuscular junction. Reduction of the disulfide bonds that link the two chains causes complete loss of toxicity.[50,120] Crude crystallin toxin is produced by E. J. Schantz in Madison, Wisconsin, and then purified under the supervision of Allergan. The preparation process includes dilution, drying, and purification, which results in a variable reduction of potency.[112] The toxin is also manufactured and marketed in England as Dysport.

The mouse assay has been the standard when measuring potency of commercially available toxin.[112,113] One unit of botulinum toxin type A is equivalent to the amount of toxin found to kill 50% of a group of 18- to 20-g female Swiss-Webster mice (LD_{50}) inoculated intraperitoneally. The dose of the British preparation is reported by weight. One nanogram of the British toxin is reported to contain

40 mouse units, where as 1 ng of the US toxin contains 2.5 mouse units.[105] Clinically, however, it appears as though one unit of American toxin may be equivalent to 4 to 5 Dysport units. The differences in measurement between the two forms of the toxin have been somewhat confusing and may explain the differences in results, particularly the higher incidence of side effects with the more potent British version.

Mechanism of Action

The therapeutic effect of botulinum toxin type A results from its action at the neuromuscular junction. The toxin exerts its potent neuroparalytic effect by interfering with the release of acetylcholine.[50,120,129] There are three steps involved in toxin-mediated paralysis: binding, internalization, and inhibition of neurotransmitter release. Toxin binding is by the heavy-chain subunit and may be to a ganglioside component of the membrane of the presynaptic cholinergic nerve terminal. After binding, the toxin is then internalized via the mechanism of receptor-mediated endocytosis, an energy-dependent process independent of nerve activity. The intracellular action of the toxin does not effect the synthesis or storage of the acetylcholine. The current consensus is that the toxin inhibits calcium-dependent exocytosis of acetylcholine quanta by decreasing the frequency of acetylcholine release.

The treatment of muscle with botulinum toxin type A results in an accelerated loss of junctional acetylcholine receptors. Paralysis and a nearly complete decline of miniature endplate potential occurs within a few hours of injection. The muscle becomes functionally denervated, it atrophies, and develops extrajunctional acetylcholine receptors. Days after exposure, the axon fibrils begin to sprout and form junction plates on new areas of the muscle cell walls. Weakness is fully reversible over a period of 3 months. Pathways of degradation of the toxin are not well established.

Clinically, there is typically a 24- to 72-hour delay between the administration of toxin and the onset of clinical effect. It is likely that the clinical effect of toxin is due primarily to the peripheral effect. There are clinical, pharmacologic, and physiologic reasons to believe that the toxin could also have central action. Botulinum toxin type A can enter the central nervous system and bind to brain synaptosomes and nonspecifically inhibit release of neurotransmittors in animal preparations.[47,132] Radiolabeled toxin injected into the gastrocnemius muscles of both the rat and the cat is transported to the spinal cord by retrograde transport through the ventral roots, and radioactivity is detected in the cord segments from which the innervation of the injected muscle arises. Intraspinal transfer is evidenced by the subsequent appearance of botulinum toxin in the cord contralateral to the injection. In the cord, the toxin appears to block recurrent inhibition mediated by the Renshaw cell, presumably by an action of the toxin between the Renshaw cell and α-motoneuron.[130]

Antibodies

Following high doses and repeated injections of botulinum toxin type A, some patients will develop antibodies.[61,129] The only apparent symptom of the antibody development is the clinical resistance to repeated injections. This complication is a significant problem for patients with chronic disorders who benefit from repeated treatment. A crude in vivo mouse neutralization bioassay has been used to detect serum antibodies to botulinum toxin type A.[51,61] A positive assay result occurs when mice inoculated with both the toxin and serum remain healthy after the injection; death of the unprotected mice constitutes a negative assay result. Enzyme-linked immunosorbent assays (ELISA) for the detection of antibody have been developed, but their specificity and clinical correlation with resistance to treatment have not yet been demonstrated.[27] Some patients seem to develop unresponsiveness without apparent antibody formations; the explanation for this is unknown.

At the National Institutes of Health, Hallet has begun to use botulinum toxin type F in experimental trials.[84] They found that type F can be effective for the patients with antibodies to type A. The effective dose is about the same as that of type A measured in mouse units. The duration of action may be modestly reduced.

Complications (Toxicity)

The treating physician should be knowledgeable in relevant anatomy and pathokinesiology and have a basic understanding of electromyography (EMG) prior to chemical denervation use. All peripheral paralytic agents that have the potential to weaken muscles may as a consequence worsen function. A thorough understanding of the TBI patient's course of recovery, time since injury, and muscles contributing to the dynamic deformity must be known prior to injection. Preinjection evaluation may include visual analysis, palpation of muscles, dynamic EMG and diagnostic anesthetic nerve blocks. The routine use of dynamic EMG and injection using EMG guidance is unsettled.[19,134] Our experience has been to individualize evaluation and treatment. When patterns of movement are atypical, and offending muscles are not palpable, we do not hesitate to use dynamic, wire-electrode EMG for identifying affected muscles and EMG-guided hollow-tipped needles for injection. As pointed out in prior studies, EMG recording may be no better in identifying dystonic muscles than clinical evaluation by a skilled observer with experience. EMG guidance of the actual injection, however, is clearly useful in the treatment of limb dystonias.[134]

The level of toxic dose in humans is not known. Scott and Suzuki[116] determined the LD_{50} to be approximately 39 U/kg for monkeys given botulinum toxin type A intramuscularly. Extrapolating data from monkeys to a 70-kg human suggests an LD_{50} of 2730 to 2800 U.

The long-term consequences of chronic injections into muscles is unknown as well. This can be a potential problem in unremitting conditions such as blepharospasm, spasmodic dysphonia, and other dystonias that require repeat injections every 3 months. This is less of a concern following TBI, where patients with abnormal tone generally improve over time and require fewer injections. Weakness or routine EMG changes in muscles distal to the site of injection have not been reported. However, there are detectable abnormalities on single-fiber EMG with cumulative intramuscular doses.[111] This typically manifests as increased jitter in limb muscles distant to those injected. The effect is probably universal in patients treated for cervical dystonia; there has been no objective weakness in these patients.[77] The clinical relevance and duration of these fidings is unclear.

Further studies are needed to investigate the distant effects of the toxin. Weakness of adjacent muscles is the most common side effect. Dysphagia occurs, probably from spread of the toxin to the pharyngeal muscles, particularly after bilateral sternocleidomastoid injections.[61] This adverse effect needs to be observed very carefully to prevent aspiration. Dysphagia may last up to 6 weeks. Women, possibly because of their thinner necks, are at higher risk for dysphagia. TBI patients frequently have both clinical and videofluoroscopic evidence of abnormal swallowing and as a consequence, may be at increased risk for aspiration if deep neck muscles are injected. Caution is recommended in treating patients with pre-existing disorders affecting neuromuscular transmission function. Eaton-Lambert syndrome, myasthenia gravis, and motor neuron disease are not usually seen in young adult males who are at greatest risk for TBI.

Aminoglycosides interfere with neuromuscular transmission and may potentiate the effect of botulinum toxin type A therapy.[110] Patients who are concurrently being treated with aminoglycosides should not be injected or should be injected with caution. There are no absolute contraindications to injection of botulinum toxin type A except a history of hypersensitivity to the toxin (none yet reported) and infection at the site of injection. Women, however, should not be injected during pregnancy or lactation.

It is seldom necessary to emphasize that injection of the toxin be administered only by clinicians thoroughly knowledgeable about the physiologic as well as clinical effects of the toxin. Familiarity with anatomy is necessary to ensure the proper and safe administration. Finally, it is a prudent clinical practice to inform patients and families about the alternative therapies, limited duration of benefit, possibility of poor or no response, potential complications, and lack of information as to the effects of long-term treatment with botulinum toxin.

Technical Considerations

Preparation prior to injection requires the following: toxin, standard freezer, saline without preservative, syringe with small-gauge needles, Teflon-coated needles, alcohol swabs, gauze, and in many circumstances, an EMG machine. Toxin is supplied by the manufacturer Allergan (Irvine, CA) and is marketed as Botox. A standard vial of Botox contains 100 units of toxin. Toxins are supplied in lyophilized form and must be stored in a freezer below $-5°$C and warmed to room temperature before use. The manufacturer recommends that once diluted, the solution should be stored in the refrigerator between $2°$ to $8°$C and used within 4 hours. Frozen lyophilized toxin is reconstituted with sterile nonpreserved saline to various concentrations, depending on the injection site. The dilution is influenced by the size of the muscles to be injected. For injection of extremity muscles in TBI patients, adding 1 or 2 mL of sodium chloride 0.9% to the lyophilized powder yields corresponding doses of 10 and 5 U/0.1 mL, respectively).

Few studies evaluating the effect of botulinum toxin type A on spasticity have been published. Snow et al. injected nine patients with multiple sclerosis in a randomized crossover study to reduce leg adductor spasticity.[122] They chose 400 mouse units as a standard dose, based on their previous experience. No patient developed side effects attributed to the toxin. The toxin produced a significant reduction in spasticity and improvement in nursing care. Lux et al.[85] reported a single case study using botulinum toxin type A to treat hamstring spasticity following a pontine hemorrhage. A total of 300 U was injected into multiple sites in three separate series of injections over 6 weeks. It produced both subjective and objective improvement.[85] In addition to lower limb spasticity, others have reported favorable results with injection of spastic elbow, wrist, and long-finger flexors. Therefore, the optimal dose of botulinum toxin type A to be injected is based on the extent to which the muscles appear to be involved on clinical or electromyographic grounds.

Our usual beginning dose of toxin is 20 to 40 U/elbow flexor, wrist flexor, and finger flexors (60 to 120 U/limb). Approximately 60 to 80 U/plantar flexor, and 100 U/adductor and knee flexor are given. This again depends on the size of the muscle and degree of electrophysiologic overactivity. Each patient builds his or her own portfolio of response to therapy.

A tuberculin syringe equipped with a 27-gauge 0.25 inch needle is used to carefully withdraw toxin from the vial. The toxin is denatured by bubbling or similar violent agitation. After withdrawing the toxin into the syringe, the needle is changed to a fresh 27-gauge 1.25-inch needle, which is not as painful as bigger-bore needles and is still able to reach some of the deep muscles of the leg and arm. Although each vial contains 100 U of toxin, it is usually impossible to withdraw the entire solution, so 90 U are typically harvested from the bottle. The surface area is prepared with alcohol swab before injections are made.

The number of injection sites for each muscle does not make a significant difference in the final outcome. For example, two sites are adequate for the sternocleidomastoid.[19] However, for large muscles, such as the biceps femoris, we use several sites. Pain at the local injection site may be seen but is never serious. Increased spasms are occasionally noted.

For treatment of deep muscles not readily palpable, Teflon-coated injection EMG needles connected to an EMG machine via an alligator clip attached to the hub of the needle is recommended. The appropriate muscle is identified by hearing the muscle interference pattern on EMG. Once the muscle is identified, the syringe barrel is withdrawn slightly to insure that a vessel has not been impaled, and then the toxin is slowly injected. The average latency between the injection and the onset of effect is 1 week, and the average duration of maximal improvement is 3 months.[61,129] One exception may be laryngeal injections, which are usually effective within 12 to 24 hours.

Conclusions

Botulinum toxin represents a new approach for the treatment of hypertonicity following TBI. Patient acceptance of this form of therapy so far has been high. Compared to alternative methods of therapy, including systemic medications and phenol neurolysis, treatment with botulinum toxin type A may be preferred. The toxin is easily administered and is not associated with adverse effects other than temporary weakness. Improvements in its application for hypertonicity following TBI may be expected as more experience is gained.

REFERENCES

1. Adams JH, Brierley JB, Connor RCR, Triep CS: The effects of systemic hypotension on the human brain. Brain 89:235–268, 1966.
2. Adams JH, Doyle D, Graham DI, et al: Deep intracerebral haematomas in fatal nonmissile head injury in man. J Neurol Neurosurg Psychiatry 49:1039–1043, 1986.
3. Adams JH, Graham DI, Murray LS, et al: Diffuse axonal injury due to nonmissile head injury in humans: An analysis of 45 cases. Ann Neurol 12:557–563, 1982.
4. Adams RD, Victor M: Principles of Neurology. New York, McGraw-Hill, 1989, p 62.
5. Alexander MP: Traumatic brain injury. In Benson DF, Blumer D (eds): Psychiatric Aspectts of Neurologic Disease, vol 2. New York, Grune and Stratton, 1982, pp 219–249.
6. American Academy of Neurology Therapeutics and Technology Assessment Subcommittee: Assessment: The clinical usefulness of botulinum toxin-A in treating neurologic disorders. Neurology 40:1332–1336, 1990.
7. Apolinario E, Pominelli JC, Fernandez M, Sotelano F: Follow-up of a series of phenol spinal blocks. Paraplegia 4:162–164, 1966.
8. Auerbach SH: Neuroanatomical correlates of attention and memory disorders in traumatic brain injury: An application of neurobehavioral subtypes. J Head Trauma Rehabil 1:1–12, 1986.

9. Awad EA: Phenol block for control of hip flexor and adductor spasticity. Arch Phys Med Rehabil 53:554–557, 1972.
10. Binet A: Valeur de la sympathectomie chemique en gynecologie. Gynecol Obstet 27:393–415, 1933.
11. Bond MR, Brooks DN: Understanding the process of recovery as a basis for the investigation of rehabilitation for the brain injured. Scand J Rehabil Med 8:127–133, 1976.
12. Botte MJ, Keenan MAE: Percutaneous phenol blocks of the pectoralis major muscle to treat spastic deformities. J Hand Surg 13:147–149, 1988.
13. Brattstrom M, Moritz U, Svantesson G: Electromyographic studies of peripheral nerve block with phenol. Scand J Rehabil Med 2:17–22. 1970.
14. Braun RM, Hoffer MM, Mooney V, et al: Phenol nerve block in the treatment of acquired spastic hemiplegia in the upper limb. J Bone Joint Surg 55:580–585, 1973.
15. Brink JD, Imbus C, Woo-Sam J: Physical recovery after severe closed head trauma in children and adolescents. J Pediatr 97:721–727, 1980.
16. Brooks N, Campsie L, Symington C, et al: The five year outcome of severe blunt head injury: A relative's view. J Neurol Neurosurg Psychiatry 49:764–770, 1986.
17. Cain HD, Glass A, Spiegler J, et al: Peripheral nerve and motor point phenol blocks for spasticity. Paraplegia 4:166–167, 1966.
18. Cameron MM: Chronic subdural haematoma: A review of 114 cases. J Neurol Neurosurg Psychiatry 41:834–839, 1978.
19. Comella CL, Buchman AS, Tanner CM, et al: Botulinum toxin injection for spasmodic torticollis: Increased magnitude of benefit with electromyographic assistance. Neurology 42:878–882, 1992.
20. Cooper IS, Hirose T, Matsuoka S, et al: Specific neurotoxin perfusion: A new approach to selected cases of pain and spasticity. Neurology 15:985–993, 1965.
21. Cooper KR: Respiratory complications in patients with serious head injuries. In Becker DP, Gudeman SK (eds): Textbook of Head Injuries. Philadelphia, WB Saunders, 1989, pp 255–277.
22. Copp EP, Keenan J: Phenol nerve and motor point block in spasticity. Rheumatol Phys Med 11:287–292, 1972.
23. Courville CB: Essentials of neuropathology. A brief account of the more common lesions of the nervous system, the mechanism of their formation and the course of their development. Los Angeles, San Lucas Press, 1953, p 144.
24. Dam M: Side effects of drug therapy in epilepsy. Acta Neurol Scand 78(suppl 11F):34–40, 1988.
25. Das TK, Park DM: Effect of treatment with botulinum toxin on spasticity. Postgrad Med J 65:208–210, 1989.
26. Deichmann WB, Keplinger ML: Phenols and phenolic compounds. In Patty FA (ed): Industrial Hygiene and Toxicology. New York, Interscience Publishers, 1963, pp 1363–1375.
27. Dezfulian M, Bartlett JG: Detection of clostridium botulinum type A toxin by enzyme-linked immunosorbent assay with antibodies produced in immunologically tolerant animals. J Clin Microbiol 19:645–648, 1984.
28. Doppler K: Die sympathikodiaphtherese (chemische sympathikusausschaltung) an der anteria femoralis. Med Klin 22:1954–1956, 1926.
29. Dubovsky SL, Ringel SP: Psychopharmacologic treatment in neurological practice. J Neuro Rehab 2:51–66, 1987.
30. Dykstra DD, Sidi A: Treatment of detrusor-sphinctor dyssynergia with botulinum A toxin: A double blind study. Arch Phys Med Rehabil 71:24–26, 1990.
31. Dykstra DD, Sidi A, Scott AB, et al: Effects of botulinum A toxin on detrusor-sphinctor dyssynergia in spinal cord injury patients. J Urol 139:912–922, 1988.
32. Erb DE, Povlishock JT: Axonal damage in severe traumatic brain damage: An experimental study in cat. Acta Neuropathol (Berl) 76:347–358, 1988.
33. Esplin DW: Phenols, cresols, and resorcinols. In Gilman AG, Rall TW, Nies AS, Taylor P (eds): The Pharmacological Basis of Therapeutics. New York, McMillan, 1970, pp 1035–1038.
34. Fahn S: Concept and classification of dystonia. Adv Neurol 50:1–7, 1988.
35. Felsenthal G: Pharmacology of phenol in peripheral nerve blocks: A review. Arch Phys Med Rehabil 55:13–15, 1974.
36. Fusfeld RD: Electromyographic findings after phenol block. Arch Phys Med Rehabil 49:217–220, 1968.
37. Garland DE, Lilling M, Keenan MAE: Percutaneous phenol blocks to motor points of spastic forearm muscles in head-injured adults. Arch Phys Med Rehabil 65:243–245, 1984.
38. Garland DE, Lucie SR, Waters RL: Current uses of open phenol nerve block for adult acquired spasticity. Clin Orthop 165:217–222, 1982.

39. Garland DE, Rhoades M: Orthopedic management of brain injured adults. Clin Orthop 131:111, 1978.

40. Gennarelli TA, Thibault LE, Adams JH, et al: Diffuse axonal injury and traumatic coma in the primate. Ann Neurol 12:564–574, 1982.

41. Glass A, Cain HD, Liebgold H, Mead S: Electromyographic and evoked potential responses after phenol blocks of peripheral nerves. Arch Phys Med Rehabil 49:455–459, 1968.

42. Glenn MB: Nerve blocks. In Glenn MB, Whyte J (eds): The Practical Management of Spasticity in Children and Adults. Philadelphia, Lea and Febiger, 1990, pp 227–258.

43. Graham DI, Adams JH: Ischaemic brain damage in fatal head injuries. Lancet i:265–266, 1971.

44. Graham DI, Ford I, Adams JH, et al: Ischaemic brain damage is still common in fatal non-missile head injury. J Neurol Neurosurg Psychiatry 52:346–350, 1989.

45. Graham DI, Lawrence AE, Adams JH, et al: Brain damage in non-missile head injury secondary to high intracranial pressure. Neuropathol Appl Neurobiol 13:209–217, 1987.

46. Gudeman SK, Kishore KS, Becker DP, et al: Computed tomography in the evaluation of incidence and significance of post-traumatic hydrocephalus. Radiology 141:397–402, 1981.

47. Habermann E: 125 I-labeled botulinum neurotoxin from clostridium botulinum A: Preparation, binding to synaptosomes and ascent to the spinal cord. Naunyn Schmeidebergs Arch Pharmacol 281:47–56, 1974.

48. Hallan RI, Williams NS, Melling J: Treatment of anismus in intractable constipation with botulinum A toxin. Lancet ii:714–717, 1988.

49. Halpern D, Meelhuysen FE: Phenol motor point block in the management of muscular hypertonia. Arch Phys Med Rehabil 47:659–664, 1966.

50. Hambelton P, Shone CC, Melling J: Botulinum toxin—Structure, action and clinical uses. In Jenner P (ed): Neurotoxins and Their Pharmacological Implications. New York, Raven Press, 1987, pp 233–260.

51. Hatheway CH, Snyder JD, Seals JE, et al: Antitoxin levels in botulism patients treated with trivalent equine botulism antitoxin to toxin types A, B, and E. J Infect Dis 150:407–412, 1984.

52. Hecht JS: Subscapular nerve block in the painful hemiplegic shoulder. Arch Phys Med Rehabil 73:1036–1039, 1992.

53. Heiden JS, Small R, Caton W, et al: Severe head injury and outcome: A prospective study. In Popp AJ (ed): Neural Trauma. New York, Raven Press, 1979, pp 181–193.

54. Henderson VW: Outcome prediction after severe closed head injury in adults. Bull Clin Neurosci 52:47–63, 1987.

55. Holbourn AHS: Mechanisms of brain injuries. Lancet ii:438–441, 1943.

56. Hufschmidt A, Mauritz KH: Chronic transformation of muscle in spasticity: Peripheral contribution to increased tone. J Neurol Neurosurg Psychiatry 48:676–685, 1985.

57. Hughes-Davies DI, Rechman LR: Clinical lumbar sympathectomy. Anesthesia 31:1068, 1970.

58. Iggo A, Walsh EG: Selective block of small fibers in the spinal roots by phenol. J Physiol 146:701–708, 1959.

59. Jackson MD, Davidoff G: Gastroparesis following traumatic brain injury and response to metoclopramide therapy. Arch Phys Med Rehabil 70:553–555, 1989.

60. Jankovic J, Brin MF: Therapeutic uses of botulinum toxin. N Engl J Med 324:1186–1194, 1991.

61. Jankovic J, Schwartz KS: Clinical correlates of response to botulinum toxin injections. Arch Neurol 48:1253–1256, 1991.

62. Jellinger K, Seitelberger F: Protracted post-traumatic encephalopathy. Pathology, pathogenesis and clinical implications. J Neurol Sci 10:51–94, 1970.

63. Jennett B, Teasdale G: Management of head injuries in the acute state: Circulation management of head injuries. Philadelphia, FA Davis, 1981, pp 228–229.

64. Kasdon DL, Abramovitz JN: Neurosurgical approaches. In Glenn MB, Whyte J (eds): The Practical Management of Spasticity in Children and Adults. Philadelphia, Lea and Febiger, 1990, pp 259–267.

65. Katz DI, Alexander MP, Seliger GM, Bellas DN: Traumatic basal ganglia hemorrhage: Clinicopathologic features and outcome. Neurology 39:897–904, 1989.

66. Katz J, Knott LW, Feldman DJ: Peripheral nerve injections with phenol in the management of spastic patients. Arch Phys Med Rehabil 48:97–99, 1967.

67. Keane JR, Itabashi HH: Locked-in syndrome due to tentorial herniation. Neurology 35:1647, 1985.

68. Keenan MAE: The orthopedic management of spasticity. J Head Trauma Rehabil 2:62–67, 1987.

69. Kelly RE, Gautier-Smith PC: Intrathecal phenol in the treatment of reflex spasms and spasticity. Lancet ii:1102–1105, 1959.

70. Khalili AA, Benton JG: A physiologic approach to the evaluation and the management of spasticity with procaine and phenol nerve block: Including a review of the physiology of the stretch reflex. Clin Orthop 47:97–104, 1966.

71. Khalili AA, Betts HB: Peripheral nerve block with phenol in the management of spasticity. JAMA 200:1155–1165, 1967.

72. Khalili AA, Harmel MH, Forster S, Benton JG: Management of spasticity by selective peripheral nerve block with dilute phenol solutions in clinical rehabilitation. Arch Phys Med Rehabil 45:513–519, 1964.

73. Koppang K: Intrathecal phenol in the treatment of spastic conditions. Acta Neurol Scand (suppl 3):63–68, 1962.

74. Koyama H, et al: Phenol block for hip flexor muscle spasticity under ultrasonic monitoring. Arch Phys Med Rehabil 73:1040–1043, 1992.

75. Kraus JK, Black MA, Hessol N, et al: The incidence of acute brain injury and serious impairment in a defined population. Am J Epidemiol 119:186–201, 1984.

76. Lance JW: Symposium synopsis. In Feldman RG, Young RR, Koella WP (eds): Spasticity: Disordered Motor Control. Chicago, YearBook Publishers, 1980, pp 485–494.

77. Lange DJ, Brin MF, Fahn S, Lovelace RE: Distant effects of locally injected botulinum toxin: Incidence and course. Adv Neurol 50:609–613, 1988.

78. Levin HS, Benton AL, Grossman RG: Neurobehavioral Consequences of Closed Head Injury. New York, Oxford Press, 1982, pp 123–139.

79. Levin HS, Meyers CA, Grossman RG, et al: Ventricular enlargement after closed head injury. Arch Neurol 38:623–629, 1981.

80. Levin HS, Williams D, Crofford MJ, et al: Relationship of depth of brain lesions to consciousness and outcome after closed head injury. J Neurosurg 69:861–866, 1988.

81. Lister J: On a new method of treating compound fractures, abscesses, etc. Lancet i:326–329, 1967.

82. Liversedge LA, Maher RM: Use of phenol in relief of spasticity. BMJ 2:31–33, 1960.

83. Lourie H, Vanasupa P: Comments on the use of intra-spinal phenol-pantopaque for relief of pain and spasticity. J Neurosurg 20:60–63, 1963.

84. Ludlow CL, Hallett M, et al: Therapeutic use of type F botulinum toxin [letter]. N Engl J Med 326:350–351, 1992.

85. Lux WE, Rome S, McCarthy AD: Use of botulinum toxin in the treatment of spasticity in large muscles [abstract]. Arch Phys Med Rehabil 73(suppl):1008, 1992.

86. Macek K: Medical news: Venous thrombosis results from some phenol injections. JAMA 249:1807, 1983.

87. MacPherson P, Graham DI: Arterial spasm and slowing of the cerebral circulation in the ischaemia of head injury. J Neurol Neurosurg Psychiatry 36:1069–1072, 1973.

88. Maher NH, Griffith ER: Hypertonicity and movement disorders. In Rosenthal M, Griffith ER, Bond MR, Miller JD (eds): Rehabilitation of the Adult and Child with Traumatic Brain Injury. Philadelphia, FA Davis, 1980, pp 127–147.

89. Maher RM: Relief of pain in incurable cancer. Lancet i:18–20, 1955.

90. Meelhuysen FE, Halpern D, Quast J: Treatment of flexor spasticity by paravertebral lumbar spinal nerve block. Arch Phys Med Rehabil 49:717–722, 1968.

91. Miller JD: Pathophysiology of human head injury. In Becker DP, Gudeman SK (eds): Textbook of Head Injuries. Philadelphia, WB Saunders, 1989, pp 507–524.

92. Miller JD, Becker DP, Ward JD, et al: Significance of intracranial hypertension in severe head injury. J Neurosurg 47:503–516, 1977.

93. Miller JD, Butterworth JF, Gudeman SK, et al: Further experience in the management of severe head injury. J Neurosurg 54:289–299, 1981.

94. Mooney V, Frykman G, McLamb J: Current status of intraneural phenol injections. Clin Orthop 63:122–131, 1969.

95. Morrison JE, Matthews D, Washington R, et al: Phenol motor point blocks in children: Plasma concentrations and cardiac dysrhythmias. Anesthesiology 75:359–362, 1992.

96. Muizelaar JP: Cerebral blood flow, cerebral blood volume, and cerebral metabolism after severe head injury. In Becker DP, Gudeman SK (eds): Textbook of Head Injuries. Philadelphia, WB Saunders, 1989, pp 221–240.

97. Nathan PW: Intrathecal phenol to relieve spasticity in paraplegia. Lancet ii: 1099–1102, 1959.

98. Nathan PW, Sears TA, Smith MC: Effects of phenol solutions on the nerve roots of the cat: An electrophysiological and histological study. J Neurol Sci 2:7–29, 1965.

99. O'Shanick GJ: Emergency psychopharmacology. Am J Emerg Med 2:164–170, 1984.

100. Pacult A, Gudeman SK: Medical management of head injuries. In Becker DP, Gudeman SK (eds): Textbook of Head Injuries. Philadelphia, WB Saunders, 1989, pp 195–198.

101. Pederson E, Juul-Jenson P: Intrathecal phenol in the treatment of spasticity. Acta Neurol Scand 38(suppl 3):69–77, 1962.
102. Penn RD: Intrathecal baclofen for severe spinal spasticity. N Engl J Med 320:1517–1521, 1989.
103. Prigatano G, Altman IM, O'Brien KP: Behavioral limitations that brain injured patients tend to underestimate. Clin Neuropsychol 163–176, 1990.
104. Putnam TJ, Hampton AO: A technique of injection into the gasserian ganglion under roentgenographic control. Arch Neurol Psychiatr 35:92–98, 1936.
105. Quinn N, Hallet M: Dose standardization of botulinum toxin. Lancet i:964, 1989.
106. Reid W, Watt JK, Gray TG: Phenol injection of the sympathetic chain. Br J Surg 57:45–50, 1970.
107. Roper B: Evaluation of spasticity. Hand 7:11–14, 1975.
108. Rosenblum WI: Pathology of human head injury. In Becker DP, Gudeman SK (eds): Textbook of Head Injuries. Philadelphia, WB Saunders, 1989, pp 525–537.
109. Rosenblum WI, Greenberg RP, Seelig JM, Becker DP: Midbrain lesions: Frequent and significant prognostic feature in closed head injury. Neurosurgery 9:613–620, 1981.
110. Sande MA, Mandell GL: Antimicrobial agents: The aminoglycosides. In Gilman AG, Rall TW, Nies AS, Taylor P (eds): The Pharmacological Basis of Therapeutics. New York, MacMillan, 1990, pp 1098–1116.
111. Sanders DB, Massey EW, Buckley EG: Botulinum toxin for blepharospasm: Single-fiber EMG studies. Neurology 36:545–547, 1986.
112. Schantz EJ, Johnson EA: Dose standardization of botulinum toxin. Lancet 335:421, 1990.
113. Schantz EJ, Kautter DA: Standardized assay for clostridium botulinum toxins. J Assoc Anal Chem 61:96–99, 1978.
114. Schaumburger HN, Byck R, Weller RO: The effect of phenol on peripheral nerve. A histologic and electrophysiologic study. J Neuropathol Exp Neurol 29:615–630, 1970.
115. Scott AB: Botulinum toxin injection into extraocular muscles as an alternative to strabismus surgery. Ophthalmology 87:1044–1049, 1980.
116. Scott AB, Suzuki D: Systemic toxicity of botulinum toxin by intramuscular injection in the monkey. Mov Disord 3:333–335, 1988.
117. Scott BA, Weinstein ZRW: The neurosurgical management of spasticity. S Afr Med J 60:849–850, 1981.
118. Scott BA, Weinstein ZRW, Chiteman R, Pulliam MW: Intrathecal phenol and glycerin in metrizamide for treatment of intractable spasms in paraplegia. J Neurosurg 63:125–127, 1985.
119. Seliger GM, Katz DI, Seliger M, Ditullio M: Late improvement in closed head injury with a low-pressure valve shunt. Brain Inj 6:71–73, 1992.
120. Simpson LL: The origin, structure, and pharmacologic activity of botulinum toxin. Pharmacol Rev 33:155–188, 1981.
121. Smith MC: Histological findings following intrathecal injections of phenol solutions for the relief of pain. Br J Anaesth 36:387, 1964.
122. Snow BJ, Tsui JKC, Bhatt MH, et al: Treatment of spasticity with botulinum toxin: A double-blind study. Ann Neurol 28:512–515, 1990.
123. Sorenson PS, Jansen EC, Gjerras F: Motor disturbance in normal-pressure hydrocephalus: Special reference to stance and gait. Arch Neurol 43:34–38, 1986.
124. Stewart WA, Lourie H: An experimental evaluation of the effects of subarachnoid injection of phenol-pantopaque in cats. J Neurosurg 20:64–72, 1963.
125. Sunderland S: Nerves and Nerve Injuries. Baltimore, Williams & Wilkins, 1978.
126. Suvansa S: Treatment of tetanus by intrathecal injection of carbolic acid. Lancet i:1075–1078, 1981.
127. Sweet WH: The treatment of trigeminal neuralgia (tic douloureux). N Engl J Med 315:174, 1986.
128. Tardieu G, Hariga J: Traitement des raideurs musculaires d'orgine cerebrale par infiltration d'alcohol dilue. Arch Fr Pediatr 21:25–41, 1964.
129. Van Ermengen E: Euber einen never anaeroben bacillus und seine beziehunger zum botulismus. Z Hyg infektionskrankn 26:1–56, 1987. English translation, Rev Infect Dis 1:701–719, 1978.
130. Weigard H, Wellhoner HH: Type A botulinus toxin in cats: Neural ascent and action on spinal cord reflexes. Naunyn Schmiedebergs Arch Pharmacol 282:R106, 1974.
131. Whyte J, Robinson KM: Pharmacologic management. In Glenn MB, Whyte J (eds): The Practical Management of Spasticity in Children and Adults. Philadelphia, Lea and Febiger, 1990, pp 201–226.

132. Williams RS, Tse C-K, Dolly JO, et al: Radioiodination of botulinum neurotoxin type A with retention of biologic activity and its binding to brain synaptosomes. Eur J Biochem 131:437–445, 1983.
133. Wood KM: The use of phenol as a neurolytic agent: A review. Pain 5:205–229, 1978.
134. Yoshimura DM, Aminoff MJ, Olney RK: Botulinum toxin therapy for limb dystonias. Neurology 42:627–630, 1992.
135. Zierski J, Miller H, Dralle D, Wurdlinger T: Implanted pump system for treatment of spasticity. Acta Neurochir Suppl (Wien) 43:94–99, 1988.

SUSAN J. HERDMAN, PhD, PT
JANET O. HELMINSKI, MS, PT

VESTIBULAR DEFICITS IN THE HEAD-INJURED PATIENT

From the
Department of Otolaryngology–
  Head and Neck Surgery
Johns Hopkins University
Baltimore, Maryland (SJH)
  and
Institute for Neuroscience
Northwestern University
Chicago, Illinois (JOH)

Correspondence to:
Susan J. Herdman, PhD
Department of Otolaryngology–
  Head and Neck Surgery
P.O. Box 41402
Baltimore, MD 21203-6402

Vestibular dysfunction is a common sequelae of closed-head trauma; up to 78% of patients complain of vertigo during the acute stage and 20% still have symptoms 6 months after their injury.[20] Head trauma can result in a fracture of the petrous bone, affecting the bony and membranous labyrinth or the internal auditory canal, which houses the vestibular, auditory, and facial nerves; in microvascular changes, affecting the eighth nerve or the hair cells in the labyrinth; or in damage to central vestibular pathways.[9,11,19,20] Patients with head trauma, therefore, can present with multiple vestibular deficits, including unilateral or bilateral vestibular loss, postconcussional Meniere's disease, benign paroxysmal positional vertigo (BPPV), perilymphatic fistula, or central vertigo.

There often is a delay before vestibular deficits are recognized in the head trauma patient. Immediately after a head injury, patients often have life-threatening injuries that must be treated before vestibular studies can be performed. Furthermore, some vestibular lesions do not result in complaints of vertigo, an illusionary sense that the world is turning or tilting, which would typically be associated with a vestibular deficit. Patients may instead report a sense of being off balance. Because disequilibrium can occur from many nonvestibular causes, vestibular deficits can be overlooked. Disequilibrium, however, is the primary complaint in patients with bilateral vestibular deficits or in patients in the chronic stage following unilateral vestibular lesions.

Because many patients with head trauma also have central nervous system (CNS) deficits, the diagnosis of a vestibular problem can be very difficult. CNS lesions and multiple medications can make the patient feel dizzy without an underlying vestibular lesion. A careful clinical examination and vestibular function testing are usually needed to identify the type and extent of vestibular deficit. This assessment may have to be deferred or modified if the patient has cognitive problems or is agitated and confused. Given the high incidence of vestibular injury, it is important to assess the vestibular system in patients with complaints of vertigo or disequilibrium.

BENIGN PAROXYSMAL POSITIONAL VERTIGO

Probably the most common vestibular disorder following head trauma is BPPV. Patients with BPPV complain of brief spells of vertigo associated with lying down, rolling over, or gazing upward. This disorder is believed to be due to debris, probably fragments of otoconia, which either adhere to the cupula of the posterior semicircular canal or are floating in the endolymph of the posterior canal.[3,8,16] When the patient moves into certain positions, the debris causes an inappropriate response from the posterior canal, which results in vertigo and nystagmus. The nystagmus and vertigo last only a brief time, usually less than 60 seconds.[1] Pharmacologic treatment does not help except to relieve the nausea these patients may experience. BPPV can occur immediately, within a few days, or even several weeks after the injury. In most patients, BPPV resolves spontaneously within 6 to 8 weeks. In patients in whom the disorder does not resolve, specific physical therapy exercises are the treatment of choice.[10] Two single-treatment approaches have been used successfully in the management of patients with BPPV.[4,10,17]

In the Semont maneuver, the patient is first rapidly moved into a side-lying position with the affected ear undermost.[10] The patient is maintained in that position for 4 minutes and then is rapidly moved into the opposite side-lying position, with the head in the same orientation on the body. Most patients experience a brief period of vertigo in this second position. If the patient does not complain of vertigo, the head is abruptly "jostled" through a small range of motion, with the goal of dislodging the debris in the posterior canal. The patient is maintained in the second position for 4 minutes and then gradually sits up. For the next 48 hours, the patient cannot lie down, roll over, or look up or down with the head. For 5 days afterward, the patient should avoid lying on the affected side.

In the second approach, based on a treatment developed by Epley,[4] the patient is moved first into the Hallpike position with the affected ear down.[4] After 3 minutes, the patient's head is moved into extension and turned to the opposite Hallpike position. The patient then rolls onto his shoulder, and the head is turned further so that the nose is pointed down. After 3 minutes, the patient slowly sits up. The post-treatment protocol is the same as that described for the Semont maneuver. These maneuvers are 70 to 85% successful after only one treatment.[4,10,15,17] The following case study illustrates the management of a brain-injured patient with BPPV who was untreated for several years after her original injury.

CASE REPORT

The patient, a 49-year-old woman, was in a motor vehicle accident 2 years prior to vestibular evaluation. She was admitted through the emergency room with a severe closed-head injury and a perforated transverse colon. Some time during the acute period following her injury, she had had a respiratory arrest and developed anoxic encephalopathy. She was comatose for 2 months and in a confusional state for an additional 3 months. As her awareness returned, she complained of episodic vertigo, diplopia, and disequilibrium. Her diagnosis at that time included traumatic and anoxic encephalopathy, left third-nerve palsy, right hemiataxia and numbness, and vertigo and disequilibrium. She was transferred to a rehabilitation center for intensive therapy and at the time of her discharge, she was walking independently. It was recommended that she use a cane; however, she preferred not to and relied instead on occasionally steadying herself on furniture, walls, and her husband. She was independent in all self-care activities.

Two years after the accident, she was referred to the neurology department for evaluation of her vertigo. She had no further history of trauma, exposure to ototoxic medication, or surgery to ears, eyes, or head. There was no history of cardiovascular disease or diabetic or thyroid disorders.

Her primary complaint was vertigo lasting less than 60 seconds that occurred whenever she would lie down or if she stood quickly. She described her dizziness as very intense and stated that it interfered with her daily activities. For example, she had difficulty transferring in and out of bed. She also complained of gait imbalance and stiffness and numbness in her right upper and lower extremities.

Previous Diagnostic Test Results. Normal results were obtained on magnetic resonance imaging of head, without gadolinium. Although posterior fossa views were taken, the eighth cranial nerve was not visualized. Normal results were obtained on electroencephalography and auditory brainstem evoked responses. Electronystagmography revealed an up-beating nystagmus when the patient was supine or in the left lateral position. Caloric responses were normal.

Neurologic Examination. On mental status evaluation, impaired memory, attention, and calculation ability were noted. Her right pupil was 4 mm and reactive to light; her left pupil was 6 mm and nonreactive. There was full extraocular right eye movement. The left fourth and sixth cranial nerves were normal, but she had a complete left third-nerve palsy. This resulted in torsional eye movements of the left eye when she looked down to the left. Normal results were obtained for eye grounds, optic nerve head, and venous pulsations. Full visual fields were revealed by confrontation testing, with no visual extinction. Visual acuity was 10/15-1 in the right eye and 20/60-1 in the left (corrected) when her head was stationary, and was 20/25-1 in both eyes during gentle oscillations of her head (2 Hz). The gain of vestibulo-ocular reflex (VOR) appeared to be normal based on the visualization on the optic nerve head during head movement and in her ability to maintain gaze stability during rapid head thrusts. She had normal smooth pursuit, saccades, and VOR cancellation (taking the third-nerve palsy into consideration). There was no spontaneous nystagmus, no tragal pressure–induced or Valsalva maneuver–induced nystagmus and no head shaking–induced nystagmus as determined by the use of Frenzel lenses.

When the patient was moved into the right Hallpike position, she developed a torsional and up-beating nystagmus, with the fast phases counterclockwise, after a latency of 5 seconds. Concurrent with the appearance of the nystagmus, she complained of severe vertigo. The nystagmus and vertigo lasted for 20 seconds. As the torsional nystagmus resolved, a sustained right-beating nystagmus appeared. Hearing was normal as well as the results of the remainder of her cranial nerve exam.

Motor Examination. Increased tone in right upper and lower extremities during passive muscle stretch was noted. She had hyperactive deep tendon reflexes on the left and bilateral up-going toes. There was normal strength in all four extremities. Normal sensory threshold to vibration in feet was also noted. The patient had normal upper extremity coordination and ataxic heel to shin on the left side. She could toe-and-heel walk. She had increased sway during the Romberg test with her eyes closed but did not lose her balance. She could not perform the tandem Romberg with her eyes closed; with her eyes open, the test result was normal. Her gait was slow when she was tandem walking.

Other Assessments. Electro-oculography was performed (measuring right eye only because of the left third-nerve palsy), and it revealed (1) normal saccade latency, amplitude, and velocity; (2) normal smooth pursuit and optokinetic nystagmus to the right and left; (3) normal VOR gain and time constant for 60-second rotations to right and left; and (4) no significant directional preponderance of the vestibular response.

Dynamic posturography was also performed. It revealed an inability to maintain balance when both visual and somatosensory cues were absent or inappropriate. This may indicate a decreased ability to use vestibular cues for balance, although patients with balance problems from other disorders may also have difficulty on these tests. Posturography also revealed delayed long-latency responses bilaterally, as measured by surface-electrode electromyography. Delays in the long-latency responses occur when there is damage to the supraspinal pathways.

Comments.   The appearance of a torsional and up-beating nystagmus, with concurrent complaints of vertigo, when the patient was moved into the right Hallpike position is consistent with BPPV involving the right posterior canal. There was a brief latency before the onset of the nystagmus, and the duration of the nystagmus and vertigo was less than 60 seconds. BPPV is common following head trauma but must be distinguished from other forms of positional vertigo, such as central positional vertigo, cervical vertigo, and vertigo from perilymphatic fistula.[2,6,7,13,18] In this patient, the appearance of the nystagmus of BPPV is confounded by the presence of a geotropic nystagmus and her third-nerve palsy, both also due to her head trauma.

Central positional vertigo is characterized by vertigo, which begins as soon as the patient is moved into the provoking position. Unlike BPPV, however, central vertigo persists as long as the patient stays in that position. Furthermore, the nystagmus that occurs with central vertigo often does not have the torsional component that is typical of BPPV. Cervical vertigo occurs with extension of the neck rather than with movement of the head into a position that places the posterior canal in the plane of gravity. Presumably, cervical vertigo is due to abnormal inputs from the joint and muscle receptors of the neck.[2] Perilymphatic fistula, an abnormal communication between the inner and middle ears, is also common after head trauma and can closely resemble BPPV. It is often difficult to diagnose perilymphatic fistula, and the final diagnosis often cannot be confirmed until surgical exploration of the middle ear is performed. This patient, however, had no nystagmus triggered by tragal pressure or by Valsalva maneuver, and she had normal hearing. The patient's balance problems could be related to the BPPV but probably were secondary to her cerebellar and brainstem injuries.

There was no evidence for vestibular hypofunction because her vestibular-ocular reflex gain was normal both clinically and with quantitative testing, and her VOR time constant was normal. In patients with unilateral vestibular deficits, both VOR gain and the time constant are decreased during the acute stage of the injury. VOR gain will improve with time (and adaptation) but VOR time constant will not change significantly.

Treatment.   The patient was referred to physical therapy for treatment of her right BPPV, which consisted of the Semont maneuver, a single-treatment approach that theoretically can be effective whether the debris is adherent to the cupula or free-floating in the long arm of the posterior canal. This patient tolerated the treatment well. When she was reassessed several weeks later, she had no vertigo when moved into the right Hallpike position and, with Frenzel lenses, there was no evidence of a torsional nystagmus. She still had complaints of balance problems when walking and was placed on a balance exercise program; however, no significant improvement occurred in her positional stability.

UNILATERAL VESTIBULAR LOSS

Unilateral and even bilateral vestibular hypofunction are less common than BPPV following closed-head trauma. The incidence increases dramatically in the presence of skull fractures. In head-injured patients without skull fracture, vestibular hypofunction occurs in 28% of the cases; if there is a skull fracture but not of temporal bone, the incidence increases to 50%; when the temporal bone is involved, the incidence has been reported to be as high as 87 to 100%.[19,20] The following case illustrates the diagnosis and treatment of an agitated patient with a unilateral vestibular deficit.

CASE REPORT

A 53-year-old man was found unconscious, lying on his basement floor at the foot of the steps, with blood running from the left ear and a left periorbital laceration and hematoma. Initially, he was responsive only to pain, pupils were equal and reactive, and vital signs were stable. On admission to the hospital, the patient was agitated. In the emergency room, he lapsed into coma, with a Glasgow coma score of 6. Blood alcohol level was found to be 0.132. Computed tomographic scanning revealed a left temporal lobe hematoma with multiple skull fractures, including the left occiput, left maxillary sinus, left lateral orbit, and left zygomatic arch. The patient underwent a left craniotomy and hematoma evacuation. He was hospitalized for 3 months and then was discharged to a rehabilitation center.

On admission to the rehabilitation center, he was independent in bed mobility, feeding, orofacial hygiene, bathing, and dressing, and he was continent. Because of his imbalance, he required supervision with transfers and ambulation on level surfaces and required minimal to moderate physical assistance with ambulation on uneven surfaces. The patient displayed moderate-to-severe cognitive and behavioral problems and could only function with structure or physical assistance. He was agitated, clinically depressed, and had no concept of time. His speech was verbose and confabulatory. He exhibited difficulty expressing his needs and had dysnomia. The patient understood simple sentences and could follow up to three-step commands. Due to his disorientation and confusional state, the patient was at high risk for elopement. Therefore, for patient safety, a 24-hour attendant supervised the patient, and he was not allowed to leave the premises. Hearing was found to be minimally reduced on the right and severely impaired on the left. His medications included carbamazepine, haloperidol, and midazolam.

Initially, the patient complained of blurred vision and decreased visual acuity. He expressed vague complaints of dizziness in environments with increased visual stimulation and with activities requiring changes in head position, such as moving from a standing position to the floor. A neuro-otology consultation was requested. Due to the patient's impaired cognition and behavior, specific vestibular function tests, such as rotary chair tests or the caloric test, could not be performed.

Visual examination revealed a pale, left optic disc. The patient had peripheral and nasal visual field cuts with left-eye viewing. No nystagmus was noted in room light, but the patient had a right-beating, spontaneous nystagmus noted with the patient wearing Frenzel glasses (magnifying glasses designed to enable the examiner to see the patient's eyes while preventing visual fixation by the patient). The patient was able to fixate on a stationary target during gentle horizontal and vertical oscillations of the head and during rapid head movements to the right. With rapid head movements toward the left, however, he was unable to keep his eyes on the target. The patient did not develop nystagmus or vertigo when moved into the right or left Hallpike position.

Comments. Unilateral vestibular deficits are characterized during the acute stage by spontaneous nystagmus in room light, a skew deviation, postural instability, and complaints of vertigo. These deficits reflect the asymmetry in the tonic firing rate of the vestibular system created by the unilateral lesion. Compensation is due to a rebalancing of the tonic firing rate of the vestibular system and to the use of visual fixation to suppress the nystagmus. The disturbances in the tonic vestibular function usually recover within 1 to 2 weeks after the injury. Persistence of the spontaneous nystagmus in room light or of the other symptoms would suggest the presence of a cerebellar lesion or a lesion of the vestibular nuclei. Disruption of the dynamic vestibular responses (those occurring in response to head movement) results in a decrease in the gain of the VOR and in a gait ataxia. Recovery of the dynamic vestibular responses requires both visual input and movement.[5,14]

This patient did not have a spontaneous nystagmus in room light, indicating that the static vestibular responses had compensated, but he did have a spontaneous, right-beating nystagmus when visual fixation was prevented. The direction of the fast phase of the nystagmus (to the right) is due to the imbalance in the vestibular system. The spontaneous discharge of the normal (right) side produces a slow-phase eye movement to the left with a quick corrective saccade to the right and is evidence of a left vestibular deficit. The gain of his vestibular response was decreased, as indicated by the fact that he could not maintain fixation during rapid head movements to the left. The findings of both of these clinical tests suggest that the patient had a unilateral peripheral vestibular deficit on the left.

Treatment. Physical therapy was initiated specifically for vestibular rehabilitation with the goals of decreasing the patient's disequilibrium and improving his gaze stability during head movements. The patient was instructed in exercises designed to increase the gain of his vestibular system through vestibular adaptation. These exercises were performed with the patient seated using a small (foveal) visual target (Table 1). Initially, he was able to perform the exercises in horizontal and vertical planes three times per day for only 15 seconds at a time. Movements were slow and deliberate. The patient required constant verbal cuing to attend to the task. The duration and progression of the exercises at any given session were based on level of agitation. With increased stimulation, an increase in his level of agitation was noted. His attendant was instructed in the exercises and supervised the exercise program on the nursing floor.

Assessment of his balance was performed through the use of the Balance Master (Neurocom International). The patient stood with feet together, arms folded across chest, and eyes open for 20 seconds on a firm force plate with 1.50% sway. With eyes closed, sway increased to 3.68%. The patient was unable to stand in tandem but was able to stand with single-limb support. Loss of balance was noted with quick pivot turns during ambulation. When the patient was ambulating with his eyes opened and when moving his head, he reduced the speed of movement, had a lateral deviation of approximately 2 feet, and occasionally lost his balance. The patient required contact guarding to minimal physical assistance for safety. The patient was started on a program of exercises to improve postural stability, including balance activities with reduced and conflicting sensory information and varied base of supports (Table 2).

Following 6 weeks of therapy, gaze-stabilization exercises had been progressed to standing with feet together with full visual field stimulation. The patient was able to perform exercises in horizontal and vertical planes three times per day for 2 minutes. Exercises were performed at moderate speed. Increased agitation was no longer noted with exercises. The patient was able to attend to the task without redirection. The attendant had been discontinued, and the family was instructed in a home exercise program.

TABLE 1. Gaze Stabilization Exercises

Goal
  Increase the gain of the central vestibular system.

Activity
  Fovea visual stimulation: Sit facing a plain wall, an arm's length away. Tape a business card or lettering to the wall at eye level. Continuously turn your head as quickly as possible 45° to the right and left, keeping the words in focus. Continue moving head 1–2 minutes as tolerated. Rest. Repeat moving your head 30° up and down.

Progression
  Visual stimulation:
    Fovea visual stimulation: Tape business card to plain wall.
    Full visual stimulation: Place business card in center of patterned background, e.g., a checkerboard, painting, or loud wallpaper.
  Postural Control: Perform activity while
    Sitting
    Standing
      On a firm surface
      On a conforming surface
      On a reduced base of support

TABLE 2.   Balance Exercises

Goals
   Substitution of one sense for another
     Vision for vestibular
     Somatosensory or proprioception for vestibular
   Enhancement or suppression of sensorimotor reflexes
     Vision
     Somatosensory

Activities
   Static activities: decrease base of support
     Feet together
     Semi-heel-toe
     Heel-toe
     Single limb support
   Dynamic activities
     Active weight shift
     Ambulation forward and backwards
     Ambulation with abrupt stops
     Ambulation with sharp-pivot turn
     Ambulation turning head right and left every third step
     Ambulation moving head up and down every third step
   Functional activities

Sensory Environments Activities Performed
   Visual
     Visual conditions
       Eyes opened
       Intermittent eyes opened and eyes closed
       Eyes closed
     Environment
       Room without clutter and plain walls
       Hallway
       Moving environment
   Somatosensory
     Somatosensory conditions
       On a firm surface
       On a conforming surface
         Carpet
         2-inch medium density Sunmate foam
         Grass
         Gravel
         Sand
       Uneven terrain
       Upper extremity tactile cues
         Touching surface
         Use of assistive device

A marked improvement in balance was noted. The patient was able to stand for 20 seconds with feet together, arms folded across chest, and eyes opened or closed on firm and conforming surfaces. A marked improvement in sway was noted. On the SMART Balance Master System (Neurocom International), the patient was able to stand on a firm platform with eyes opened with 0.17% sway and could stand on a firm surface with eyes closed with only 0.18% sway. The patient was able to stand in tandem for 60 seconds with eyes opened and 3 seconds with eyes closed. He was able to walk in tandem for 20 ft with standby assistance. The patient was able to ambulate 30 ft with eyes closed and standby assistance. The patient deviated 1 ft laterally toward the left, as compared with 2 ft initially. He ambulated with eyes opened while moving his head in horizontal and vertical planes with standby assistance. Only a minimal lateral deviation was noted, and the patient never lost his balance. The patient required standby assistance for quick pivot turns to the left. He ambulated on uneven surfaces with standby assistance. Community ambulation was not assessed because of the patient's high risk for elopement. He exhibited difficulty negotiating in crowded treatment areas. Therefore, he would probably have difficulty ambulating in settings with increased visual stimulation and variations in supporting surface.

CENTRAL LESIONS

Patients with central lesions affecting the vestibular system may have complaints of both vertigo and disequilibrium. The following case study illustrates a patient who had both a central and a peripheral vestibular deficit. As noted earlier, the treatment of this patient was more difficult, and the outcome was not as good as would be expected if the patient had only a peripheral vestibular deficit.

CASE REPORT

The patient was a 53-year-old who fell 18 ft, landing on his head. Although he was alert and oriented at the scene of the accident and denied any neurologic symptoms, he was taken to a trauma hospital for evaluation. The results of his examination were normal except for scalp lacerations and lower back abrasions and contusions. Radiographs were normal and laboratory test results were negative. The patient was admitted for observation and then discharged following normal results on a second neurologic examination.

Five days later, he was readmitted to the hospital with complaints of dizziness, blurred vision, diplopia, headache, vomiting, and ataxia. On examination, he had a sixth-nerve palsy and a gaze-evoked nystagmus. Electronystagmography showed right vestibular paresis. The patient was diagnosed as having a postconcussional syndrome and labyrinthitis. He was treated with meclizine hydrochloride.

Two years later, the patient was referred for reassessment of his dizziness and possible treatment. He had become less active, walked with a cane, and rarely left his home. He required help in self-care activities, such as bathing and dressing. The patient complained of vertigo and disequilibrium. Medications included amitriptyline hydrochloride, diazepam, and kaolin. He had increased his dose of both the amitriptyline hydrochloride and the diazepam in an attempt to decrease his vertigo.

At the time of his initial examination, he was lethargic, apathetic, and poorly attentive, with difficulty following simple commands. Rotary chair testing showed a normal VOR gain (0.5) but a decreased time constant (6.4 seconds). His saccadic eye movements were slow and hypometric. Smooth pursuit eye movements were poor, especially to the right. He had decreased optokinetic nystagmus. Caloric tests revealed a left vestibular paresis. Dynamic posturography showed that the patient had normal stability only when standing on a stable support surface with his eyes open. When he closed his eyes, he had increased anterior-posterior sway, and on all other test conditions (moving visual world, moving support surface, or altered visual and somatosensory cues) he lost his balance.

Comments. The results of the rotary chair test (decreased time constant) and of the caloric test indicated a unilateral vestibular deficit. Normal time constants are higher than 10 seconds. Unilateral lesions result in a decrease of the time constant to between 5 and 10 seconds, whereas bilateral vestibular lesions would result in a time constant of less than 5 seconds. The eye movement tests also showed abnormalities in saccadic and smooth pursuit eye movements and in optokinetic nystagmus. These findings could have been related to the medications he was taking or to the presence of a central lesion.

Most patients with peripheral vestibular lesions recover within 6 months after head injury.[20] This patient's continued difficulties may have been related to medications, to his relative level of inactivity, or to the presence of a central lesion affecting the structures involved in compensation. Medications intended to decrease the symptoms of vertigo and disequilibrium often act by suppressing the vestibular system and therefore may also delay or slow vestibular adaptation.[21] Vestibular adaptation is the ability of the vestibular system to make long-term changes in the response of the neurons to an input, that is, to change the gain of the vestibular response. Adaptation is one of the primary mechanisms for recovery following peripheral vestibular lesions. This patient had also self-limited his daily activities; from experience, movement made him dizzy; therefore, he stopped moving. He was also less active because of the sedation produced by the combination and dosages of his medications. Studies have shown that if movement is restricted, especially during the early period following a peripheral vestibular loss, the onset of recovery can be delayed, the recovery period may be prolonged, and the final level of recovery may be lessened.[12] This patient had attempted to decrease his symptoms by avoiding the movements that provoked them, but unfortunately, this strategy may also limit the final level of recovery. Finally, this patient may have a central lesion affecting the structures that are involved in recovery, such as the cerebellum or the vestibular nuclei. Abnormal saccadic and smooth pursuit eye movements may occur with lesions in the cerebellum, brainstem, or cerebral cortex.

Treatment. The initial treatment approach was to taper the patient's medications. He was able, ultimately, to discontinue taking the amitriptyline hydrochloride and diazepam and as a result became more alert and active. He was then started on a home program of exercises designed to induce adaptation of his vestibular system and to improve his postural stability. Studies on nonhuman primates support the notion that both visual input and movement are necessary for recovery following unilateral vestibular lesions.[5,12] Although these studies suggest that exercises might be more effective if given during the early stage after the vestibular loss, anecdotal evidence on human subjects suggests that the exercises can be beneficial even when started several years after the onset.

The patient continued to perform the exercises, which were modified to make them more challenging. After 6 months of training, he no longer used a cane while walking and had become more active. Posturography testing showed considerable improvement. The patient was able to maintain his balance under all conditions except when both visual and somatosensory cues were altered. He still had complaints of vertigo, however, and would lie down and nap during the day to avoid the sensation. Rotary chair testing was repeated after the medication withdrawal. The patient still had abnormal saccadic eye movements indicating that there was a central lesion. The presence of a CNS lesion perhaps explains why this patient had failed to fully recover from his unilateral, peripheral vestibular lesion.

CONCLUSIONS

Persistent complaints of vertigo or of disequilibrium often indicate involvement of the vestibular system in patients with closed-head injury. Formal vestibular function studies and a clinical examination should be performed to identify the underlying cause of these complaints. Some vestibular problems, such as BPPV, do not respond to medication but can be easily treated with simple exercises in most patients. Unilateral and even bilateral vestibular paresis or paralysis are also common, frequently associated with fractures through the labyrinth. The recovery from these deficits is often quite good, but the final level of recovery is dependent on whether there is a central lesion affecting the structures involved in compensation.

REFERENCES

1. Baloh RW, Honrubia V, Jacobson K: Benign positional vertigo: Clinical and oculographic features in 240 cases. Neurology 37:371–378, 1987.
2. de Jong JMBV, Bles W: Cervical dizziness and ataxia. In Bles W, Brandt T (eds): Disorders of Posture and Gait. Amsterdam, Elsevier, 1986.
3. Epley JM: New dimensions of benign paroxysmal positional vertigo. Otolaryngol Head Neck Surg 88:599–605, 1980.
4. Epley JM: The canalith repositioning procedure: For treatment of benign paroxysmal positional vertigo. Otolaryngol Head Neck Surg 107: 1992.
5. Fetter M, Zee DS, Proctor LR: Effect of lack of vision and of occipital lobectomy upon recovery from unilateral labyrinthectomy in rhesus monkey. J Neurophysiol 59:394–407, 1988.

6. Glasscock ME, McKennan FX, Levine SC: Persistent traumatic perilymphatic fistulas. Laryngoscope 97:860–864, 1987.
7. Gulya AJ: Perilymphatic fistulas. In Nadol JB, Schuknecht HF (eds): Surgery of the Ear and Temporal Bone. New York, Raven Press, 1993.
8. Hall SF, Ruby RRF, McClure JA: The mechanisms of benign paroxysmal vertigo. J Otolaryngol 8:151–158, 1979.
9. Healy GB: Current concepts in otolaryngology: Hearing loss and vertigo secondary to head injury. Med Intell 306:1029–1031, 1982.
10. Herdman SJ, Tusa RJ, Zee DS, et al: Single treatment approaches to benign paroxysmal positional vertigo. Arch Otolaryngol Head Neck Surg 119:450–454, 1993.
11. Kirtane MV, Medikeri SB, Karnik PP: ENG after head injury. J Laryngol Otol 96:521–528, 1982.
12. LaCour M, Roll JP, Appaix M: Modifications and development of spinal reflexes in the alert baboon. (*Papio papio*) following an unilateral neurectomy. Brain Res 113:255–269, 1976.
13. Lehrer JF, Rubin RC, Poole DC, et al: Perilymphatic fistula—A definitive and curable cause of vertigo following head trauma. West J Med 141:57–60, 1984.
14. Maoli C, Precht W: On the role of vestibulo-ocular reflex plasticity in recovery after unilateral peripheral vestibular lesions. Exp Brain Res 59:267–272, 1985.
15. Pagnini P, Vannucchi P, Vicini C: La Rieducazione vestibolare: aspetti clinici e risultati. G Ital Otoneurol 8:81–94, 1989.
16. Schuknecht HF: Cupulolithiasis. Arch Otolaryngol 90:765–778, 1969.
17. Semont A, Freyss G, Vitte E: Curing the BPPV with a Liberatory maneuver. Adv OtoRhino-Laryngol 42:290–293, 1988.
18. Snow JB: Positional vertigo. N Engl J Med 310:1740–1741, 1984.
19. Toglia JU: Acute flexion-extension injury of the neck. Neurology 26:808–814, 1976.
20. Tuohima P: Vestibular disturbances after acute mild head injury. Acta Otolaryngol Suppl (Stockh) 359:7–67, 1978.
21. Zee DS: Vertigo. In Current Therapy in Neurological Disease. Philadelphia, DC Decker, 1985.

JAMES R. HANSEN, MD
JENNIFER S. COOK, MD

POST-TRAUMATIC NEUROENDOCRINE DISORDERS

From
Pediatric Endocrinology and
    Diabetes (JRH)
Emanuel Children's Hospital
Portland, Oregon
    and
Pediatric Endocrinology
Blank Children's Hospital
    and
Iowa Physician's Clinic
Des Moines, Iowa (JSC)

Correspondence to:
James R. Hansen, MD
Pediatric Endocrinology and
    Diabetes
Emanuel Children's Hospital
2801 N. Gantenbein Avenue
Portland, OR 97227

Endocrine abnormalities following head trauma are not commonly reported. This observation is surprising, given that hormonal regulation of homeostasis is carefully controlled by the orchestrated release of multiple hormones from the pituitary. The pituitary, in turn, responds to finely tuned neuropeptide signals that originate in the hypothalamus when electrical inputs from various regions of the brain are converted into chemical information. Transduction of this information involves many neuronal pathways and the delicate hypothalamic-pituitary portal system, which provides a conduit for the flow of neuropeptides into the pituitary. The pituitary is protected within the sella turcica of the sphenoid bone, but the other components of this important regulatory system are vulnerable to the forces that are applied when head trauma is sustained. It is likely that endocrine disturbances following traumatic brain injuries have been overlooked. Early recognition of hormone imbalances is desirable because normalization of endocrine function may facilitate the recovery and rehabilitation of these individuals. Consequently, we hope that this review will lead to an increased awareness of possible neuroendocrine dysfunction as a result of brain injury.

ANATOMIC STUDIES

Postmortem examination following fatal head trauma has revealed a high prevalence of hypothalamic and pituitary lesions. Abnormalities of the pituitary have included anterior lobe necrosis, posterior lobe hemorrhage, and complete as well as partial transection of the hypothalamic-pituitary stalk. Depending on the series, anterior pituitary infarction occurred in 9 to 38% of cases, posterior pituitary hemorrhage in 12 to 45%, and damage to the stalk in 5 to 30%.[8,14,24,29] In their studies, Daniel et al.[12,13,14] observed anterior pituitary necrosis similar to that seen after surgical division of the pituitary stalk in humans and animals. They concluded that traumatic rupture of the pituitary stalk damaged the portal blood supply and thus led to anterior lobe infarction. Kornblum,[29] however, has proposed an alternate mechanism for anterior pituitary necrosis: as the pituitary swells after injury, the portal vessels are compressed between the stalk and diaphragm, and the portal blood supply to the anterior lobe of the pituitary is subsequently interrupted. Depending on the nature of the trauma, it is possible that both mechanisms may lead to deprivation of portal blood flow to the pituitary.

Hypothalamic injury has also been observed during postmortem inspection of the brain. Crompton[11] reported ischemic or hemorrhagic lesions of the anterior hypothalamus in 45 of 106 cases of acute, closed-head injury. The lesions were often associated with hemorrhage or infarction of the pituitary.

While hypothalamic and pituitary lesions are commonly reported after fatal head injury, anatomic evaluation of the hypothalamus and pituitary in survivors of head trauma is often not done or is limited by available imaging modalities. In general, magnetic resonance imaging has been superior to computed tomographic scanning in showing soft tissue damage. Limitations of resolution, however, may preclude identification of damaged areas. Consequently, evaluation of hypothalamic-pituitary function following head injury should include hormone measurements.

NORMAL HYPOTHALAMIC-PITUITARY FUNCTION

Monitoring for abnormalities of the hypothalamic-pituitary axis requires knowledge of normal neuroendocrine physiology. Figure 1 shows the location of the pituitary, the hormones that it secretes in response to hypothalamic neuropeptides, and the target sites for these chemical messengers. With the exception of prolactin, the release of anterior pituitary hormones is stimulated by hormones that are synthesized by hypothalamic neurons and secreted in bursts into the hypothalamic-pituitary portal system. Intermittent exposure of the pituitary to stimulatory neuropeptides leads to the pulsatile pattern of release that is typical of the anterior pituitary hormones. Posterior pituitary hormones, arginine vasopressin and oxytocin, are carried by long axonal projections from the hypothalamus to the pituitary. Because these axons project along the pituitary stalk, damage to the stalk may disturb the normal secretion of arginine vasopressin and oxytocin. Table 1 summarizes the pituitary hormones, their functions, and the hypothalamic neuropeptides that trigger their release.

Anterior Pituitary Hormones

GROWTH HORMONE

Growth hormone is stimulated by growth hormone–releasing hormone (GHRH) and inhibited by somatostatin. GHRH is mainly secreted by neurons in the region of the arcuate nucleus and at the periphery of the ventromedial nucleus. Neurons that secrete somatostatin, however, are localized primarily to the paraventricular nucleus with projections into the median eminence.

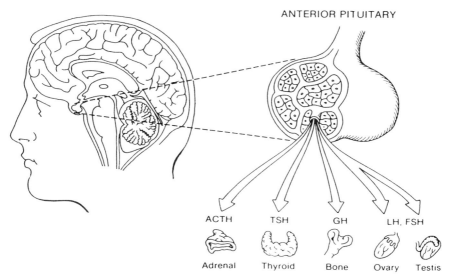

FIGURE 1. The anterior pituitary gland and its hormones (prolactin is not shown because its release is primarily under the inhibitory influence of dopamine). The release of corticotropin (ACTH), thyrotropin (TSH), growth hormone (GH), luteinizing hormone (LH), and follicle-stimulating hormone (FSH) is regulated by stimulatory hypothalamic neuropeptides (releasing hormones). (From Hansen JR, Cook JS, Conn PM: Effects of head injury on pituitary function. *J Head Inj* 2:6–10, 1990; with permission.)

The synchronized secretion of GHRH and somatostatin results in pulsatile growth hormone release during stages III and IV of deep sleep. Growth hormone release in a normal 10-year-old boy is shown in Figure 2. Following its release, growth hormone plays an important role in regulating growth and metabolism.

TABLE 1. Pituitary Hormones and Regulatory Hypothalamic Hormones

Pituitary Hormone	Main Functions	Regulatory Hormone*
Anterior Pituitary		
Growth Hormone	Linear growth, metabolic processes	GHRH (+)
		Somatostatin (–)
Thyrotropin (TSH)	Iodide uptake by thyroid, release of thyroxine and T$_3$	TRH (+)
Corticotropin (ACTH)	Adrenal androgen and cortisol production	CRH (+)
Gonadotropins (LH, FSH)	Gonadal steroid secretion, gametogenesis	GnRH (+)
Prolactin	Lactation	Dopamine (–)
Posterior Pituitary		
Vasopressin	Antidiuresis	None
Oxytocin	Smooth muscle contraction (uterus, mammary gland)	None

* The *plus* sign indicates stimulatory, the *minus* inhibitory.
CRH = corticotropin-releasing hormone; FSH = follicle stimulating hormone; GHRH = growth hormone–releasing hormone; GnRH = gonadotropin-releasing hormone; LH = luteinizing hormone.

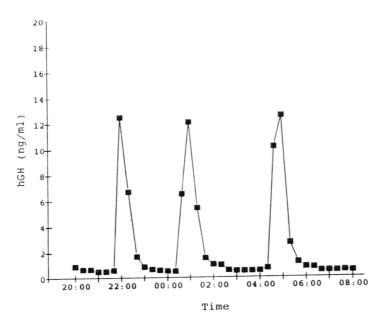

FIGURE 2.   Overnight pattern of human growth hormone (hGH) release in a normal prepubertal 10-year-old boy. (From Hansen JR, Cook JS, Conn PM: Effects of head injury on pituitary function. *J Head Inj* 2:6–10, 1990; with permission.)

Growth hormone has traditionally not been replaced following epiphyseal fusion and the completion of normal linear growth. Because it is becoming increasingly clear that growth hormone regulates many other functions besides growth, studies are beginning to establish optimal replacement doses in adults. Given its potent anabolic effects, treatment of growth hormone inadequacy may prove useful in the rehabilitation of head injury patients.

THYROTROPIN

Thyrotropin, which is also called thyroid-stimulating hormone (TSH), is released from the pituitary by thyrotropin-releasing hormone (TRH). Secretory neurons for TRH are located in the preoptic hypothalamus and in the paraventricular nucleus. Following its release, TSH stimulates iodide uptake by the thyroid gland and the release of thyroid hormones. These hormones, in turn, are critical for normal growth and development as well as many other important metabolic processes, including protein synthesis and degradation.

Serious, nonthyroidal illnesses are often associated with low 3,4,3'-triiodothyronine (T_3) levels. Subnormal levels of T_3 are typically not recognized since serum T_3 is not usually measured. TSH and thyroxine (T_4) levels are within normal ranges, but reverse T_3 levels are elevated. These findings are thought to reflect a protein-sparing tendency as a result of the catabolic state associated with these illnesses. Because T_3 is the biologically active form of thyroid hormone, the question frequently arises of whether decreased T_3 levels produce thyroid hormone deficiency at the tissue level in these patients. Normal TSH levels and normal TRH-stimulated TSH release, however, argue against thyroid hormone inadequacy.

Consequently, replacement therapy is not needed unless decreased TSH release in response to TRH is observed or thyroxine levels are subnormal.

CORTICOTROPIN

Corticotropin (adrenocorticotropic hormone, ACTH) controls the production of cortisol and adrenal androgens. Cortisol affects metabolic, immune, and inflammatory processes. It also plays an essential role in the conversion of norepinephrine, which is produced by the adrenal medulla, into epinephrine. This catecholamine prepares the body for "fight or flight" during times of physical stress. Adrenal androgens produce masculine characteristics. The principal adrenal androgen is dehydroepiandrosterone (DHEA), which mainly circulates as a sulfated derivative (DHEA-S). DHEA is converted into more potent androgens at target sites and thus contributes to the development of pubic hair and axillary hair, as well as the pathogenesis of acne. DHEA-S levels begin to rise between 5 and 8 years of age during the adrenarchal phase of puberty and may play a role in the mid-childhood growth spurt and the onset of gonadarche. ACTH release from the pituitary is regulated by corticotropin-releasing hormone, which is produced by neurons in the paraventricular nucleus.

GONADOTROPINS

Luteinizing hormone (LH) and follicle-stimulating hormone (FSH) are collectively known as gonadotropins. LH and FSH regulate the production of gonadal steroids and gametogenesis. Estrogen and testosterone produce secondary sexual characteristics and have effects on behavior, metabolic processes, and body composition. LH and FSH are released from the pituitary by gonadotropin-releasing hormone (GnRH). This neuropeptide is secreted by neurons located in the medial preoptic and infundibular areas of the hypothalamus. The pattern of GnRH release is a critical determinant of LH and FSH secretion. GnRH is secreted during fetal development and for up to 2 years after birth.[25] Reactivation of pulsatile release at the time of puberty (gonadarche) leads to an increase in the amplitude and frequency of nocturnal LH pulses,[7] and thus heralds the onset of this important biologic event. Disorders ranging from infertility to precocious puberty may occur as a result of disturbed GnRH release.

PROLACTIN

Prolactin bears a striking structural resemblance to growth hormone. Both hormones probably evolved through duplication of a common ancestral gene. Even though prolactin is probably the oldest of our hormones, its possible function in humans beyond its role in lactation remains poorly understood. Prolactin release from the pituitary is primarily under the inhibitory influence of dopamine.[20] TRH and oxytocin stimulate prolactin release, but their roles in physiologic regulation of prolactin secretion are not fully understood. Cell bodies for the neurons that produce dopamine are located in the arcuate of the hypothalamus. These neurons project axons to the median eminence through the infundibular dopaminergic tract.

Posterior Pituitary Hormones

ARGININE VASOPRESSIN

Arginine vasopressin, which is also known as antidiuretic hormone, is secreted by neurons located in the supraoptic and paraventricular nuclei. Long axonal projections carry these hormones to the posterior pituitary. Arginine vasopressin–containing fibers also project to the median eminence. Arginine vasopressin that is secreted into the hypophyseal portal system may have regulatory effects in the anterior pituitary, given its ability to stimulate the release of ACTH. Arginine vasopressin has many actions throughout the body. It signals the kidneys to retain water in response to increases in plasma osmolality that are sensed by osmoreceptors located in the vascular organ of the lamina terminalis and the subfornical organ. Arginine vasopressin also increases blood pressure through receptors in peripheral arterioles. Other effects of arginine vasopressin may include stimulation of gluconeogenesis in the liver and avoidance behavior.

OXYTOCIN

Oxytocin stimulates milk ejection as a result of smooth muscle contraction in the alveoli and ducts of the mammary gland, and it also contributes to the delivery of the fetus by stimulating uterine contractions. Apprehension, fear, and changes in environment stimulate oxytocin secretion, whereas loud noise, pain, and fever may inhibit its secretion. Oxytocin is produced by neurons located in the supraoptic and paraventricular nuclei. Like arginine vasopressin, it is carried by long projections into the posterior pituitary. Both arginine vasopressin and oxytocin travel to the pituitary in association with neurophysins, which were once thought to be carrier proteins but are actually portions of arginine vasopressin and oxytocin precursors.

ASSESSMENT OF NEUROENDOCRINE FUNCTION

Although the concentration of hypothalamic hormones in the hypothalamic-pituitary portal circulation is sufficient to measure using available assays, their concentrations in the systemic circulation are usually too low to detect. Serum levels of pituitary hormones are measured instead because they typically reflect the secretory patterns of hypothalamic neuropeptides. The pulsatile nature of their secretion, however, usually prevents definitive assessment with a single, random serum sample.[39] As a result, multiple tests have been developed to assess the adequacy of pituitary function.

Stimulation Testing

These tests have traditionally involved the use of agents that are known to stimulate the release of pituitary hormones. This type of testing is known as tolerance testing or stimulation testing. In many cases, the test actually involves infusion of the hypothalamic releasing hormone that is known to stimulate the particular pituitary hormone of interest. For example, TRH may be given to assess the normalcy of TSH release. Other tolerance tests, however, involve the use of other secretagogues that are able to elicit pituitary hormone release. Traditional testing for growth hormone adequacy, for example, involves the infusion of arginine followed by another agent, such as insulin or clonidine. During these tests, the hormone of interest is measured at baseline and at frequent time intervals over the succeeding 1 to 3 hours. An absent or decreased response in pituitary hormone release is usually interpreted as evidence of pituitary insufficiency.

The problem with this approach, however, is that the acute response of the pituitary to secretagogues simply tests the ability of the relevant cells in the pituitary to produce receptors and release the hormone of interest. Tolerance testing does not, however, provide insight into the normalcy of hypothalamic neuropeptide pulsatility.[5,46] Table 2 summarizes commonly used tolerance tests.

TABLE 2. Commonly Used Tolerance Tests

Pituitary Hormone	Stimulus
Growth hormone	Arginine
	Insulin
	Clonidine
	L-Dopa
TSH	TRH
ACTH	Insulin
	Metyrapone
LH, FSH	GnRH
Prolactin	TRH
Arginine vasopressin	Water deprivation
Oxytocin	Nipple stimulation

Serial Sampling

To better assess the normalcy of hypothalamic regulation of pituitary hormone secretion, a newer method that involves frequent blood sampling has been tried.[16,33,36,38,39,42] Measurement of hormone levels in these serial blood samples permits one to assess the pulse pattern of a given hormone. This approach, however, has been limited by numerous factors, including the costs associated with an overnight admission and multiple assays, a lack of normative data, problems associated with defining what constitutes a pulse, and variability of hormone release patterns within the same person on different testing days. Monitoring of hormone pulsatility, however, has led to the realization that many problems such as growth hormone inadequacy are often due to differences in hypothalamic neuropeptide signaling of the pituitary rather than abnormalities within the pituitary itself.

Symptoms and Signs of Pituitary Insufficiency

Because hormone testing involves a significant amount of time, expense, and sometimes discomfort, it is desirable to do a careful history, physical examination, and screening studies prior to doing stimulation tests. Disordered pituitary hormone secretion often produces characteristic symptoms and signs. Typical symptoms and signs are shown in Table 3.

TABLE 3. Symptoms and Signs of Pituitary Hormone Disturbances

Pituitary Hormone	Symptoms and Signs
Growth hormone	Short stature, slow growth, hypoglycemia, increased body fat, delayed bone age
TSH	Short stature, slow growth, weight gain, bradycardia, dry skin, coarse hair, fatigue, hypothermia, constipation, hypercholesterolemia, menstrual irregularities
ACTH	Hypoglycemia, fatigue, anemia, fainting, hypotension, weakness, weight loss, delayed adrenarche
LH, FSH	Delayed or arrested puberty, decreased libido, impotence, infertility, irregular menses
Prolactin	Decreased milk production, galactorrhea, impotence
Vasopressin	Polyuria, increased thirst, fever

Screening Studies

If these symptoms and signs are present, then screening studies should be performed. In some cases, however, it is not possible to obtain a reliable history, or other problems are occurring that may preclude the recognition of physical signs. Screening studies may be very useful in these situations. Table 4 summarizes measurements that are helpful screening tests of pituitary hormone adequacy.

HYPOTHALAMIC-PITUITARY FUNCTION FOLLOWING HEAD TRAUMA

Most of the information regarding endocrine function after head trauma is from case reports. These reports indicate that head trauma severity does not predict which patients will develop pituitary dysfunction,[2,10,17] nor whether the disturbance will be temporary or permanent. Survivors may experience the loss of one or multiple hormones. Both children and adults have exhibited decreased pituitary function after head trauma.[17,18,23,32,34,35] Although many patients have had a period of unconsciousness,[17,30,35,45] others have not. Reports of skull fractures are common, and they may involve single or multiple sites.[1,17,28,30,32,35,43,44] There may be associated neurologic abnormalities.[1,10,17,18,30,35,43,44] Blindness with various field defects is commonly reported. The diagnosis of hormone abnormalities in these case reports occurred weeks to years after the head injury was sustained. In many patients, symptoms and signs of pituitary insufficiency had been present for long periods but had gone unrecognized.

Limited prospective studies have investigated the effects of head injury on specific pituitary hormones. Most of these studies, however, have been done during the early recovery period. In many cases, patients were still in intensive care settings.

LUTEINIZING HORMONE AND FOLLICLE-STIMULATING HORMONE

Hypogonadism is one of the most common endocrine disturbances reported after head trauma. Kinnunen and Iauppinen[27] found amenorrhea in 26 of 78 women who had suffered head injury. Normal menses returned by 3 months in all patients. Hansen et al.[23] reported on a 14-year-old adolescent male who had a temporary arrest of puberty development after a moderately severe closed-head injury with deep facial and scalp lacerations and a comminuted left tripod fracture of the cheek. No loss of consciousness was reported. In the six cases of traumatic hypopituitarism reported by Edwards and Clark,[17] all six survivors developed permanent hypogonadism.

TABLE 4.   Screening Assessment of Pituitary Hormone Adequacy

Pituitary Hormone	Measurement
Growth hormone	Height, weight, bone age ($<$18 years); somatomedin C, IGFBP-3
TSH	Free thyroxine, T_3 by RIA
ACTH	Serum cortisol (1600 hr)
LH, FSH	Serum estradiol or testosterone
Prolactin	Serum prolactin
Vasopressin	Serum sodium, urine output

IGFBP-3 = insulin-like growth factor binding protein 3; RIA = radioimmunoassay.

Investigators have observed low basal gonadotropin and testosterone concentrations immediately after head trauma.[37,47] In a prospective study, Clark et al.[10] evaluated hypothalamic-pituitary-gonadal function in 33 men who had a history of loss of consciousness for at least 24 hours following a head injury. GnRH stimulation tests were performed on admission, 1 week later, and after 3 to 6 months in 21 patients. Initial testing showed low basal gonadotropin levels and low serum concentrations of testosterone. Exaggerated LH and FSH release in response to exogenous GnRH occurred in a pattern typical of hypothalamic dysfunction. After 3 to 6 months, 5 of 21 patients continued to have low serum testosterone concentrations. Three of the 5 patients had persistently elevated LH and FSH levels in response to GnRH.

Precocious puberty has also been observed in children following head trauma.[6] When secondary sex characteristics occur in females younger than 8 years of age and males younger than 9 years, than puberty is early in its onset. Central, or true, precocious puberty occurs when it is dependent on gonadotropin release in response to endogenous GnRH secretion. Gonadal steroid production occurs and may lead to premature epiphyseal fusion and adult short stature. Early puberty may also produce behavioral problems. In a report by Blendonohy and Philip,[6] two girls who were 3 and 5 years of age developed pubertal changes following head trauma. Both girls had physical findings and laboratory test results that were typical of central precocious puberty. These tests included a GnRH stimulation test, which showed a pubertal (i.e., LH predominant) pattern of response.

THYROID-STIMULATING HORMONE

Both normal and abnormal thyroid function have been reported after head trauma.[19] King et al.[26] found normal basal serum concentrations of TSH, and Matsuura[31] et al. observed normal serum TSH levels before and after TRH stimulation at the time of admission following head injury. In another study, though, TSH responses to TRH were diminished. Exaggerated responses of TSH to TRH have also been seen.

Two studies have shown a relationship between the severity of head trauma and TSH levels. Chiolero et al.[9] observed TSH concentrations that directly correlated with the Glasgow coma scale and indirectly with the 5-day maximum intracranial pressure. In a study by Gottardis et al.,[21] patients who died had an absent response of TSH to TRH; survivors exhibited normal responses. In a subsequent study, however, these investigators showed that TSH abnormalities were not predictive of an individual patient's course.

Several factors may explain the differences that were observed in the above studies. The severity of the head trauma, the time of the study after the head injury, and the dosages and types of medication that the patients were receiving may have affected the results. Furthermore, methods used to assess thyroid function varied between investigators. Adequate assessment of thyroid function is important, however, because abnormal thyroid hormone levels may affect pituitary hormone release.

PROLACTIN

Disturbances in TRH release may also be expressed as abnormalities in prolactin secretion. High basal serum prolactin levels were seen in patients following severe head injuries in two studies: one group of patients exhibited normal TRH-stimulated prolactin levels, whereas the other group showed diminished prolactin responses. In a prospective study, Clark et al.[10] observed elevated prolactin levels at admission and 1 week later. Prolactin levels decreased but remained elevated after 3 to 6 months. Disturbances in prolactin secretion may not become evident until patients present with galactorrhea, amenorrhea, or impotence.

GROWTH HORMONE

Growth hormone levels are not typically evaluated in patients following head injury. This lack of assessment may be related to the conventional thinking that growth hormone replacement is not necessary once linear growth is complete. This approach is inconsistent with our practice of replacing other pituitary hormones. Now that supplies permit, studies to define growth hormone effects and replacement doses in adults are being undertaken. It is becoming clear that this potent anabolic hormone has many other effects besides the stimulation of growth.

Elevated basal growth hormone levels have been observed following head injury in two studies. In another study, Barreca et al.[2] found decreased growth hormone responses during stimulation testing in 5 of 10 patients with central diabetes insipidus after head trauma. In another study, patients who survived head injuries had stimulated growth hormone levels that were significantly higher than those who died.[21] A subsequent study, however, indicated that growth hormone secretory abnormalities were not predictive of the course of an individual patient.[22] Growth disturbances may be seen in children many years after head trauma.

CORTICOTROPIN

The hypothalamic-pituitary-adrenal axis is often difficult to assess immediately after head injury because many patients receive corticosteroids as part of their management. Serum concentrations of ACTH have been measured, however, prior to the initiation of glucocorticoid therapy. Barton et al.[3] found increased serum levels of cortisol and ACTH 2 hours after injury. In another study, normal serum ACTH concentrations were observed during the first 5 days after head trauma.[9] ACTH release in response to insulin-induced hypoglycemia was decreased in 3 of 10 patients with central diabetes insipidus following head injury.[2] Two of these patients also had decreased basal serum cortisol concentrations. Although typically seen in association with other pituitary hormone insufficiencies, there are reports of isolated ACTH deficiency after head trauma.[40]

ARGININE VASOPRESSIN

Decreased and increased levels of arginine vasopressin have been commonly reported after head injury; these abnormalities result in central diabetes insipidus and the syndrome of inappropriate antidiuretic hormone secretion (SIADH), respectively.[4,15,34]

Based on studies to date, central diabetes insipidus is the most common neuroendocrine disorder following head injury. The onset and duration of symptoms, however, is highly variable.[4] In eight pediatric patients with head trauma, Padilla et al.[34] observed increased urinary arginine vasopressin levels during the first 3 days of hospitalization. Two patients met the clinical criteria for the diagnosis of SIADH. No correlation existed between vasopressin levels and the Glasgow coma score or the occurrence of cerebral edema. In a review of

1800 cases of head trauma in adults, Doczi et al.[15] found that SIADH occurred in 0.6% of patients with minor head trauma, 10.6% of those with moderate head trauma, and 4.7% with severe head injuries. Recognition of SIADH led to more frequent evaluation of other pituitary hormones.

CONCLUSIONS AND RECOMMENDATIONS

Healthcare providers who manage patients following head injury need to be aware that neuroendocrine disturbances may occur. Because abnormalities may be masked by other problems, it is important that one have a high index of suspicion and do appropriate screening studies to assess pituitary function. Early recognition of hormone disturbances may promote the rehabilitation and recovery of head injury survivors. Improved imaging methods may eventually facilitate the identification of disturbed hypothalamic-pituitary function. Until then, one must rely on careful clinical observation and hormone testing. Additional prospective studies are needed to further define the mechanisms and effects of head trauma on neuroendocrine function.

REFERENCES

1. Altman R, Pruzanski W: Post-traumatic hypopituitarism and anterior pituitary insufficiency following skull fracture. Ann Intern Med 55:149–154, 1961.
2. Barreca T, Perrea C, Sannia A, et al: Evaluation of anterior pituitary function in patients with posttraumatic diabetes insipidus. J Clin Endocrinol Metab 51:1279–1282, 1980.
3. Barton R, Stoner H, Watson S: Relationships among plasma cortisol, adrenocorticotropin, and severity of injury in recently injured patients. J Trauma 27:384–392, 1987.
4. Barzilay Z, Somekh E: Diabetes insipidus in severely brain damaged children. J Med 19:47–xx, 1988.
5. Bercu B, Shulman D, Root A, Spilliotis B: Growth hormone (GH) provocative testing frequently does not reflect endogenous GH action. J Clin Endocrinol Metab 63:709, 1986.
6. Blendonohy PM, Philip PA: Precocious puberty in children after traumatic head injury. Brain Inj 5:63–68, 1991.
7. Boyar R, Finkelstein J, Roffwarg H, et al: Synchronization of augmented luteinizing hormone secretion with sleep during puberty. N Engl J Med 287:582–586, 1972.
8. Ceballos R: Pituitary changes in head trauma. Ala J Med Sci 3:185–198, 1966.
9. Chiolero R, Lemarchand T, Schutz Y, et al: Plasma pituitary hormone levels in severe trauma with or without head injury. J Trauma 28:1368–1374, 1988.
10. Clark J, Raggatt P, Edwards O: Hypothalamic hypogonadism following major head injury. Clin Endocrinol 29:153–165, 1988.
11. Crompton M: Hypothalamic lesions following closed head injury. Brain 94:165–172, 1971.
12. Daniel P, Prichard M, Smith B: The extent of the infarct in the anterior pituitary found soon after pituitary stalk section in the baboon and rhesus monkey. J Physiol 146:2P–4P, 1959.
13. Daniel P, Prichard M, Treip C: Traumatic infarction of the anterior lobe of the pituitary gland. Lancet ii:927–930, 1959.
14. Daniel P, Treip C: Acute massive traumatic infarction of the anterior lobe. In Gardiner-Hill H (ed): Modern Trends in Endocrinology, 2nd series. New York, Hoeber, 1961, pp 55–68.
15. Doczi T, Tarjanyi J, Huszka E, Kiss J: Syndrome of inappropriate secretion of antidiuretic hormone (SIADH) after head injury. Neurosurgery 10:685–688, 1982.
16. Donaldson D, Pan F, Hollowell J, et al: Reliability of stimulated and spontaneous growth hormone (GH) levels for identifying the child with low GH secretion. J Clin Endocrinol Metab 72:647–652.
17. Edwards O, Clark J: Post-traumatic hypopituitarism: Six cases and a review of the literature. Medicine (Baltimore) 65:281–290, 1986.
18. Eichler I, Frisch H, Eichler H, Soukop W: Isolated growth hormone deficiency after severe head trauma. J Endocrinol Invest 11:409–411, 1988.
19. Fleischer A, Rudman D, Payne N, et al: Hypothalamic hypothyroidism and hypogonadism in prolonged traumatic coma. J Neurosurg 49:650–657, 1978.
20. Foreman M, Porter J: Prolactin augmentation of dopamine and norepinephrine release from superfused medial basal hypothalamic fragments. Endocrinology 108:800–803, 1981.

21. Gottardis M, Nigitsch C, Schutzhard E, et al: The secretion of human growth hormone stimulated by human growth hormone releasing factor following severe cranio-cerebral trauma. Intensive Care Med 16:163–166, 1990.

22. Hackl J, Gottardis, Wieser C, et al: Endocrine abnormalities in severe traumatic brain injury—A cue to prognosis in severe craniocerebral trauma? Intensive Care Med 17:25–29, 1991.

23. Hansen J, Cook J, Conn PM: Effects of head injury on pituitary function: Pediatric case study. J Head Inj 2:6–10, 1990.

24. Harper C, Doyle D, Adams J, Graham D: Analysis of abnormalities in pituitary gland in non-missile head injury: Study of 100 consecutive cases. J Clin Pathol 39:769–773, 1986.

25. Kaplan S, Grumbach M: Pathogenesis of sexual precocity. In Grumbach M, Sizonenko P, Aubert M (eds): Control of the Onset of Puberty. Baltimore, Williams & Wilkins, 1990, pp 620–628.

26. King L, Knowles H, McLaurin R, et al: Pituitary hormone response to head injury. Neurosurgery 9:229–235, 1981.

27. Kinnuen I, Iauppinen M: The effect of brain injury on the menstrual cycle. Acta Endocrinol 6:183–187, 1951.

28. Klachko D, Winer N, Burns T, White E: Traumatic hypopituitarism occurring before puberty: Survival 35 years untreated. J Clin Endocrinol 28:1768–1772, 1968.

29. Kornblum R, Fisher R: Pituitary lesions in craniocerebral injuries. Arch Pathol Lab Med 88:242–248, 1969.

30. Landau H, Adin I, Spitz I: Pituitary insufficiency following head injury. Isr J Med Sci 14:785–788, 1978.

31. Matsuura H, Nakazawa S, Walabayashi I: Thyrotropin-releasing hormone provocative release and prolactin and thyrotropin in acute head injury. Neurosurgery 16:791–795, 1985.

32. Miller W, Kaplan S, Grumbach M: Child abuse as a cause of post-traumatic hypopituitarism. N Engl J Med 302:724–728, 1980.

33. Oerter K, Guardabasso V, Rodbard D: Detection and characterization of peaks and estimation of instantaneous secretory rate for episodic pulsatile hormone secretion. Comput Biomed Res 19:170–191, 1986.

34. Padilla G, Leake J, Castro R, et al: Vasopressin levels and pediatric head trauma. Pediatrics 83:700–705, 1989.

35. Paxson C, Brown D: Post-traumatic anterior hypopituitarism. Pediatrics 57:893–896, 1976.

36. Rose S, Ross J, Urigate M, et al: The advantage of measuring stimulated as compared with spontaneous growth hormone levels in the diagnosis of growth hormone deficiency. N Engl J Med 319:201–207, 1988.

37. Rudman D, Fleischer A, Kutner M, Raggio J: Suprahypophyseal hypogonadism and hypothyroidism during prolonged coma after head trauma. J Clin Endocrinol Metab 45:747–754, 1977.

38. Saini S, Hindmarsh P, Matthews D, et al: Reproducibility of 24-hour serum growth hormone profiles in man. Clin Endocrinol 34:455–462, 1991.

39. Santoro N, Filicori M, Crowley W: Hypogonadotropic disorders in men and women: Diagnosis and therapy with pulsatile gonadotropin-releasing hormone. Endocr Rev 7:11–23, 1986.

40. Scoble J, Havard C: Anosmia and isolated ACTH deficiency following a road traffic accident. J Neurosurg 73:453–454, 1990.

41. Treip C: Hypothalamic and pituitary injury. J Clin Pathol 23(suppl 4):178–185, 1970.

42. Urban R, Evans W, Rogol A, et al: Contemporary aspects of discrete peak-detection algorithims. I: The paradigm of the luteinizing hormone pulse signal in men. Endocr Rev 9:3–37, 1988.

43. Valenta L, De Feo D: Post-traumatic hypopituitarism due to a hypothalamic lesion. Am J Med 68:614–617, 1980.

44. Weiss S, Jacobe J, Fishman L, Lemaire W: Hypopituitarism following head trauma. Am J Obstet Gynecol 127:678–679, 1977.

45. Winternitz W, Dzur J: Pituitary failure secondary to head trauma. J Neurosurg 44:504–505, 1976.

46. Woolf P, Schalch D: Hypopituitarism secondary to hypothalamic insufficiency. Ann Intern Med 78:88–90, 1973.

47. Woolf P, Hamill F, McDonald J, et al: Transient hypogonadotrophic hypogonadism after head trauma: Effects on steroid precursors and correlation with sympathetic nervous system activity. Clin Endocrinol 25:265–274, 1986.

RONALD E. SAUL, MD

NEUROBEHAVIORAL DISORDERS FOLLOWING TRAUMATIC BRAIN INJURY

Part I. Neurobehavioral Sequelae in the Early Stages of Recovery

From the
Department of Neurology
UCLA School of Medicine
Los Angeles, California
and
Adult Brain Injury Service
Rancho Los Amigos Medical
 Center
Downey, California

Correspondence to:
Ronald E. Saul, MD
550 N. Brand Boulevard, Suite 700
Glendale, CA 91203

In addition to the traditional neurologic sequelae of traumatic brain injury (TBI) which include post-traumatic headache, dizziness, and epilepsy, TBI neurobehavioral sequelae affect complex arrays of cognition, emotional expression, and behavior. These include problems with attention and memory, cognitive and executive dysfunction, personality changes, anxiety and affective disorders, psychosis, irritability, and aggression.[17] For the patient and family, such disorders often represent a significant and disabling problem, which may be alleviated by early recognition and proper management. This chapter reviews recent literature on the subacute neurobehavioral sequelae of moderate to severe closed TBI, emphasizing the clinical features and syndromes associated with different stages of recovery, their precipitating biologic and psychosocial determinants, and appropriate intervention, in particular, new pharmacologic approaches to treatment.

BIOLOGIC AND PSYCHOSOCIAL DETERMINANTS

Of the multiple determinants precipitating neurobehavioral syndromes following head trauma, the condition of the brain at the time of injury deserves major consideration. Advanced age, previous head injuries, other structural and metabolic abnormalities, and toxic exposure, including substance abuse, are factors increasing the vulnerability of the patient with a new TBI.[25] Poor prognosis is associated with the severity of TBI, as reflected in a low initial Glasgow coma score, prolonged post-traumatic amnesia, and secondary complications (e.g., focal hematomas), and with subsequent physical underactivity, agitation, and a developing seizure disorder.[23,30] Sparadeo and Gill report that patients using alcohol at the time of injury had increased length of hospitalization, longer duration of agitation, and lower cognitive function at hospital discharge compared with patients with no detectable alcohol level at time of hospitalization.[32] Ruff et al. similarly found TBI patients with a history of alcohol abuse had a poorer outcome with increased mortality and a higher prevalence of mass lesions.[28] The presence of total anosmia, reflecting damage to olfactory nerves adjacent to orbital frontal cortex, predicted major vocational problems 2 years after medical clearance to return to work.[36]

The patient's preinjury level of psychosocial function is a critical factor in anticipating the response to head injury. Knowledge of previous coping strategies, of past psychiatric illness in both the patient and family, and of responses to therapy will avert unnecessary exacerbations and assist in planning appropriate treatment.[25] Although many victims of TBI do not have a positive psychiatric history, a significant percentage have had attentional deficits, learning disabilities, behavioral problems, and substance abuse. Preexisting socioeconomic status, level of education, and support networks will affect behavioral symptoms and the course of recovery.[30]

These biologic and psychosocial determinants have received considerable emphasis in the rehabilitation and psychiatric literature, which, to a great extent, has considered closed nonpenetrating head injury a relatively homogeneous entity. From a neurologic perspective, recent basic neuroscience research, along with more refined neuroimaging and psychological techniques, have improved our understanding of the diverse pathophysiologic processes underlying specific behavioral syndromes. Penetrating high-speed missile injuries typically produce a circumscribed cortical surface injury and familiar, highly specific lateralized deficit, such as hemiplegia, aphasia, or hemineglect. In closed-head injury (CHI), there is frequently symmetrical damage to extensive areas of the frontal and temporal lobes. Deficits in arousal, attention, memory, self-regulation, and initiation from subcortical and rostral brainstem damage occur in severe cases of both penetrating and closed-brain injuries. In CHI, however, the additive effect of cortical contusions and diffuse axonal shearing with white matter degeneration in limbic circuits may produce striking behavioral and emotional changes. They may resemble a so-called functional psychiatric disorder and are often superimposed on more easily defined motor, linguistic, and cognitive deficits.[1,17] Effective management requires an understanding of how these different areas of deficit interact and compound in the CHI patient at various stages of recovery.[3]

PATHOPHYSIOLOGY AND STAGES OF RECOVERY

Alexander[2-4] has provided a useful framework for brain-behavioral correlations in subacute CHI. Clinical problems can be related to the interaction of three major pathologic processes—diffuse axonal injury (DAI), focal lesions, and hypoxic-ischemic injury—and to any secondary complications such as extracerebral hematomas, seizures, or hydrocephalus. DAI refers to the mechanical disruption of axons in the brainstem and deep white matter of the cerebral hemispheres. At times, simultaneous tearing of small blood vessels produces punctate hemorrhages in the same distribution. Focal cortical contusions are tissue abrasions localized to the brain surface and adjacent subcortical areas. Hypoxic-ischemic injury results from a critical reduction in brain arterial perfusion and oxygen supply and may take the form of neuronal dropout or frank infarction (tissue necrosis). DAI, hypoxic-ischemic injury, and focal contusions will be discussed in turn with emphasis on diagnosis, measures of severity, clinical consequences, natural history, and treatment.

DIFFUSE AXONAL INJURY

Two separate mechanical forces may produce brain injury: contact phenomena and acceleration-deceleration.[13] Rotational to a greater degree than linear acceleration results in axonal shear strain, the major cause of diffuse injury. The severity of clinical effects is directly proportional to the amount and density of DAI, which can range from temporary reversible dysfunction to complete irreversible destruction. The distribution of DAI follows a gradient from peripheral cortex to midbrain, with more severe injuries involving the corpus callosum, deep hemispheric white matter, and dorsolateral midbrain.[5]

The diagnosis of DAI is largely based on typical clinical features, extracted from the patient's history. First, the mechanism of the injury itself must be considered. Typically, a motor vehicle accident or fall from a significant height can generate the accelerational forces required for major DAI. This would rarely occur with a fall to the ground from a standing position. Second, in DAI, the patient is unconscious from the time of impact; in contrast, a lucid conscious interval followed by deterioration into coma frequently occurs with an expanding mass lesion.[19] Brain magnetic resonance imaging (MRI) may confirm the diagnosis, even months to years after injury, by demonstrating multiple small hemorrhagic lesions or generalized atrophy in severe cases.[22] The depth of white matter lesions on MRI may be a useful index of DAI severity, with the resulting clinical effects understandable in terms of cortical-cortical, cortical-subcortical, and cortical-bulbar disconnection. MRI, however, may fail to show subtle but pertinent degrees of DAI. Marked and persistent brainstem signs—disordered eye movements, explosive crying, dysphagia, as well as cerebellar, pyramidal, and central vestibular deficits—indicate particularly severe injury.

Recovery from DAI, regardless of severity, follows a predictable pattern from immediate coma or stupor, to a period of confusion with amnesia, to a more prolonged period of functional restoration. In mild DAI, there may be rapid and ill-defined transitions from one stage to another. Coma of several minutes' duration can be followed by several hours of confusion and further recovery over months, whereas in severe DAI coma may last days to weeks, confusion days to months, and overall recovery years.[19] The best indices of DAI severity and long-term outcome are (1) the early Glasgow coma scale scores; (2) the duration of coma, its termination signaled by the patient's ability to follow commands; and (3) the duration of post-traumatic amnesia (PTA), the time period until restoration of continuous day-to-day memory. A period of PTA of less than 2 weeks is compatible with a relatively favorable outcome; when the PTA is longer than 4 weeks, only a small percentage of patients achieve this result.[23]

Brain MRI is a sensitive, but not infallible, means of detecting DAI involving deep regions of the hemispheres and brainstem. These abnormalities, in particular, late ventricular enlargement, predict poor neuropsychological test performance and poor outcome.[15,37,38] Electroencephalographic recordings have not proven useful in outcome prediction; quantitative electroencephalographic analysis and topographic mapping, however, show promise in detecting areas of dysfunction not shown in the routine electroencephalogram. Newer imaging techniques, such as single-photon computed emission tomography (SPECT) and positron-emission tomography (PET) can detect areas of abnormal function in the absence of structural changes on computed tomographic scanning and MRI.[21,27]

Several scales have been developed to represent the progression of clinical recovery with severe diffuse TBI. The eight-level Rancho Los Amigos scale[18] is most commonly used, with three levels describing coma, three the confusional period, and two subsequent recovery stages (Table 1). Sbordone[29] has proposed a six-stage recovery model highlighting behavioral and cognitive features, with special emphasis on the patient's awareness of deficit. The six-stage model developed by Alexander,[2] (Table 2), however, best respects the neurophysiologic correlates of the recovery process and will be discussed in detail. Recovery may plateau at any stage, determined by severity of injury and clinical complications.[2]

Alexander and Katz[2,19] stress the importance of precise neurobehavioral diagnosis (stage of recovery and profile of impairments) in setting appropriate treatment goals. Guidelines include the selection of therapies respecting the neurologic diagnosis and expected course of recovery. The patient should be able to respond to the intervention. Therapy should be directed toward clearly specified functional goals and relevant to the patient's needs at that point in time. Deficits that are functionally irrelevant or likely to spontaneously remit should not be treated.

In *coma,* the first stage, there are no signs of wakefulness or cognitive activity. The second stage, *unresponsive vigilance,* is characterized by cognitive unresponsiveness but with resumed gross wakefulness and sleep-wake cycles. The 2% of patients who plateau here are said to be in a persistent vegetative state. The use of multimodality sensory stimulation programs for such patients remains controversial. They have not proven effective in enhancing responsiveness but may be useful in monitoring for subtle changes.[8] In the third or *mute responsive stage,*

TABLE 1.   Rancho Los Amigos Scale of Cognitive Levels*

I.	*No response to stimulation*	—
II.	*Generalized responses*	Limited, inconsistent and nonpurposeful responses, often only in pain
III.	*Localized responses*	Purposeful responses, may follow simple commands
IV.	*Confused-agitated*	Disoriented with heightened state of activity and aggressive behavior
V.	*Confused-inappropriate*	Alert but distractible, responds to commands, agitated responses to external stimuli, absence of new learning
VI.	*Confused-appropriate*	Good directed behavior with cuing, severe memory impairment, but able to relearn old skills as ADLs, aware of self and others
VII.	*Automatic-appropriate*	Oriented but robotlike in daily routine, minimal or absent confusion, shallow recall, increasing awareness of self and environmental interaction, impaired insight, problem solving, and judgment, unrealistic planning for future
VIII.	*Purposeful and appropriate*	Recalls past events, learns new activities, independent ADLs persistent defects in stress tolerance, judgment, and abstract reasoning

* Adapted from Hagen C, Malkmus D, Durham P: Levels of cognitive functioning. In *Rehabilitation of the Head Injured Adult.* Downey, CA, Rancho Los Amigos Professional Staff Assoc., 1979, p 27. ADL = activity of daily living.

TABLE 2. Alexander's Stages of Recovery from Diffuse Axonal Injury*

I.	*Coma*	Eyes closed, unresponsive
II.	*Vegetative state-unresponsive vigilance*	Sleep-wake cycles, nonpurposive wakefulness
III.	*Mute responsiveness*	Purposeful wakefulness, limited response to commands
IV.	*Confusional state*	Attention severely impaired, amnesic with recovered speech, hypoaroused or agitated state
V.	*Emerging independence*	Resolution of post-traumatic amnesia, cognition and social interaction improved, becoming independent in ADL
VI.	*Intellectual/social competence*	Recovery of cognition, goal-directed behaviors, personality and social skills

* Adapted from Alexander MP: Traumatic brain injury. In Benson DF, Blumer D (eds): *Psychiatric Aspects of Neurologic Disease*, vol 2. New York, McGraw-Hill, 1982, pp 251–278.

patients will follow commands, at first inconsistently. Patients are nonverbal or have sparse, hypophonic speech. Automatic, reflexive responses are frequently mistaken for willful cognitive responses by family and nursing staff. In this stage and the subsequent confusional state, emerging responsiveness should not be compromised by the administration of sedative, narcotic, and centrally active hypertensive agents, often mistakenly given for treatment of pain or motor restlessness. The treatment team's efforts should be directed toward delineating the dimensions of responsiveness and using methods such as intermittent graded stimulation to elicit volitional responses.

In the *confusional state,* stage IV, severely impaired attentional mechanisms compromise all previously established cognitive operations. Patients exhibit wandering attention and are unable to reliably focus, sustain, or shift attention among external stimuli and internal mental processes. Attentional disturbances severely impair new learning and day-to-day recall, characteristic of the continuing period of PTA. Perseveration, confabulation, and denial of illness frequently emerge to compensate for the cognitive deficits. The confabulation seen in this setting may have a unique, grandiose, and preposterous quality, often appearing as confusion clears. It is usually related to some event in the patient's life and may be repeatedly produced. The patient, for example, may insist he or she is attending a class at his or her high school, despite contrary physical evidence.[4] Semantic knowledge, vocabulary, praxis, and motor learning show lesser degrees of impairment at this stage. The Galveston Orientation and Amnesia Test (GOAT) is helpful in tracking the course of PTA. Formal neuropsychological testing, however, is of dubious value.

Patients frequently show rapid transitions from an underaroused, abulic, and apathetic state to a hyperaroused and agitated state, accompanied by combative and paranoid behavior. These symptoms, as well as perceptual distortions, such as delusions and frank hallucinosis, are consistent with those seen in any other delirium. As the confusion clears, reduplicative paramnesia may emerge—for example, the reduplication of place, in which a place familiar to the patient exists simultaneously in two places. Of rare occurrence but more disturbing to the patient is the delusional replacement of a familiar and important person, such as a family member or physician, by a physically similar imposter (Capgras syndrome), or the converse, the replacement of an unfamiliar person by a physically similar person (Fregoli syndrome). Persistent reduplicative paramnesia of person or place is also rare but may occur after CHI with a unique constellation of lesions: bilateral orbital-frontal contusions plus a right parietal contusion for reduplicative paramnesia of place, or plus a right temporal contusion for reduplicative paramnesia of person and Capgras syndrome.[4]

Disturbed sleep-wake cycles along with altered thirst and appetite patterns are commonly encountered, probably reflecting hypothalamic injury.[12] Decreased stage I symptoms and a greater number of awakenings than control subjects have been reported.[20,26] Although a patient may have a dense amnesia for the events of the head injury, he or she may experience intrusive anxiety-provoking dreams and feelings of being overwhelmed and placed in mortal jeopardy, which severely disturb sleep. O'Shanick believes this phenomenon, encountered in the late PTA phase, supports the added diagnosis of post-traumatic stress syndrome.[25] Elements of the Klüver-Bucy syndrome, to be subsequently reviewed with temporal lobe syndromes, are also occasionally seen during the coma recovery period in TBI patients with severe DAI. Hyper-reactivity to internal and external stimulation—tactile, olfactory, and gustatory, as well as auditory and visual—is frequently noted. A patient may interpret a novel stimulus or person as painful or terrifying; he or she may scream, utter obscenities, become assaultive, or wander off, if ambulatory.[17] Rarely, a total lack of spontaneous activity at rest evolves into a hypervigilant, intensely hyperactive manic state only under stimulation.[6]

At this stage, psychological interventions, such as frequent verbal reorientation, provision of clocks, calendars, and familiar objects from home will improve the patient's returning information processing and adaptation to a new and disturbing environment. Increasing stimulation and activity will promote initiation in the hypoaroused patient.[31] Stimulant medication, amphetamine, methylphenidate, or pemoline, as well as dopamine agonists, such as bromocriptine, may be beneficial. Some of these patients may be more abulic (lacking spontaneity) and akinetic than somnolent and unmotivated; this post-traumatic parkinsonian state responds favorably to amantadine. The use of stimulant drugs entails some risk; patients may become irritable or agitated. Rebound depression may follow their discontinuation. The dosages should always be tapered slowly. Prescribed in usual doses, they do not apparently lower seizure threshold.[10,16] The reader is cautioned that pharmacologic intervention to improve recovery from TBI is still in its infancy. The human literature consists primarily of short-duration case studies and small open trials in heterogeneous groups. The use of single-subject long-term crossovers or traditional double-blind matched-group design is needed to ensure progress in the field.[17]

A reduced level of therapeutic interaction, with emphasis on correcting the attentional disturbance, however, will be required if the patient becomes hyperaroused and agitated. There is frequently an associated disturbance in sleep-wake cycles. To prevent excessive daytime sleep as well as daytime fatigue and confusion, a sedative in adequate doses should be administered at bedtime. Repeated doses must be avoided to prevent oversedation and hangovers.[19] Neuroleptics, such as parenteral haloperidol, are most commonly prescribed for acute agitation. They provide reliable short-term sedation, but are less effective for long-term use. Undesirable side effects include rigidity, akathisia, autonomic instability, neuroleptic malignant syndrome and probable retardation of cognitive recovery. Amantadine in moderate doses (100 to 400 mg/d) is a useful alternative; it is not sedating and promotes arousal, attention, and motor performance. Troublesome side effects, such as seizures and paradoxical excitement, are rare. Other alternatives to neuroleptics include carbamazepine, valproic acid, lithium, verapamil, naltrexone, or a β-blocker. Overall, none of these have worked reliably enough to achieve established primacy. A good result is unlikely in more than 40% of treated patients; nevertheless, in a given patient, one agent may work well when prescribed in judicious doses with careful monitoring. Benzodiazepines and anticholinergic antidepressants should generally be avoided.[10,17]

Medication for treatment of post-traumatic delirium has principally been targeted toward the dopaminergic and GABA-ergic systems. Van Woerkom et al. studied neurotransmitter function during the PTA period in patients with hyperactivity or excitability following diffuse injury or frontal-temporal contusion. The focally contused patients had lower levels of the serotonin metabolite, 5-hydroxyindoleacetic acid.[35] This finding, along with several recent clinical reports, suggests that agents potentiating central serotonin, such as trazodone, may more effectively decrease agitation and normalize sleep-wake cycles in post-traumatic delirium.[9,25] Although this disorder generally results from the primary effects of the injury on brain tissue, other aggravating factors must be searched for and, if possible, corrected. These include infections, anemia and coagulopathies, hypoxia, alcohol- or benzodiazepine-abstinence syndromes, medication side effects, vitamin and mineral deficiencies, fluid and electrolyte imbalance, hydrocephalus, inadequate pain relief, and sensory deprivation.[30,31]

With clearing of confusion and resolution of post-traumatic amnesia, patients enter the *stage of emerging independence,* stage V, comparable to Rancho Level VI.[2,19] They generally have increased awareness of their physical deficits and achieve a measure of independence in mobility and activities of daily living, which allow discharge from inpatient rehabilitation facilities. Their insight, however, into coexisting behavioral and cognitive deficits with their imposed social and vocational limitations is often severely compromised. Residual problems include reduced inhibition and monitoring of thoughts and behavior, leading to inappropriate social interactions. Modality-specific deficits from focal pathology, such as aphasia, can now be clearly recognized and treated. At this stage, a comprehensive neuropsychological assessment, addressing the patient's specific needs, should be considered. The final stage, stage VI, *intellectual/social competence,* which approximates Rancho Level VII, may be quite prolonged, up to 10 years in some cases with more severe diffuse injuries.[29] Recovery, often incomplete, of cognitive abilities, goal-directed behavior, and social skills characterizes this stage.

HYPOXIC-ISCHEMIC INJURY

The diagnosis of hypoxic-ischemic injury is primarily based on the clinical history, e.g., a documented respiratory arrest, prolonged and severe increased intracranial hypertension, or a hypotensive episode. The signs of hypoxic-ischemic injury may be similar to those seen with DAI, the two often occurring together. Hypoxic-ischemic injury may be diffuse or focal. Diffuse hypoxic-ischemic injury may be suspected when there is a more prolonged period of confusion than anticipated for a given length of coma. Hypoxic-ischemic injury is probably responsible for CHI patients who remain vegetative. The presence of persistent clinical signs, representing the effects of focal hypoxic-ischemic injury in certain predisposed locations, may establish the diagnosis. An infarction in the posterior cerebral artery territory, resulting from a mass lesion and uncal (temporal lobe) herniation, may present with hemianopia and visual perceptual deficits, including alexia and anomia. Persistent amnesia suggests hippocampal injury, and ataxia, cerebellar damage. Extrapyramidal movement disorders implicate the basal ganglia. A wide variety of neurobehavioral signs occur with vascular border zone lesions, including proximal weakness, transcortical aphasia, semantic anomia, visual-spatial disorders, modality-specific agnosia, and visual-motor dissociation (Balint's syndrome).[2,4]

FOCAL BRAIN CONTUSIONS

Focal brain contusions are typically seen in CHI. Although they may underlie the site or be linearly opposite the point of impact anywhere in the brain, they most frequently involve the anterior-inferior frontal lobes or the tips and inferior aspects of the temporal lobes. The lesions may be superficial, involving only the gyral crests, or may extend deeply into the white matter with associated edema, hemorrhage, and mass effect, possibly requiring surgical evacuation.[4] Lesion location and, especially, lesion depth determine the clinical consequences. Deeper unilateral lesions and bilateral lesions in homologous areas involve more cortical-cortical and cortical-subcortical pathways, leading to more diffuse long-term effects.[37] As a secondary pressure effect on the upper brainstem, a focal lesion may impair consciousness, followed by a period of confusion and amnesia. With the clearing of the attentional disorder, the specific and expected clinical effects of the lesion become apparent, The brain MRI is the most useful diagnostic tool for detection of focal contusions; smaller lesions, especially those adjacent to bone, may be missed on a computed tomographic scan.

Focal contusions predominantly injure prefrontal and anterior temporal areas, comprising paralimbic and multimodal association cortices and their subcortical connections. Higher-order cognitive and behavioral processes, including emotion and self-awareness, are impaired, generally sparing the more posteriorly represented language, perceptual, praxic, and sensorimotor functions. Typically seen are features of the frontal lobe syndrome. One or more deficits in executive function, cognitive processing, self-monitoring, and drive may predominant, depending on the locus of the frontal lesion and the often-associated DAI, which disrupts pathways to and from the prefrontal cortex. The orbital-frontal (pseudo-psychopathic) syndrome is behaviorally expressed as disinhibition, affective lability and hyperactivity, impulsivity, distractibility, antisocial behavior, sexual preoccupation without overt sexual aggression, impaired insight, and poor interpersonal judgment. An orbital-frontal lesion that extends posteriorly to the septal area may produce a profound persistent memory loss and motivational disorder. The frontal convexity (pseudoretarded) syndrome is behaviorally expressed as a lack of will (abulia), apathy, indifference, decreased initiative, psychomotor retardation, inflexibility, perseveration, and motor impersistence. Akinesia, sparse verbal output, and incontinence characterize the medial frontal syndrome, a less common consequence of TBI.[11,19]

Abulic patients with a convexity lesion may deny their disability (anosognosia). They often get stuck in a cognitive rut, preferring simple tasks and unchanging rules as well as environmental structure and predictability. There may be associated parkinsonian signs, accounting for successful treatment with the dopamine agonist drug amantadine.[17] In contrast, the disinhibited orbital-frontal patient may exhibit a compulsion to joke (witzelsucht); this impulsive behavior may take the form of lewd talk, promiscuous behavior, substance abuse, and increased risk taking such as reckless driving, leading to arrest and other legal difficulties. Although not usually as violent as patients with temporal lobe injury, the frontal patient may lose self-control and become assaultive, especially when stressed or under the influence of alcohol or benzodiazepines. Clinically, a mixture of these syndromes is more common than any one of them. All are characterized by inability to plan, limited insight into the nature of their disability, unrealistic ambition, and poor judgment. Other features include an inability to appreciate the effects of one's remarks or behavior on others, inattention to personal appearance and hygiene, and a loss of social graces, e.g., eating manners.[2,30,33,34]

The temporolimbic syndromes frequently associated with temporal lobe contusions are even more variable than the frontal lobe syndromes.[17] Lesions in different regions with specialized functions may produce corresponding deficits in receptive language, memory, high-level sensory integration, as well as emotional regulation and expression. The predominantly temporal lobe amnestic, aphasic, and behavioral disorders, including those characterized as chronic affective and aggressive disturbances, will be subsequently reviewed under late neurobehavioral effects of CHI. Personality disorders induced by temporal lobe injury may be primary or secondary to complex partial seizures. In its most extreme form, bilateral extensive temporal damage produces the Klüver-Bucy syndrome, identified in the coma recovery stage by apathy, visual and tactile agnosia, prosopagnosia (impaired recognition of familiar faces), oral exploration with bulimia-hyperphagia, hypersexuality or altered sexual behavior, aphasia, dementia, and amnesia.[24] These symptoms contrast with the personality disturbance associated with the later emergence of complex partial seizures. Excessive talkativeness, circumstantiality, viscosity, hypergraphia, hyposexuality, and uncharacteristic philosophical and religious interests have been attributed to chronic limbic hyperexcitability.[12]

Gerstenbrand et al.[14] reported the clinical features of partial or complete Klüver-Bucy syndrome in 30 patients recovering from a post-traumatic apallic state, corresponding to Rancho stage III and Alexander's stage II—unresponsive vigilance. In the Klüver-Bucy syndrome prestage, the patient does not perceive or react to the environment but exhibits spontaneous motor activity–mass movements, stereotyped chewing and sucking automatisms, unidirectional grasping movements, and play-like genital manipulation. In the subsequent full-stage Klüver-Bucy syndrome, there is no evidence of higher cortical function, but the primitive movement patterns change into object-directed movements. The patient shows extreme distractibility and impulsively attends to and grasps every object in sight, taking them to the mouth. Objects, however, are not recognized; memory and learning are absent. There is often associated bulimia, continued autosexual behavior without shame, loss of fear, and euphoric mood.

In the Klüver-Bucy remission stage, the primitive motor patterns normalize but remain compulsive and meaningless to the patient. For example, the examiner's hand may be raised to the mouth imitating a kiss. The hypersexuality becomes more object directed, with reduced masturbation. There is generally a friendly euphoric mood with increased suggestibility; less frequently, the mood may be dysphoric and irritable, with sham-like rage outbursts when their actions are inhibited. Remnants of the complete syndrome, seen during the 1-year follow-up, included altered sexual behavior and an affective disorder, either placidity or irritability.[14] Treatment of the Klüver-Bucy syndrome with carbamazepine is occasionally successful.[17]

CONCLUSION

In summary, this chapter has stressed the role of precise neurologic diagnosis in the postacute period following moderate to severe TBI. The primary pathophysiologic processes—DAI, hypoxic-ischemic injury, and focal frontal-temporal contusion—are described and causally related to the neurobehavioral disturbances characteristically seen during each of the early stages of recovery. Existing management principles and strategies, both behavioral and pharmacologic, are critically assessed. Finally, the biopsychosocial determinants of injury and of recovery are reviewed to improve estimates of outcome following TBI.

REFERENCES

1. Adams JH, Graham DI, Murray LS, Scott G: Diffuse axonal injury due to nonmissile head injury in humans: An analysis of 45 cases. Ann Neurol 12:564–574, 1982.
2. Alexander MP: Traumatic brain injury. In Benson DF, Blumer D (eds): Psychiatric Aspects of Neurologic Disease, vol 2. New York, McGraw-Hill, 1982, pp 251–278.
3. Alexander MP: The role of neurobehavioral syndromes on the rehabilitation and outcome of closed head injury. In Levin HS, Grafman J, Eisenberg HM (eds): Neurobehavioral Recovery from Head Injury. New York, Oxford University Press, 1987, pp 191–205.
4. Alexander MP: Some neurobehavioral aspects of closed head injury. In Mueller J (ed): Neurology and Psychiatry: A Meeting of Minds. Basel, Karger, 1989, pp 175–191.
5. Blumbergs PC, Jones NR, North JB: Diffuse axonal injury in head trauma. J Neurol Neurosurg Psychiatry 52:838–841, 1989.
6. Backhine S, Lacomblez L, Benoit N, et al: Manic-like state after bilateral orbitalfrontal and right temporoparietal injury: Efficacy of clonidine. Neurology 39:777–781, 1989.
7. Blumer D, Benson DF: Personality changes with frontal and temporal lobe lesions. In Benson DF, Blumer D (eds): Psychiatric Aspects of Neurologic Disease. New York, Grune & Stratton, 1975, pp 151–170.
8. Bontke CF, Boake C: Traumatic brain injury rehabilitation. Neurosurg Clin North Am 2:473–482, 1991.
9. Cassidy JW: Pharmacological treatment of post-traumatic behavioral disorders: Aggression and disorders of mood. In Wood RLI (ed): Neuro-Behavioral Sequelae of Traumatic Brain Injury. London, Lawrence Erlbaum, 1990, pp 219–247.
10. Cope DN: Pharmacology for behavioral deficits: Disorders of cognition and affect. In Wood RLI (ed): Neuro-Behavioral Sequelae of Traumatic Brain Injury. London, Lawrence Erlbaum, 1990, pp 248–274.
11. Cummings JL: Behavioral disorders associated with frontal lobe injury. In Cummings JL (ed): Clinical Neuropsychiatry. Orlando, FL, Grune & Stratton, 1985.
12. Eames P: Organic bases of behavioral disorders after traumatic brain injury. In Wood RLI (ed): Neuro-Behavioral Sequelae of Traumatic Brain Injury. London, Lawrence Erlbaum, 1990, pp 133–152.
13. Gennarelli TA, Thibault LE, Adams JH, et al: Diffuse axonal injury and traumatic coma in the primate. Ann Neurol 12:564–574, 1982.
14. Gerstenbrand F, Poewe W, Aichner F, et al: Klüver-Bucy syndrome in man: Experiences with post-traumatic cases. Neurosci Biobehav Rev 7:413–417, 1983.
15. Godersky JC, Gentry LR, Tranel D, et al: Magnetic resonance imaging and neurobehavioral outcome in traumatic brain injury. Acta Neurochir Suppl (Wien) 51:311–314, 1990.
16. Gualtieri CT, Evans RW: Stimulant treatment for the neurobehavioral sequelae of traumatic brain injury. Brain Inj 2:273–290, 1988.
17. Gualtieri CT: The neuropsychiatric sequelae of traumatic brain injury. In Gualtieri CT (ed): Neuropsychiatry and Behavioral Pharmacology. New York, Springer-Verlag, 1991, pp 1–25.
18. Hagen C, Malkmus D, Durham P: Levels of cognitive functioning. In Rehabilitation of the Head Injured Adult. Downey, CA, Rancho Los Amigos Professional Staff Association, 1979, p 27.
19. Katz DI, Alexander MP: Neurologic diagnosis and treatment planning. In Deutsch PM, Fralish KB (eds): Innovations in Head Injury Rehabilitation. New York, Bender, 1990.
20. Kowatch RA: Sleep and head injury. Psychiatr Med 7:37–41, 1989.
21. Langfitt TW, Obrist WD, Alavi A, et al: Regional structure and function in head-injured patients: Correlation of CT, MRI, PET, CBF and neuropsychological assessment. In Levin HS, Grafman J, Eisenberg HM (eds): Neurobehavioral Recovery from Head Injury. New York, Oxford, 1987, pp 30–42.
22. Levin HS, et al: Magnetic resonance imaging after diffuse nonmissile head injury. Arch Neurol 42:963–968, 1985.

23. Levin HS, Eisenberg HM: Management of head injury—Neurobehavioral outcome. Neurosurg Clin North Am 2:457–471, 1991.
24. Lilly R, Cummings JL, Benson DF, et al: The human Klüver-Bucy syndrome. Neurology 33:1141–1145, 1983.
25. O'Shanick GJ: Closed head injury. In Michels R, Cavenar JO Jr, Cooper AM, et al (eds): Psychiatry. Philadelphia, JB Lippincott, 1988.
26. Prigatano GP, Stahl ML, Orr WC, et al: Sleep and dreaming disturbances in closed head injury patients. J Neurol Neurosurg Psychiatry 45:78–80, 1982.
27. Ruff RM, Buchsbaum MS, Troster AI, et al: Computerized tomography, neuropsychology and positron emission tomography in the evaluation of head injury. Neuropsychiatr Neuropsychol Behav Neurol 2:103–123, 1989.
28. Ruff RM, Marshall LF, Klauber MR, et al: Alcohol abuse and neurological outcome of the severely head injured. J Head Trauma Rehab 5:21–31, 1990.
29. Sbordone RJ: Overcoming obstacles in cognitive rehabilitation of persons with severe traumatic brain injury. In Kreutzer JS, Wehman PH (eds): Cognitive Rehabilitation for Persons with Traumatic Brain Injury. Baltimore, Paul H. Brookes, 1991, pp 105–116.
30. Silver JM, Hales RE, Yudofsky SC: Neuropsychiatric aspects of traumatic brain injury. In Yudofsky SC, Hales RE (eds): Textbook of Neuropsychiatry, 2nd ed. Washington, American Psychiatric Press, 1992, pp 363–396.
31. Slagle DA: Psychiatric disorders following closed head injury: An overview of biopsychosocial factors in their etiology and management. Int J Psychiatr Med 20:1–35, 1990.
32. Sparadeo FR, Gill D: Effects of prior alcohol use on head injury recovery. J Head Trauma Rehabil 4:75–82, 1989.
33. Stuss DT: Contributions of frontal lobe injury to cognitive impairment after closed head injury: Methods of assessment and recent findings. In Levin HS, Grafman J, Eisenberg HM (eds): Neurobehavioral Recovery from Head Injury. New York, Oxford, 1987, pp 166–177.
34. Stuss DT, Benson DF: The Frontal Lobes. New York, Raven Press, 1986.
35. Van Woerkom T, Teelken A, Minderhoud J: Difference in neurotransmitter metabolism in frontotemporal lobe contusion and diffuse cerebral contusion. Lancet i:812–813, 1977.
36. Varney NR: Prognostic significance of anosmia in patients with closed head injury. J Clin Exp Neuropsychol 10:250–254, 1988.
37. Wilson JTL: The relationship between neuropsychological function and brain damage detected by neuroimaging after closed head injury. Brain Inj 4:349–363, 1990.
38. Wilson JTL, Wiedmann KD, Hadley DM, et al: Early and late magnetic resonance imaging and neuropsychological outcome after head injury. J Neurol Neurosurg Psychiatry 51:391–396, 1988.

RONALD E. SAUL, MD

NEUROBEHAVIORAL DISORDERS FOLLOWING TRAUMATIC BRAIN INJURY

Part II. Late Neurobehavioral Sequelae

From the
Department of Neurology
UCLA School of Medicine
Los Angeles, California
and
Adult Brain Injury Service
Rancho Los Amigos Medical
    Center
Downey, California

Correspondence to:
Ronald E. Saul, MD
550 N. Brand Boulevard, Suite 700
Glendale, CA 91230

In patients with moderate to severe traumatic brain injury (TBI), disabling cognitive and behavioral problems often develop or become apparent some months or even a year or more after the trauma. These probably reflect unique pathophysiological processes set in motion at the time of the injury. Often insidious in onset, these neurobehavioral sequelae may be overlooked and go untreated (Table 1).[12]

COGNITIVE IMPAIRMENT

Among the most persistent and disruptive alterations in the later recovery stages following closed-head injury (CHI) are changes affecting attention, information processing, and memory and language, the basic elements of cognition. Attention can be divided into a number of component processes, some of which are regularly compromised by TBI. Clinicians frequently observe that TBI patients are highly distractible and have difficulty sustaining attention, which in turn contributes to the apparent memory deficit characteristic of the confusional stage of recovery. Reduced attentional capacity can secondarily reduce language comprehension and visual-spatial processing, because the patient's already slowed rate of information processing is limited to relatively small units. The inability to divide attention can compromise the patient's ability to attend simultaneously to task instructions and monitor his or her own performance. Similarly, impulsivity and perseveration may

PHYSICAL MEDICINE AND REHABILITATION: State of the Art Reviews—
Vol. 7, No. 3, October 1993. Philadelphia, Hanley & Belfus, Inc.

593

TABLE 1. Late Neurobehavioral Sequelae of TBI

Cognitive impairment	Affective disorders
Attention deficits	Depression
Anterograde and retrograde memory deficits	Mania
Impaired awareness of interpersonal situations	Other late complications
Language and communication disorders	Anxiety and panic disorders
Perceptual-motor deficits	Post-traumatic stress disorder
Aggression	Acquired obsessive-compulsive disorder
Psychosis	Changes in sexual behavior
	Alzheimer's disease (?)

reflect a loss of frontal goal-directed control over attention, which is easily pulled to irrelevant aspects of a task.[18,21,45]

Regarding which deficits are most likely to become permanent, neuropsychological studies have yielded variable results.[42] There is general agreement, however, that slowed information processing and disturbed maintenance of vigilance over long intervals remain impaired in the more severe cases. The role of behavioral modification and medication in treating attentional disorders is unclear. Stimulants have been used to increase alertness and reduce distractability. It is well recognized that other medications, e.g., anticonvulsants (phenobarbital and primidone), antihypertensives (methyldopa and propranolol), and antispasticity agents (diazepam, baclofen, and dantrolene) may impair arousal and attention. These drugs should be withdrawn or replaced with less sedating alternatives, e.g., carbamazepine, atenolol, hydrochlorothiazide, and phenol nerve blocks.[45]

TBI frequently results in a combination of anterograde and retrograde memory deficits. After recovery from the confusional state in moderate to severe CHI, the interval of anterograde–post-traumatic amnesia remains a gap in the patient's memory, except for preserved islands of memory. Retrograde amnesia, the period prior to injury for which the patient has no recollection, is usually briefer than the period of post-traumatic amnesia and, over time, parallel with the resolution of post-traumatic amnesia, shrinking to a few minutes preceding impact. Immediate (short-term) memory is generally preserved in TBI following emergence from the confusional state. Recent (long-term) memory and new learning on both verbal and visual tasks frequently remain impaired, despite adequate recovery of intellectual ability, in survivors of moderate or severe CHI.[3,18,21] Memory-augmenting drugs, drills, and computer-driven exercises are of questionable therapeutic value, but diaries and other compensatory measures may be useful.[45]

In addition to attentional and memory impairment, patients often have difficulty organizing thoughts and interpreting interpersonal situations, leading to paranoid suspiciousness and misunderstanding of intentions. Furthermore, they frequently fail to acknowledge deficits produced by the injury or, if acknowledged, minimize their severity, resulting in an impaired capacity for formulating goals and realistic plans. This lack of knowledge of one's cognitive processes, also called metacognition, is related to the severity of the injury and is typically associated with frontal lobe lesions.[10] A study of behavioral competency in 53 TBI patients showed a lack of correlation between impaired awareness and either neuropsychological test results or specific brain lesion sites; however, with more widespread lesions, there was a greater probability of awareness being impaired.[28]

There are two major approaches for dealing with cognitive impairment in TBI patients. The first, referred to as cognitive retraining, directly treats primary impairments, e.g., memory, by reducing them or restoring them to premorbid levels through practice or instruction in compensatory strategies. The principal support for this approach comes from encouraging results in several well-conducted individual case studies; however, results based on group studies have been modest and equivocal. The second, or functional, approach attempts to alleviate or circumvent the impact of cognitive deficits on everyday activities. For example, the emphasis may be placed on acquiring knowledge needed in the work domain. This approach has proven more successful than cognitive retraining.[19] Controversial issues in cognitive rehabilitation were recently reviewed by Berrol et al.[2]

Depending on the site and extent of pathology, language and communication disorders following closed TBI may take many forms. Classical aphasia is typically rare and usually the result of a left frontal-temporal mass lesion, but linguistic disturbances can frequently be demonstrated during the early stages of recovery. Hagen[14] attributes the preponderance of irrelevant, confabulatory, circumlocutory, and tangential responses of these patients to the disordered thought processes of the confusional state. They retain basic phonologic, syntactic, and semantic skills and thus may be characterized as showing communicative incompetence but good linguistic skills. Studies of long-term recovery of language after severe CHI indicate that two-thirds of the patients fully recover or show only residual anomia, whereas severe aphasia accompanied by global cognitive impairment persists in the remaining one-third. Anomic aphasia, defined as a word-finding or object-naming disorder accompanied by semantic errors, circumlocution, and concretism, is the most common disturbance after resolution of post-traumatic amnesia. Left frontal lesions will reduce verbal fluency, and dominant parietal lesions may produce agraphia, alexia, and acalculia along with anomia.

The most common nonaphasic speech disorder is dsyarthria, which can range from a mild articulatory deficit to nearly unintelligible but linguistically correct speech.[18,21] Other nonaphasic language disorders include talkativeness, peculiar phraseology, and socially inappropriate verbal communication with uninhibited use of four-letter expletives.[29] Expressive or receptive dysprosody, an impairment of the melody, cadence, and affective coloring of speech, can follow right hemispheric lesions. In the majority of CHI patients, basic functional communication skills recover in 6 months. The patient may appear normal to the casual observer, but communication problems frequently emerge and interfere with reentry in the more challenging school or work setting. Early referral to the rehabilitative team speech-language pathologist is advisable to facilitate recovery of communicative skills, teach compensatory techniques, and prevent secondary emotional disturbances.[21,42,45]

Although the effects of TBI on perceptual-motor skills have been considered minor, recent studies have documented that perceptual deficits occur with an unexpectedly high frequency. Impairment on complex visuoperceptive tasks, such as recognition of faces and embedded figures, occurs more frequently with right parietal-temporal lesions. CHI patients also showed a significant impairment in perception and memory of facial affect, which contributes to the occurrence of socially inappropriate behavior after severe head injury. Visuospatial disorders, such as hemineglect and visuoconstructive disorders, manifested, for example, by defective copying of designs, occur with involvement of parietal cortex. Rarely, prosopagnosia, the inability to recognize familiar faces, follows bilateral or extensive right inferior occipitotemporal lesions. DAI may also produce a disconnection syndrome by disrupting callosal pathways. Impaired interhemispheric transfer of auditory, tactile, and motor information has been documented. Levin found callosal atrophy in survivors of moderate to severe CHI.[18,20,21] These disorders have functional consequences in many areas of activities of daily living, such as dressing, grooming, meal preparation and eating, ambulation, driving, manual assembly tasks, and writing.

AGGRESSION

CHI patients frequently exhibit an excess of emotional expression in the form of uncontrolled rage attacks, sudden mood changes (emotional lability), or unprovoked crying or laughing (emotional incontinence).[12] After aphasia, such disturbances, in particular, irritability and aggression, are the most common manifestations of temporal lobe injury, with a 70% incidence in the first year after CHI. Irritability and loss of temper persist for 10 to 15 years after severe injury. Silver et al.[33] summarize the specific critical features of organic aggressive syndrome following brain injury, which allows its differentiation from long-standing personality and related psychiatric disorders. The persistent or recurrent outbursts, whether verbal or physical, are out of proportion to the precipitating stress or provocation. They are explosive, not gradual in buildup, and triggered by trivial or modest stimuli. The aggression is nonpurposeful and periodic, with brief outbursts separated by long calm periods. Furthermore, patients are upset and embarrassed, rather than blaming others or justifying their behavior.[33]

Treatment of any underlying medical illness or associated attentional, cognitive, affective, and epileptic disorder should be implemented before the use of specific measures for aggression. Behavioral therapy should be the first line of treatment. Provision of structure and routine in all activities as well as a calm nonthreatening environment, alternation of activity and rest periods, and cautious use of mechanical restraints are helpful measures.[23] Appropriate behaviors should be positively reinforced with credits or tokens and direct or indirect reinforcement for inappropriate behaviors removed.[12] Referral to a neurobehavioral program for stays of 1 month up to a year or more may be necessary in severe cases to gain control over physical aggression and gross social inappropriateness. A detailed account of behavioral approaches in management is beyond the scope of this chapter; the reader is referred to the critical reviews by Wood and Cope.[47,48]

Psychopharmacologic agents may be quite effective in the treatment of aggression and other neurobehavioral disorders. TBI patients, compared to those with an intact brain, however, are often more sensitive to both drug therapeutic and side effects. Because of the sedative and anticholinergic side effects of thioridazine, amitryptyline, and related compounds, the initial dose administered must be lower and the dose raised and lowered in small increments over protracted time periods. In addition, psychotropic medication affects the seizure threshold. Of the antipsychotics, molindone and fluphenazine have the lowest potential, and clozapine, probably one of the highest, for seizure induction. A higher incidence has also been attributed to the antidepressants maprotiline and bupropion. Seizure occurrence with tricyclic antidepressants is related to greater severity of brain injury. Usually, seizure control can be maintained with cautious drug administration and use of a concomitant effective anticonvulsant regimen.[33]

Before embarking on a therapy program for violent behavior, a method for documenting aggressive fluctuations over time in response to interventions is mandatory. The Overt Aggression Scale has proven validity and reliability for this purpose.[49] The use of many of these drugs must be time-limited to avoid seriously disabling side effects, ranging from oversedation to tardive dyskinesia. Antipsychotics, such as haloperidol, are most commonly used for acute aggressive episodes, but chronic administration should be avoided because of the risks of extrapyramidal side effects, of developing tolerance, and of increasing agitation from frequently unrecognized akathisia. Silver et al.[33] recommend the use of haloperidol only for management of brief aggressive episodes or of aggression resulting from psychotic ideation. It is initially given in a dose of 1 mg orally or 0.5 mg intravenously or intramuscularly every hour until control is achieved, then 2 mg orally or 1 mg intravenously or intramuscularly every 8 hours. After 48 hours of control, the dose should be tapered; patients should not remain on haloperidol longer than 6 weeks unless they have associated psychosis.

The sedative properties of the benzodiazepines may also be helpful in acute management, although there are reports of increased hostility and paradoxical induction of rage. Lorazepam is given initially as a dose of 1 to 2 mg orally or intramuscularly, repeating every hour if necessary until control is achieved and maintaining at 2 mg orally or intramuscularly three times a day. It should also be tapered if the patient remains calm over 48 hours. Lorazepam may be used in combination with haloperidol. Clonazepam may be effective when anxiety is also present. Long-term use of benzodiazepines must be avoided, as they will predictably interfere with memory and new learning, thereby delaying recovery.[4,33]

Various agents have proven merit in the treatment of chronic aggression. Of the antidepressants, amitryptyline and trazodone have been effective in several open studies.[25,27,35] Preliminary reports[37,38] describe the use of fluoxetine, a potent serotonergic antidepressant; it must be started with a lower-than-standard dose, 5 mg/d, and cautiously increased as tolerated. Because of its potential for neurotoxicity, lithium should be used only when the aggression is related to a manic or cyclic mood disorder. Carbamazepine can be highly effective, particularly for patients who have aggressive episodes and seizures or epileptic foci. The potential risk, however, of bone marrow suppression and hepatotoxicity requires periodic monitoring with blood-platelet counts and liver function tests. The anticonvulsant valproic acid may also be useful. The effects of buspirone are less predictable, but it has proven useful in some patients.[22] Other drugs useful for sedation include paraldehyde, chloral hydrate, and diphenhydramine.

There is a vast literature on the use of β-blockers, which have documented effectiveness in patients unsuccessfully treated with the agents described above. Those most thoroughly investigated include propranolol, nadolol, pindolol, and metoprolol. Because of the considerable time needed to titrate the drug upward and to determine its effectiveness as well as its significant hypotension, the use of propranolol has waned, and the above drugs have substituted. For once-a-day use, propranolol and nadolol are available in long-acting forms. The use of β-blockers requires a thorough medical evaluation. They cannot be used in patients with bronchial asthma, chronic obstructive pulmonary disease, insulin-dependent diabetes, hyperthyroidism, persistent angina, congestive heart failure, and peripheral vascular disease. Propranolol is generally started at a dose of 20 mg three times a day and slowly increased, while pulse rate and blood pressure are monitored, until aggression is controlled.[4,33]

AFFECTIVE DISORDERS

Affective disorders are quite common in the months following TBI. Reported rates vary from 10 to 77% for depression following severe TBI. Sadness is common, as patients describe the loss of their former self, reflecting awareness of cognitive and motor deficits. Psychiatric evaluation is often necessary to differentiate such grief reactions from major depression; patients with depressed mood also may not experience the associated somatic symptoms required for the diagnosis of major depression. In some cases, the injury itself is the direct result of severe depression, leading to substance abuse and risk taking, if not suicidal behavior. Silver et al.[33,34] hypothesize that there may be two types of depressive syndromes after TBI. The first group of patients, with reactive neurotransmitter receptor changes, are more irritable with positive symptoms and respond to antidepressants. The second have more severe injuries, with decreased neurotransmitters, leading to anhedonia, withdrawal and apathy; they preferentially respond to agonists, such as amantidine or stimulants.[33,34]

The diagnosis of depression also may be complicated by regional damage masking the expression of affective disturbance. Dysprosodic speech associated with right temporal-parietal lesions may interfere with the expression of the expected affect.[31] The lack of a depressive appearance may lead the examiner to overlook neurovegetative symptoms. Patients with aphasia cannot provide important historical information. Affective disorder often must be inferred from poor cooperation with rehabilitation, an apparent deterioration of a previously stable neurologic deficit or unusually slow recovery. In the absence of pseudobulbar palsy, excessive crying may be a helpful clue.[36] TBI increases the risk of depression over the basal rate of the general population by a factor of 5 or 10. There is also increased risk of suicide following TBI. Consequently, a high index of clinical suspicion, even with ambiguous objective signs, warrants a trial of antidepressants with careful monitoring of target symptoms.[12]

Relief of depressive symptoms with tricyclic antidepressants or carbamazepine has been reported by Varney.[43] The choice of antidepressant depends on the desired side-effect profile; those agents with the lowest incidence of sedative, hypotensive and anticholinergic side effects are preferred. Silver et al.[33,34] recommend nortriptyline (initial dose, 10 mg/d) or desipramine (initial dose, 10 mg three times a day) and careful plasma monitoring to achieve therapeutic levels. The dosage should be reduced if side effects appear. Fluoxetine has no anticholinergic effects, but some patients become sedated during treatment, and others experience restlessness and insomnia. There is also a role for stimulants and nondominant unilateral electroconvulsive therapy in intractable patients, especially those who cannot tolerate antidepressants.[13,33,36]

There has been increasing interest in manic and bipolar disorders after TBI, although they occur much less frequently than depression. They may present as pressured speech, flight of ideas, assaultive behavior, sleeplessness, grandiosity, distractability, hyperactivity, hypersexuality, and impaired insight and judgment. Irritability is more common than euphoric mood.[6,30,32,36] Starkstein et al.[39,40] reported on a series of patients who developed secondary mania after brain insults of varying etiology involving the right basotemporal and right orbital-frontal regions. In three of the eight patients studied with positron emission tomography, cerebral hypometabolism was found in the right basotemporal region. Cummings and Mendez,[8] in a study of vascular cases, maintain that diencephalic lesions are more commonly found. These manic disorders generally respond to lithium for mood stabilization and to neuroleptics, as needed, for psychotic thought disorder. Patients with cognitive deficits, however, are susceptible to the adverse CNS effects of lithium. Carbamazepine is a reasonable alternative. There have been isolated reports of successful treatment of post-traumatic bipolar disorder in patients who responded to combined lithium and carbamazepine therapy, to valproate, or to lorazepam following a failed response to lithium alone.[14,33,36]

PSYCHOSIS

Late-onset psychosis is unquestionably a severe and devastating outcome of TBI. Psychosis may develop in patients with a clear sensorium, after the coma recovery stage but within months of coma recovery. Gualtieri[13] cites cases developing abruptly as late as 3 years after injury. He suspects a prevalence rate for delayed onset psychosis as high as 5% following moderate and 10% after severe TBI. The schizophrenic-like symptoms after TBI may be indistinguishable from those of the naturally occurring disorder. Up to 15% of schizophrenic inpatients have a history of brain injury.[33] Systematized delusions involving referential thought, persecutory belief, jealousy, and fears of illness and death are related to the general cognitive functioning of the patient and have been associated with etiologically diverse lesions in basal ganglia, thalamus, and limbic structures.[7] When there is no history of prior thought disorder and the psychosis is limited to such positive symptoms as delusions and hallucinations, the diagnosis of organic delusional syndrome or organic hallucinosis is appropriate. The presence of predominantly negative symptoms, such as affective blunting, apathy, social withdrawal, and intellectual impairment justifies criteria for dementia or organic personality syndrome. In TBI patients, positive symptoms, however, may occur without the eventual development of negative symptoms, and negative symptoms may be present without positive symptoms. An imprecise and mixed clinical picture, which does not meet DSM-IIIR criteria for any specific organic disorder, is frequently seen.[12] Studies of treatment are scarce. Psychiatric consultation and the careful use of neuroleptics at the lowest effective dose is recommended.

Post-traumatic epilepsy, especially when limbic in origin, is associated with psychosis in about 7% of cases. The psychosis can be either brief or persistent, is most commonly paranoid in content, and often occurs in a state of clear consciousness. Atypical features characteristically seen in epileptic psychosis include precipitous onset, confusion and agitation, rapid fluctuations in mood with intense affect, and an intermittent course with symptom-free intervals. Suicidal ideation and suicide attempts constitute a major management risk. Attempts at classifying such psychoses emphasize level of consciousness and whether events occurred in close approximation to a well-defined epileptic attack. Delineation, however, is difficult because patients are frequently unaware of having seizures. Unusual spells, varying in duration from minutes to days, and consisting of uncharacteristic behavior, accompanied by marked lability of affect, depression, mania, delusions, and hallucinations, may occur in repetitive stereotyped episodes. It is not clear whether these are real seizures, but anticonvulsive treatment with carbamazepine, dilantin, and valproate has been effective.[24,26,41]

OTHER LATE COMPLICATIONS

Severe anxiety and panic disorders have been reported after TBI, persisting as long as 5 years. Patients are also at increased risk of developing post-traumatic stress disorder, with typical symptoms of social withdrawal, re-experiencing the traumatic event (flashback) and autonomic hyperactivity.[10] Rare cases of acquired obsessive-compulsive disorder have also been described.[9,16] Changes in sexual behavior frequently occur following TBI. Both increased and decreased sexual activity as well as preoccupation and disinterest have been reported. Kreutzer and Zasler,[17] however, in a study of 21 male patients, found predominantly negative changes: decreased sex drive, self-confidence, erectile function, and frequency of intercourse. Family members, in particular wives and mothers, of male patients often describe associated adverse behavioral changes: increased dependency, impatience and irritability, childishness, and temper tantrums with verbal and physical aggression directed at caretakers.[17] Two cases of Kleine-Levin syndrome, apparently responsive to lithium, have recently been reported. The onset of symptoms, alternating hypersomnia and hyperphagia, was temporally related to the head injury.[46]

Several studies suggest that Alzheimer's disease should be placed among the long-term sequelae of TBI,[1,11] although others dispute a relationship.[5] Henderson[15] reported that 15% of probable Alzheimer's patients had a previous history of TBI, compared with 3% of control subjects. Those patients who were 60 years of age or older or who had a severe injury, multiple head injuries, or concurrent illness such as alcoholism were at higher risk for development of post-traumatic dementia.[44] Gualtieri maintains that a patient who has sustained a severe brain injury is four or five times likelier to develop a late-life dementia and that it generally will arise at an earlier age.[12]

CONCLUSIONS

This chapter has summarized the late neurobehavioral sequelae of moderate to severe TBI. A coordinated diagnostic evaluation of neurologic, cognitive, affective, and behavioral disturbances by the rehabilitation team is essential for appropriate management. Treatment measures will generally include both behavioral approaches and pharmacotherapy. When individually tailored to each patient's unique circumstances and symptoms, the patient's capacity for recovery can be maximized.

Acknowledgment

The author thanks D. Frank Benson for reviewing the early chapter drafts and providing helpful suggestions.

REFERENCES

1. Amaducci LA, Fratiglioni L, Rocca WA, et al: Risk factors for clinically diagnosed Alzheimer's disease: A case control study of an Italian population. Neurology 36:922–931, 1986.
2. Berrol S, Volpe BT, McDowell FH, et al: Controversies in neurology: Issues in cognitive rehabilitation. Arch Neurol 47:219–224, 1990.
3. Brooks DN: Cognitive deficits. In Rosenthal M, Griffith ER, Bond MR, et al (eds): Rehabilitation of the Adult and Child with Traumatic Brain Injury. Philadelphia, FA Davis, 1990, pp 163–178.
4. Cassidy JW: Pharmacological treatment of post-traumatic behavioral disorders: Aggression and disorders of mood. In Wood RLI (ed): Neuro-Behavioral Sequelae of Traumatic Brain Injury. London, Lawrence Erlbaum, 1990, pp 219–247.
5. Chandra V, Kokmen E, Schoenberg BS, et al: Head trauma with loss of consciousness as a risk factor for Alzheimer's disease. Neurology 39:1576–1578, 1989.
6. Clark AF, Davison K: Mania following head injury: A report of two cases and a review of the literature. Br J Psychiatry 150:841–844, 1987.
7. Cummings JL: Organic psychoses: Delusional disorders and secondary mania. Psychiatr Clin North Am 9:293–308, 1986.
8. Cummings JL, Mendez MF: Secondary mania with focal cerebrovascular lesions. Am J Psychiatry 141:1084–1087, 1984.
9. Drummond LM, Gravestock S: Delayed emergence of obsessive-compulsive neurosis following head injury: Case report and review of its theoretical implications. Br J Psychiatry 153:839–842, 1988.

10. Goldstein FC, Levin HS: Manifestations of personality change after closed head injury. In Perecman E (ed): Integrating Theory and Practice in Clinical Neuropsychology. London, Lawrence Erlbaum, 1989, pp 217–243.

11. Graves AB, White E, Koepsell TD, et al: The association between head trauma and Alzheimer's disease. Am J Epidemiol 131:491–501, 1990.

12. Gualtieri T: The delayed neurobehavioral sequelae of traumatic brain injury. In Gualtieri T (ed): Neuropsychiatry and Behavioral Pharmacology. New York, Springer-Verlag, 1991, pp 26–36.

13. Gualtieri T: The psychopharmacology of traumatic brain injury. In Gualtieri T (ed): Neuropsychiatry and Behavioral Pharmacology. New York, Springer-Verlag, 1991, pp 37–88.

14. Hagen C: Language disorders in head trauma. In Holland A (ed): Language Disorders in Adults. San Diego, College Hill Press, 1983.

15. Henderson AS: The epidemiology of Alzheimer's disease. Br Med Bull 42:3–10, 1986.

16. Jenike MA, Brandon AD: Obsessive-compulsive disorder and head trauma: A rare association. J Anxiety Dis 2:353–359, 1988.

17. Kreutzer J, Zasler ND: Psychosexual consequences of traumatic brain injury: Methodology and preliminary findings. Brain Inj 3:177–186, 1989.

18. Levin HS: Outcome after head injury. Part II: Neurobehavioral recovery. In Becker DP, Povlishock JT (eds): Central Nervous System Trauma Report—1985. Washington, DC, National Institute of Neurological and Communicative Disorders and Stroke, 1985, pp 281–302.

19. Levin HS, Dikmen SS, McLean A: Long-term sequelae of head injury. Curr Opin Neurol Neurosurg 3:722–728, 1990.

20. Levin HS, Eisenberg HM: Management of head injury—Neurobehavioral outcome. Neurosurg Clin North Am 2:457–471, 1991.

21. Levin HS, Goldstein FC: Neurobehavioral aspects of traumatic brain injury. In Bach Y Rita P (ed): Traumatic Brain Injury. New York, Demos, 1989, pp 53–72.

22. Levine AM: Buspirone and agitation in head injury. Brain Inj 2:165–167, 1988.

23. Ludwig BI: Conference summary: Psychopharmacological management of the difficult patient. J Neurol Rehabil 3:147–149, 1989.

24. Monroe RR: Limbic ictus and atypical psychoses. J Nerv Ment Dis 170:711–716, 1982.

25. Mysiw WJ, Jackson RD, Corrigan JD: Amitryptyline for post-traumatic agitation. Am J Phys Med Rehabil 67:29–33, 1988.

26. Neppe VM, Tucker GJ: Neuropsychiatric aspects of seizure disorders. In Yudofsky SC, Hales RE (eds): Textbook of Neuropsychiatry, 2nd ed. Washington, DC, American Psychiatric Press, 1992, pp 397–426.

27. Pinner E, Rich CL: Effects of trazodone on aggressive behavior in seven patients with organic mental disorders. Am J Psychiatry 145:1295–1296, 1988.

28. Prigatano GP, Altman IM: Impaired awareness of behavioral limitations after traumatic brain injury. Arch Phys Med Rehabil 7:1058–1064, 1990.

29. Prigatano GP, Pepping M, Klonoff P: Cognitive, personality and psychosocial factors in the neuropsychological assessment of brain-injured patients. In Uzzell B, Gross Y (eds): Clinical Neuropsychology of Intervention. Boston, Martinus Nijhoff, 1986, pp 135–166.

30. Riess H, Schwartz CE, Klerman GL: Manic syndrome following head injury: Another form of secondary mania. J Clin Psychiatry 48:29–30, 1987.

31. Ross E, Rush J: Diagnosis and neuroanatomical correlates of depression in brain-damaged patients. Arch Gen Psychiatry 38:1344–1354, 1981.

32. Shukla S, Cook BL, Mukherjee S, et al: Mania following head trauma. Am J Psychiatry 144:93–96, 1987.

33. Silver JM, Hales RE, Yudofsky SC: Neuropsychiatric aspects of traumatic brain injury. In Yudofsky SC, Hales RE (eds): Textbook of Neuropsychiatry, 2nd ed. Washington, DC, American Psychiatric Press, 1992, pp 363–396.

34. Silver JM, Yudofsky SC, Hales RE: Depression in traumatic brain injury. Neuropsychiatry Neuropsychol Behav Neurol 4:12–23, 1991.

35. Simpson DM, Foster D: Improvement in organically disturbed behavior with trazodone treatment. J Clin Psychiatry 47:191–193, 1986.

36. Slagle DA: Psychiatric disorders following closed head injury: An overview of biopsychosocial factors in their etiology and management. Int J Psychiatry Med 20:1–35, 1990.

37. Sloan RL, Brown KW, Pentland B: Fluoxetine as a treatment for emotional lability after brain injury. Brain Inj 4:315–319, 1992.

38. Sobin P, Schneider L, McDermott H: Fluoxetine in the treatment of agitated dementia [letter]. Am J Psychiatry 146:1636, 1989.

39. Starkstein SE, Fedoroff P, Berthier ML, et al: Manic-depressive and pure manic states after brain lesions. Biol Psychiatry 29:149–158, 1991.
40. Starkstein SE, Mayberg HS, Berthier ML, et al: Mania after brain injury: Neuroradiologic and metabolic findings. Ann Neurol 27:652–659, 1990.
41. Trimble MR: The psychoses of epilepsy and their treatment. In Trimble MR (ed): The Psychopharmacology of Epilepsy. Chichester, UK, John Wiley, 1985, pp 83–94.
42. Van Zomeren AH, Saan RJ: Psychological and social sequelae of severe head injury. In Braakman R (ed): Handbook of Clinical Neurology: vol 13(57). Head Injury. New York, Elsevier, 1990, pp 397–420.
43. Varney NR, Martzke JS, Roberts RJ: Major depression in patients with closed head injury. Neuropsychology 1:7–9, 1987.
44. Violon JA, Demol J: Psychological sequelae after head trauma in adults. Acta Neurochir 85:96–102, 1987.
45. Whyte J, Rosenthal M: Rehabilitation of the patient with head injury. In Delisa JA (ed): Rehabilitation Medicine. Philadelphia, JB Lippincott, 1988, pp 599–611.
46. Will RG, Youns JP, Thomas DJ: Kleine-Levin syndrome: Report of two cases with onset of symptoms precipitated by head trauma. Br J Psychiatry 152:410–412, 1988.
47. Wood RLI: Brain Injury Rehabilitation: A Neurobehavioral Approach. London, Croom Helm, 1987.
48. Wood RLI, Cope DN: Behaviour problems and treatment after head injury. Phys Med Rehabil State Art Rev 3:123–143, 1989.
49. Yudofsky SC, Silver JM, Jackson W, et al: The overt aggression scale for the objective rating of verbal and physical aggression. Am J Psych 143:35–39, 1986.

JOEL R. SAPER, MD

POST-TRAUMATIC HEADACHE SYNDROME

From the
Michigan Head Pain and
  Neurological Institute
Ann Arbor, Michigan

Correspondence to:
Joel R. Saper, MD
Michigan Head Pain and
  Neurological Institute
3120 Professional Drive
Ann Arbor, MI 48104-5199

The post-traumatic syndrome, also called post-concussion syndrome, reflects a constellation of symptoms that may follow mild-to-moderate cranial impact and even flexion-extension injury, absent of cranial contact. According to one review,[17] mild-to-moderate head injury accounts for the vast majority of cases seen in the neurosurgery service and at least 90 to 95% of the survivors of head injury.[3,12]

Symptoms of this syndrome are so typical from patient to patient that the consistency alone has given credibility to its legitimacy. Among the most typical of complaints are head, neck, or facial pain; sleep disturbance; cognitive symptoms; depression, anxiety, or other mood disturbances; and nonspecific dizziness with or without vertigo. Although once considered a psychological disturbance, increasing data now support the belief of most authorities that the syndrome represents a neurologic, neuropsychiatric condition that can occur even in the absence of true altered consciousness following impact.[47]

Head pain occurs in most patients, persisting for more than 2 months in over 60% of cases, independent of the degree of trauma.[20,23,31,51] Moreover, the symptoms do not correlate well with the degree of injury, and in fact an inverse relationship may exist between the severity of head injury and the incidence of headache.[31] The view that litigation is the sole reason for the persistence of these symptoms is not supported by the literature.[15,18,44,47]

KEY CLINICAL FEATURES

Key clinical features of the post-traumatic syndrome may occur immediately or may be delayed in onset. Many symptoms, which in reality developed immediately after trauma, are not recognized by the patient for weeks or months later, thereby giving a false impression of a delayed onset. The most striking example of this is the neurocognitive complaints, whereby the use of a more taxing mental maneuver that would make deficits apparent may not occur during the weeks of convalescence.

Headache Patterns

Typically, head, neck, and shoulder pain are present within a few days after the injury. Neuralgic-like syndromes can develop months later. Moreover, the patterns of pain may evolve, further giving rise to the impression that symptoms have developed much later than at the time of onset.

Several head and neck pain syndromes occur[16,21,26,27,31,37]:

1. Generalized daily headache or "background headache" most typical of tension-type headache
2. Sharp or shooting-like neuralgic pain in the occipitocervical or frontal region
3. Migraine-like headaches with or without aura
4. Cluster headache–like syndromes
5. Cervical pain and upper shoulder pain
6. Cervical radiculopathy secondary to root injury
7. A spinal headache or low-pressure headache-like pattern
8. Brachioplexis-like syndromes
9. Cranial syndromes that can reflect styloid process trauma or true craniomandibular dysfunction

Other Clinical Features

Cognitive and Mood Disturbance. Cognitive impairment can be as disabling and distressing for some patients as head pain. Typically, patients report reduced ability to concentrate or stay on task. Easy distractibility and inability to pay attention to reading materials are common. Other features of the cognitive impairment seen in patients with mild-to-moderate closed head injury can be found in the references.[1,7,10,12,15,17–20,32,43,44,47]

Mood disturbance represents another important, and at times disabling, feature. Depression, anxiety, or even panic occurs in many patients. Anhedonia and reduced libido are common. Irritability, "orneriness," or "anger spells" are frequently reported and noted by family members and friends.

Reduced ambition, motivation, and social interaction are noted frequently and may reflect various factors, including pain, depression, cognitive dysfunction, and brain disturbances. More dramatic neuropsychiatric phenomena, such as rage attacks, hypomania, and impulsive behavior are also noted. Starkstein et al. recently identified positron-emission tomography (PET) scanning abnormalities in patients with post-traumatic hypomania.[42] In children, enuresis is common. Loss of attention, hyperkinesis, and loss of sense of humor are sometimes present.[3,8]

Lightheadedness, Nonspecific Dizziness, and Vertigo. Lightheadedness and nonspecific dizziness are common. Positional vertigo and true vertigo with or without positional features are also reported frequently. These symptoms seem accentuated during acute headache attacks but are present even between painful episodes.

Sleep Disturbance. Sleep disturbance is a commonly reported symptom. Early morning awakening and daytime sleepiness, as well as insomnia, are bothersome in and of themselves but also aggravate other factors, including headache, the ability to concentrate, and mood.

Spells. Various seizure-like episodes are reported. These include true syncope, true major motor epilepsy, staring spells, fuguelike states, brief episodes of disorientation and confusion, and nonepileptic loss of consciousness during acute episodes of pain. Narcolepsy and cataplexy-like spells also occur.[4,25,33,36,45,46]

Diagnostically, few of these spells exhibit sufficient criteria to diagnose true epilepsy. Moreover, electroencephalography is frequently not useful in defining these events, although there is little doubt to experienced clinicians as to the legitimacy and biologic basis of many of these attacks. Patients may be at risk during driving or when carrying out activities during which altered attention or loss of consciousness would impose a particular safety hazard.

Family Dynamic Interruption. The sudden onset of chronic, persistent illness in a formerly healthy, functional person can create rather dramatic changes within the family structure. This is particularly troublesome when the chronicity of the symptoms brings doubt as to the legitimacy and validity of the complaints. Education of family members and support for the patient are essential.

Other Symptoms. Numerous other symptoms are commonly encountered in patients with closed-head injury and postconcussion syndrome. These include weight loss or weight gain, change in appetite, increased thirst, alcohol intolerance, menstrual irregularities, and other soft neurologic findings. Endocrinologic and hypothalamic disturbances may be responsible for these complaints.[34,50]

PATHOPHYSIOLOGY

The exact mechanism for pain and its accompaniments, including neurocognitive impairment, is not known, but structural changes within the nervous system have been seen. Gross and microscopic abnormalities, including brain hemorrhage, occur in animals following carefully controlled head trauma approximating minor head injury in humans.[30,49,50] Though few human autopsy reports are available, together with animal studies the following pathology observations are noted[2,6,29]: nerve cell loss and alteration; vascular disturbances in subcortical, cortical, and brainstem regions; and degeneration and damage to microglia and axons.

Head rotation during attack may be a critical factor in determining injury and sequelae. Even in the absence of direct impact, concussion may be produced by rotational displacement.[5,9,11,28,51] The precise mechanism for head pain remains elusive. It is most likely that both extracranial and intracranial injury result in the symptoms that are noted. The pain-producing factors appear to be

1. Extracranial and cervical soft tissue injury (muscle, tendon, blood vessels, or nerve)
2. Intracranial disturbances (physiological or microstructural) of brainstem pain-modulating mechanisms
3. Cervical root, spinal cord, facet joint, atlantoaxial vertebrae, and temporomandibular joint injuries, among others, in addition to other soft tissue and bony alterations, including those of the stylomandibular ligament area
4. Ischemic brainstem and vestibular disturbance, perhaps secondary to vertebral artery spasm.

Neurobiologic and neuropsychiatric predispositional factors may explain why some patients subjected to mild-to-moderate head injury experience one or more of the sequelae, and others do not.

ASSESSMENT
The most reliable studies involve neurocognitive evaluation, which often demonstrates impaired neurocognitive function. No other practical, widely available studies so consistently demonstrate a basis for many of the features of this condition.[7,12,15,20,32,43,47] Other specific studies that are recommended include

1. Visual evoked potentials, brainstem auditory evoked potentials.
2. Electroencephalography (altered in 10 to 30% of patients but nonspecific in form).
3. Magnetic resonance imaging or computed tomographic scan of the head and neck.
4. Special sleep studies, which may demonstrate pattern abnormalities of sleep staging.
5. Dental and jaw evaluations.
6. Otolaryngologic and vestibular evaluation, including electronystagmography and other vestibular testing.
7. Diagnostic nerve blockade (vertebral, supraorbital, paravertebral, and suboccipital regions).
8. Positron-emission tomography testing. Although not yet of practical value, this study has demonstrated changes that could explain post-traumatic behavioral disturbances.[41]

Although these tests in general may not prove or establish the diagnosis with certainty, they are essential to rule out either coexistent disease from another origin or sequelae to the closed-head injury. These include such conditions as subdural or epidural hematoma; cerebrospinal fluid hypotension (from traumatic leakage); cerebral vein thrombosis or cavernous sinus thrombosis, fistula, or aneurysms; cerebral hemorrhage; true epilepsy; post-traumatic hydrocephalus; vertebral or cervical root or suboccipital injury; and jaw, temporomandibular joint, styloid ligament or process, and facial injury.

PRINCIPLES OF TREATMENT
Patients with post-traumatic syndrome are generally seriously distressed and seriously misunderstood. Appropriate treatment requires an objective approach to the complaints. Most patients are neither embellishing nor malingering. An objective, unbiased (neutral) appraisal is essential. A comprehensive data collection process and a detailed, well-designed diagnostic evaluation are necessary. Neurodiagnostic testing and the performance of sufficient other studies to rule out coexistent or mimicking illness may then support the presence of the syndrome by exclusion.

Treatment of Headache
The primary treatment for headache consists of identifying the headache pattern and treating it according to standard treatment protocols. Acute attacks of migraine should be treated with appropriate symptomatic therapies, including ergot derivatives, Sumatriptan, Midrin (isometheptene, acetaminophen, and dichloralphenazone), nonsteroidal antiinflammatory drugs, and phenothiazines (for nausea and pain).[16,22,31,34,38,39] The symptomatic approach to migraine requires restriction of treatment to no more than 2 days/week and combining symptomatic treatment with preventive treatment when the frequency of headache exceeds 2 days/week.

Preventive treatment relies on the use of various preventive agents, including β-adrenergic blockers, calcium channel blockers, antidepressants, nonsteroidal antiinflammatory agents, and anticonvulsants, such as valproate, phenytoin, and carbamazepine.

Cluster headache forms require the use of various agents found useful in cluster headache (see *Handbook of Headache Management.*[39])

A major treatment dilemma in patients with recurring headache is the "rebound" headache phenomenon. The excessively frequent use of symptomatic medications for the relief of head or neck pain can lead to increasingly frequent headaches and refractoriness to other forms of therapy. Patients who use over-the-counter or prescribed analgesics or ergot derivatives more than 2 days/week are often vulnerable to the development of this syndrome. Close questioning of patients regarding their use of over-the-counter medications is important because many patients erroneously do not consider these agents to be "true medicines."

Rebound headache[22,31,37-39,40] is a clinical phenomenon that is self-sustaining and requires complete discontinuance of the analgesics or other types of rebound-provoking medication before preventive medications will be effective. Key features of rebound include

1. The use of increasing amounts of analgesics or certain other medications at regular, predictable intervals
2. The failure of preventive medications to be effective
3. Psychological or physiologic dependence on certain medications
4. A predictable pattern of head pain between medication doses
5. Predictable awakening with headache when this has not been a pattern in the past

Nonmedicinal Interventions. Nonmedicinal interventions include biofeedback, stress management, and avoidance of provoking risk factors. Stabilizing eating and sleeping patterns, regular exercise, avoidance of foods and circumstances that provoke headaches, and discontinuance of smoking and drinking are all recommended.[22,31,38,39]

Treatment of Other Symptoms. Traumatic neuralgias may occur following head or neck injury and can result from direct trauma of nerve through compression or neuroma formation. Myofascial pain syndromes involving the upper neck and shoulders with or without trigger points are also common. Local anesthetic blockade[3,31,41] can be helpful, both diagnostically and therapeutically. Caution must be exercised, however, in that resolution of pain from a block does not indicate the diagnosis because for reasons that remain unclear, local blockade brings about relief of pain in various nonneuralgic or soft tissue injuries.

Physical therapeutic measures can be helpful but often aggravate conditions in patients with coexistent headache. Aggressive physical therapy and range-of-motion exercise should not occur until it is clear that bone and soft tissue regions of the neck have been carefully evaluated and not aggravated by physical therapeutic measures. Pharmacologic therapy for true neuralgia includes the use of various medications, including carbamazepine, phenytoin, baclofen, valproate, and clonazepam.

The reader is referred to a recently published book by these authors entitled *Handbook of Headache Management*[39] for specific therapeutic regimens, as well as for a more detailed discussion of management of pain arising from the neck.

REFERENCES

1. Carlsson GS, Svardsudd K, Wellin L: Long-term effects of head injury sustained during life in three male populations. J Neurosurg 67:197–205, 1987.
2. Dila C, Bouchard L, Myer E, et al: Microvascular response to minimal brain trauma. In McLaurin R (ed): Head Injuries. New York, Grune & Stratton, 1976.
3. Dillon H, Leopold RL: Children and the post-concussion syndrome. JAMA 175:86–92, 1961.

4. Feinsod M, Hoyt WF, Wilson WG, Spire JP: Visual evoked response: Use in neurological evaluation of post-traumatic subjective visual complaints. Arch Ophthalmol 94:237–240, 1976.
5. Fisher CM: Whiplash amnesia. Neurology 32:667–668, 1982.
6. Gennareli TA: Cerebral concussion and diffuse brain injuries. In Cooper PR (ed): Head Injury. Baltimore, Williams & Wilkins, 1982, pp 83–97.
7. Gronwall D, Wrightson P: Delayed recovery of intellectual function after minor head injury. Lancet ii:605–609, 1984.
8. Haas DC, Pineda GS, Lourie H: Juvenile head trauma syndromes and their relationship to migraine. Arch Neurol 32:727–730, 1975.
9. Jacome DF: Basilar artery migraine after uncomplicated whiplash injuries. Headache 26:515–516, 1986.
10. Jakobsen J, Daadsgaard SE, Thomsen S, et al: Prediction of post-concussional sequelae by reaction time test. Acta Neurol Scand 75:341–345, 1987.
11. Keith WS: Whiplash injury of the second cervical ganglion and nerve. Can J Neurolog Sci 13:133–137, 1986.
12. Kelly R: The post-traumatic syndrome. Proc R Soc Med 24:242–244, 1981.
13. Kerr FWL: A mechanism to account for frontal headache in a case of posterior fossa tumors. J Neurosurg 18:605–609, 1961.
14. Khurana RK, Nirankari VW: Bilateral sympathetic dysfunction in post-traumatic headache. Headache 26:183–188, 1986.
15. Klonoff PS, Snow WE, Costa LD: Quality of life in patients 2–4 years after closed head injury. Neurosurgery 19:735–743, 1986.
16. Lance JW: Mechanism and Management of Headache, 4th ed. London, Butterworth Scientific, 1982.
17. Levin HS: Treatment of post-concussional symptoms with CDP-choline. J Neurol Sci 103:S39–S42, 1991.
18. Leininger BE: Neuropsychological deficits in symptomatic minor head injury patients after concussion and mild concussion. J Neurol Neurosurg Psychiatry 53:293–296, 1990.
19. MacFlynn G, Montgomery EA, Fenton GW, Rutherford DW: Measurement of reaction time following minor head injury. J Neurol Neurosurg Psychiatry 47:1326–1331, 1984.
20. McKinley WW, Brooks DN, Bond MR: Post-concussional symptoms, financial compensation, and outcome of severe blunt head injury. J Neurol Neurosurg Psychiatry 46:1084–1091, 1983.
21. Markus DA: Migraine and tension-type headaches: The questionable validity of current classification systems. Clin J Pain 8:28–36, 1992.
22. Mathew NT (ed): Headache. Neurol Clin 8(4): 1990.
23. Matthews WB: Footballer's migraine. BMJ 2:326–327, 1972.
24. Merskey H, Woodforde JM: Psychiatric sequelae of minor head injury. Brain 95:521–528, 1972.
25. Noseworthy JH, Miller J, Murray TJ, Regan D: Auditory brainstem responses in post-concussion syndrome. Arch Neurol 389:275–278, 1981.
26. Olesen J: Classification and diagnostic criteria for headache disorders, cranial neuralgias, and headache pain. Cephalalgia 8(suppl 7):1–96, 1988.
27. Olesen J, Edvinson L (eds): Basic Mechanisms of Headache. Amsterdam, Elsevier Science Publishers, 1988.
28. Ommaya AK, Faas F, Yarnell P: Whiplash injury and brain damage: An experimental study. JAMA 204:275–289, 1968.
29. Oppenheimer DR: Microscopic lesions in the brain following head injury. J Neurol Neurosurg Psychiatry 31:299–306, 1968.
30. Povlishok JT, Becker DP, Cheng CLY, et al: Axonal changes in minor head injury. J Neuropathol Exp Neurol 42:225–242, 1983.
31. Raskin NH: Headache, 2nd ed. New York, Churchill Livingstone, 1988.
32. Rimel RW, Giordani B, Barth JT, et al: Disability caused by minor head injury. Neurosurgery 9:221–228, 1981.
33. Rizzo PA, Pierelli F, Pozzessere G, et al: Subjective post-traumatic syndrome: A comparison of visual and brainstem auditory evoked responses. Neuropsychobiology 9:78–82, 1983.
34. Rose FC (ed): Handbook of Clinical Neurology. Amsterdam, Elsevier Science Publishers, 1986.
35. Rowe JM, Carlson C: Brainstem auditory evoked potential in post-concussion dizziness. Arch Neurol 37:679–683, 1980.
36. Sackallares JC, Giordani B, Berent S, et al: Patients with pseudoseizures: Intellectual and cognitive performance. Neurology 35:116–119, 1985.
37. Saper JR: Headache Disorders: Current Concepts and Treatment Strategies. Littleton, MA, Wright-PSG Publishers, 1983.

38. Saper JR: Changing perspectives on chronic headache. Clin J Pain 2:19–28, 1986.
39. Saper JR, Silberstein SD, Gordon CD, Hamel RL: Handbook of Headache Management. Baltimore, Williams & Wilkins, 1992.
40. Silberstein SD (ed): Intractable headache: Inpatient and outpatient treatment strategies. Neurology (suppl 2), March 1992.
41. Smith RG, Cherry JE: Traumatic Eagle's syndrome: Report of a case and review of the literature. J Oral Maxillofac Surg 46:606–609, 1988.
42. Starkstein SE, Mayberg HS, Bertwier ML, et al: Mania after brain injury: Neuroradiological and metabolic findings. Ann Neurol 27:652–659, 1990.
43. Stuss DT, Ely P, Hugenholtz H, et al: Subtle neuropsychological deficits in patients with good recovery after closed head injury. Neurosurgery 17:41–47, 1985.
44. Tarsh MJ, Royston C: A follow-up study of accident neurosis. Br J Psychiatry 146:18–25, 1985.
45. Toglia JU, Rosenberg PE, Ronis ML: Post-traumatic dizziness. Arch Otolaryngol 92:485–492, 1970.
46. Torres F, Shapiro SK: Electroencephalograms and whiplash injury. Arch Neurol 5:40–47, 1961.
47. Trimbell MR: Post-traumatic Neurosis: From Railway Spine to the Whiplash. New York, John Wiley & Sons, 1981.
48. Vijayan N, Dreyfus PM: Post-traumatic dysautonomic cephalgia. Arch Neurol 32:649–652, 1975.
49. Wei EP, Dietrich WD, Polvichek JT, et al: Functional, morphological, and metabolic abnormalities of the cerebral microcirculation after concussive brain injury in cats. Circ Res 46:37–47, 1980.
50. West M, LaBella FS, Havlicek V, et al: Cerebral concussion in rats rapidly induces hypothalamic-specific effects on opiate and cholinergic receptors. Brain Res 25:271–277, 1981.
51. Winston KR: Whiplash and its relationship to migraine. Headache 27:452–457, 1987.

DOUGLAS E. GARLAND, MD

HETEROTOPIC OSSIFICATION

From the
Central Nervous System Division
Department of Surgery
Rancho Los Amigos Medical
  Center
Downey, California
  and
Department of Orthopaedics
University of Southern California
Los Angeles, California

Correspondence to:
Douglas E. Garland, MD
Central Nervous Division
Department of Surgery
Rancho Los Amigos Medical
  Center
7601 E. Imperial Highway
Downey, CA 90242

The term *heterotopic ossification* (HO) is preferred to such terms as ectopic ossification or paraosteoarthropathy when discussing the formation of new bone about joints as a consequence of head injury. Heterotopic refers to the occurrence of bone in more than one area. Microscopically, the bone is a true "ossific" process, progressing *de novo* to new bone formation rather than to calcification of soft tissue. HO associated with head injury is labeled *neurogenic.*

The majority of heterotopic bone associated with head injury is around joints, although it has been noted in the thigh. Neurogenic HO is commonly para-articular and usually occurs in one plane about the joint, although it may occur in more than one plane. The bone itself lies within a well-defined tissue plane and usually does not involve the joint capsule or muscles. Patients exhibiting marked spasticity, especially extensor rigidity, are the most likely candidates to develop this bone. Multiple sites are common in patients with marked neurologic compromise. The new bone frequently forms in the vicinity of the spastic musculature. The position of the extremity often allows early prediction of the future location of the HO. It is rare for a patient with only cognitive dysfunction to develop neurogenic HO.

Traumatic HO results from major trauma to a joint and is truly periarticular in that it may form in one or all planes around a joint.[8,15,16] This bone does not lie in well-defined tissue planes and may involve ligaments, joint capsules, and muscles. HO in the vicinity of the medial or ulnar collateral ligament of the elbow should alert the examiner to the possibility of tardy ulnar palsy.[19] Spasticity about the joint is not always present, and it may occur even in patients with only cognitive dysfunction.

GENETICS AND PATIENT PREDISPOSITION

Strong support for some type of genetic predisposition to HO formation comes from the hereditary disorder fibrodysplasia ossificans progressiva.[3] This disorder is inherited as an autosomal dominant trait with full penetrance and variable expression. It is a disorder of connective tissue, with skeletal malformations and HO. The natural history of HO associated with fibrodysplasia ossificans progressiva has similarities to the natural history of HO from other causes, especially neurogenic HO. Although the majority of cases of fibrodysplasia ossificans progressiva–associated HO are spontaneous, some cases also occur after trauma. A predilection of HO for certain locations (i.e., the axial musculature and proximal limbs) is documented that is common in both traumatic and neurogenic HO. HO frequently recurs after surgical resection and is commonly noted after resection of neurogenic HO and occasionally after traumatic HO resection.

The association of human leukocyte antigens (HLAs) with neurogenic HO has been documented. An increased prevalence of HLA-B18 and HLA-B27 antigens has been reported in patients with HO in comparison to normal subjects.[21,24] However, follow-up studies from other centers have not confirmed these findings, and this system cannot at present predict susceptibility to HO.[12,18,33]

PREVALENCE AND ONSET

The reported prevalence varies for most types of HO, but much of this difference may be the result of methodology and institutional variations. The type of center (acute care versus rehabilitation) and type of patient (with hemiplegia, paraplegia, or quadriplegia) influence the results. Methodology also affects study outcomes. Prospective versus retrospective studies, whole-body radiographs versus hip-only, and 6-month versus 1-year follow-ups have the potential to influence final data.

The prevalence of clinically significant HO—that which limits joint motion— as opposed to HO of purely academic interest or that which is solely a radiographic observation, is similar when studies from similar institutions and methodologies are compared, regardless of its cause. The most commonly reported prevalence of clinically significant HO is 10 to 20%.[13,22,23,30] Joint ankylosis occurs in fewer than 10% of the lesions.

DIAGNOSIS

Physical Examination

Limited joint motion is the most common physical finding and frequently the earliest sign of HO. An increase in spasticity commonly occurs. Joint erythema and warmth occasionally require differentiation from a septic joint. Lower limb swelling may mimic thrombophlebitis. The most common symptom of HO is pain. An increase in pain, relative increase in spasticity, or muscle guarding should alert the examiner of the possibility of HO.

Serum Alkaline Phosphatase Determination

Early reports on HO failed to detect elevated serum alkaline phosphatase (SAP) levels. However, follow-up studies have demonstrated that elevated levels of SAP are associated with clinically significant HO. SAP levels begin to rise, although remain in the normal range, within 2 weeks of injury.[25] Elevated levels may occur by 3 weeks, and the duration of persistent high levels averages 5 months. The majority of patients who develop so-called clinically significant HO will have an elevated SAP levels, especially if the HO is around the hip. This may not be true at the elbow, where small amounts of HO may decrease motion. SAP concentration does not correlate with inactivity, peak activity, or number of HO lesions. SAP determination is nonspecific and not absolute, but it may constitute the earliest and, certainly the most convenient and least expensive, laboratory test for early detection of HO. In addition, many patients are in intensive care units and cannot undergo special studies. SAP level is easy to determine and is an excellent presumptive test for HO. Medical treatment may be initiated solely on the basis of SAP elevation if fractures are not present.

Radionuclide Bone Imaging

Radionuclide bone imaging (RNBI) became efficient as a diagnostic tool in the late 1960s and early 1970s. Early bone scan technique employed injection of ^{99m}Tc polyphosphate, with follow-up scans obtained approximately 4 to 5 hours after injection. At present, the three-phase bone scan is the best method for early detection as well as confirmation of HO.[7] This test involves injection of ^{99m}Tc-labeled methylene diphosphonate followed by imaging in three phases:

Phase I—a dynamic blood flow study with frequent photoscans for approximately 1 minute

Phase II—a static scan for blood pool after the completion of phase I

Phase III—a 2- to 4-hour bone scan to determine the degree of the labeled radionuclide in bone

The first two phases are the most sensitive for the earliest detection of HO and may show abnormal results within 2 to 4 weeks after injury, even though the osseous tissue uptake may be normal (phase III). The period of positive uptake in phases I and II with a negative result in phase III may range from 2 to 4 weeks. Likewise, phase III may yield positive results up to 4 weeks before HO is observed radiographically.

A large definitive prospective or even retrospective study of the RNBI phase III evaluation of HO is not available. Correlation of RNBI and evolution of radiographic features has not been performed. It does appear that the majority of bone scans return to baseline within 7 to 12 months, while a slowly downward activity occurs in many of the remainder of the scans. A few scans remain fully active during the first year. The RNBI may become reactivated after a quiescent period.

Quantitative radionuclide bone scans compare the ratio of uptake in normal versus heterotopic bone. Because HO uptake decreases with time, serial decreases or a steady state in the ratio of uptake between normal and heterotopic bone is assumed to be an indication of HO maturity. The incidence of recurrence of HO may be decreased after resection if HO is removed during a radionuclide steady state. Unfortunately, this premise has not been adequately verified in a large homogeneous series. Our large surgical resection series demonstrated that this steady state was not a predictor of recurrence.[14] Patients with persistently active scans predictably had recurrence, whereas patients with baseline scans commonly had recurrence. Consequently, neither the natural history of HO nor treatment guidelines based on radionuclide bone imaging activity have been adequately established.

Radiography

Before RNBI became available, radiographs provided confirmatory evidence of HO. Although plain films may detect HO as early as 3 weeks after injury, radiographic detection generally is not confirmatory until 2 months after the stimulus.

Radiographs offer other benefits. They can identify the site of HO at the joint and are an easy, inexpensive, and reliable method for evaluation of treatment. Radiographs permit evaluation of maturation of HO, especially when coupled with results of SAP determinations and physical examination (showing decrease in spasticity).

Computed Tomography

The precise role of computed tomography (CT) scanning as a clinical tool for diagnosis and a measure of maturation of HO is not established.[2] CT may aid in preoperative surgical planning. Multiple sites of HO at a joint may be more readily delineated by CT than by standard radiographs. CT scanning may more clearly define localization of HO and its relationship to muscle, vessel, and nerve.

LOCATION

A retrospective review of 496 patients revealed 57 patients (11%) with 100 joints that had HO neurogenic involvement.[13] Thirty of the patients had single-joint involvement, whereas 27 patients had multiple-joint involvement. The ratio of the involved male and female patients was similar to the ratio of male to female in the total population. This finding is significant because some people suggest that, based on spinal cord injury patients wherein female HO occurrence is uncommon, HO is a disease of males. Eighty-one of the involved joints were located on spastic extremities. The other extremities may have been previously spastic but had no spasticity at transfer to our unit.

The 11% incidence may not indicate the true incidence. A routine radiographic survey of major joints was not undertaken. Only clinically significant HO, bone associated with pain and decreased range of motion, was detected. A routine radiographic survey would probably increase the incidence of HO, as has been noted. Furthermore, although the series was consecutive, the population was selected. Patients with mild head injuries are not transferred to our unit. The incidence of HO in these patients may be low or may occur in a mild, clinically insignificant form. Patients with severe neurologic involvement are frequently not candidates for rehabilitation and are not transferred to our unit. The incidence in this group as well as the amount of HO may be increased.

Hip. Forty-four hips developed HO in 33 patients. Three main locations were identified. The site of HO could frequently be predicted from the abnormal posture of the extremity. Occasionally, HO developed in more than one plane.

Heterotopic bone located anterior to the hip may result in swelling of the thigh with a palpable visual mass (Fig. 1A). The lower extremity often assumes a mildly reflexed position with external rotation of the leg. The massive amount of HO present in spinal cord–injured patients at this location is seldom observed in the head-injured population.

HO occurring posterior to the hip may be associated with hip flexion contractures. This location of HO may not result in great limitation of motion and is uncommon in the spinal cord injury population.

The most common location of HO at the hip was the inferomedial location (Fig. 2A). HO in this location is frequently associated with adductor spasticity.

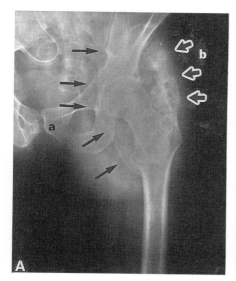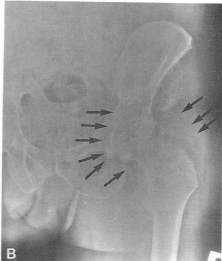

FIGURE 1. *A*, Anteroposterior radiograph of the hip. Anterior HO (*a*) is noted between the anterior-inferior iliac spine and the lesser trochanter. This site is most commonly observed in spinal cord injury HO. Head trauma anterior HO usually courses toward the greater trochanter. HO is also noted in the region of the abductor muscles (*b*). HO in this location most commonly occurs after surgery to the hip. *B*, Anteroposterior radiograph of the hip. At 1.5 years after head injury, both sites of HO were removed through an anterior approach. Radiation was given for prophylaxis. The patient had a class II neurologic recovery—voluntary muscle control with mild limb deformity and residual spasticity.

Ankylosis is uncommon unless the patient has a severe neurologic insult. Small losses of hip flexion and extension normally occur. If a large amount of HO is present, adduction range is compromised due to a mechanical block.

   Elbow. Two sites of new bone formation generally occur in the elbow, although HO may form in any or all planes, especially in the traumatized elbow. HO anterior to the elbow is often associated with flexor spasticity, as noted in the hemiplegic limb (Fig. 3). If ankylosis results, the bone usually bridges the distal humerus and proximal radius.

   New bone occurring posteriorly at the elbow is often associated with extensor posturing (rigidity) (Fig. 4). This posturing presents early after the head injury. Because extensor rigidity resolves with neurologic improvement, the elbow may assume a more flexed position at the time ankylosis is occurring. This explains the paradoxic picture of posterior bone formation in a normal, hemiplegic or flexed extremity with posterior HO. Ankylosis of all types of heterotopic bone most commonly occurs posteriorly at the elbow. Ankylosis is usually between the distal humerus and olecranon.

   Shoulder. The rate of occurrence of HO in the shoulder is similar to that in the elbow. The new bone is generally located inferomedial to the joint. The shoulder position is internal rotation and adduction (Fig. 5). Ankylosis is uncommon unless the patient sustains a severe neurologic insult.

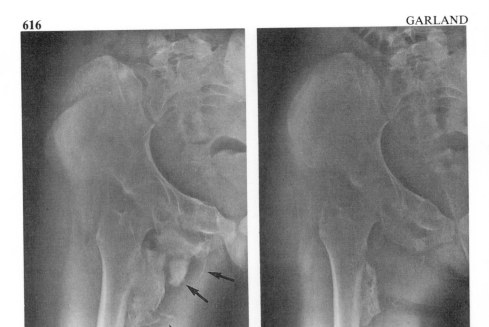

FIGURE 2. *A*, Anteroposterior radiograph of the hip. The HO is inferomedial. Ankylosis is not present, but the limb is positioned in external rotation and abduction. *B*, Anteroposterior radiograph of the hip. The HO was removed through a slightly modified anterior approach 1 year after head injury. Indomethacin was given for 3 months after resection for this class I patient.

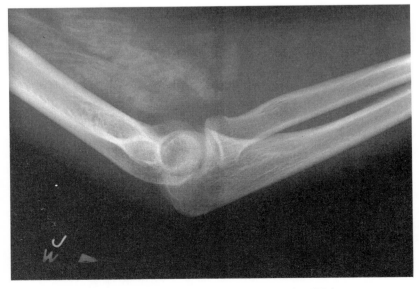

FIGURE 3. Lateral radiograph of elbow. Anterior HO is present.

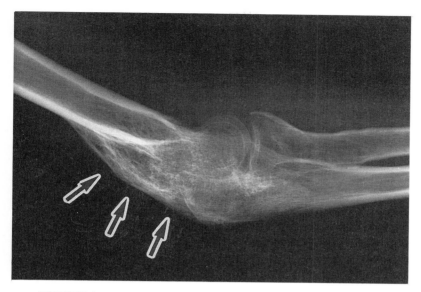

FIGURE 4. Lateral radiograph of the elbow, showing posterior HO.

Knee. HO about the knee and the quadriceps muscle is uncommon. It may appear anywhere in the distal thigh or about the knee.

NATURAL HISTORY

The natural history of HO is defined mainly through radiographs and is infrequently emphasized.[8,9] The natural radiographic history is similar and predictable in the majority of patients. It also closely parallels the elevation of SAP level and the presence of spasticity.

In a retrospective review of 23 traumatically brain-injured patients who underwent resection of HO at an average of 28 months after injury, patients were classified as belonging to classes I to V, according to their neurologic recovery. Class I patients had near-normal neurologic recovery, whereas class V patients had severe cognitive deficits and spasticity. Class I patients rarely had recurrence after resection. In contrast, every class V patient had recurrence regardless of the site of HO. Radiographic progression subsided by 6 months, and SAP levels and RNBI activity were normal or significantly decreased in patients who were making an early normal neurologic recovery (class I). Patients with severe motor compromise had larger amounts of ossific bone. This HO progressed in some instances for more than 1 year, with elevated SAP levels for 2 years or longer and occasionally, persistent activity on RNBI.[14]

TREATMENT

HO runs a gamut from being undetected and therefore untreated to having a poor response to all treatment methods. Some patients with minimal HO require no treatment, whereas others may require physical therapy, medicine, manipulation, surgical excision, or all of these. The majority of patients with HO maintain functional joint motion with standard physical therapies, medicines, and

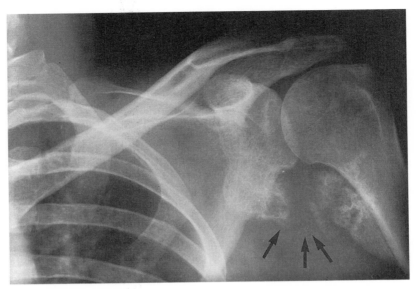

FIGURE 5.   Anteroposterior radiograph of the shoulder. A pseudoarthrosis is present, which is common and allows motion.

occasionally, forceful manipulations. A small group require surgery, and some develop recurrence of HO.

Medical Treatment

Medical treatment, including radiation, is used prophylactically in two general situations: (1) to prevent HO formation after the primary insult and (2) to prevent recurrence of HO after its surgical resection.

Ethylhydroxydiphosphonate (Etidronate Disodium)

In the early 1960s, research with polyphosphates and their inhibitory activity on calcium phosphate precipitation led to evaluation of diphosphonates, most specifically ethylhydroxydiphosphonate (EHDP), for similar effects. Definitive studies demonstrated that diphosphonates inhibited the precipitation of calcium phosphate from clear solutions, delayed aggregation of apatite crystals into layer clusters, blocked transformation of amorphous calcium phosphate into hydroxyapatite, and delayed dissolution of crystals. All effects seemed related to their affinity for hydroxyapatite. The ability of EHDP to inhibit experimental soft tissue ossification as well as normal mineralization of bone led to the clinical use of EHDP to prevent HO.[5,29]

Clinical research has not irrefutably proved or disproved the effectiveness of EHDP, but none has been able to prove absolute arrest of HO when the studies are subjected to strict scientific scrutiny.[7,11,32] Other authors have stated that EHDP is not effective in preventing HO.

Efficacious response to EHDP dictates the proper dosage and duration of treatment. Simplistically speaking, EHDP prevents conversion of amorphous calcium phosphate compounds into hydroxyapatite crystals, which is one of the final steps of bone formation. Because the majority of HO evolves radiographically over a period of 6 months, EHDP should generally be taken for this 6-month span.[8,9] Lower EHDP doses are adequate to inhibit crystal resorption, but they are less effective in inhibiting crystal growth. Therefore, the 20 mg/kg dosage is necessary to prevent HO formation. Treatment for this duration and at this dosage should prevent HO lesions in the majority of patients and also decrease the incidence of the so-called recovery phase of "rebound" calcification. Prolonged treatment at high doses of EHDP produces undesirable side effects, such as long bone fractures in dogs.[6] Therefore, dosages of 20 mg/kg for longer than 6 months' duration may not be warranted, and continued treatment may be deleterious. EHDP will not be effective for the massive heterotopic bone–forming patient, regardless of dosages and duration of treatment.

Quantitative histomorphometry demonstrates an increased number of osteo-clasts, as well as osteoblasts, in the HO lesion when compared with normal bone.[26] EHDP at a much lower dosage than that necessary for the inhibition of ossification interrupts osteoclastic function but does not destroy the osteoclasts. They eventually recover full function but over a prolonged period. This effect, although somewhat overlooked in the treatment of HO by EHDP, is extremely undesirable because resorption is an important aspect in HO maturation, which involves partial or even complete resorption of the HO lesion. With cessation of treatment, the osteoid may ossify immediately while the resorptive capability remains impaired until osteoclastic function returns. This effect may influence the rebound phenomenon as well as resorption. The effect of EHDP on osteoclasts, the recovery or rebound phase, the length of treatment, patient compliance, and the cost of the medication may eventually contribute to the selection of another drug for treatment of HO.

INDOMETHACIN

Dahl is generally credited with demonstrating the prophylactic effects of indomethacin on HO formation after total hip replacement.[27] Other studies have verified its effectiveness, including one double-blind study.[20,31] The ability of indomethacin to inhibit prostaglandin synthetase is proposed as the primary mechanism for HO prevention, although many effects on bone formation are known. Prostaglandins are mediators of inflammation, and part of indomethacin's effect is due to inhibition of the inflammatory response or suppression of mesenchymal cell proliferation. Indomethacin dosage is 25 mg three times a day for 6 weeks after total hip replacement. Ibuprofen and aspirin may also be effective when used in a similar fashion. The effectiveness of nonsteroidal anti-inflammatory drugs to prevent HO in the neurologic patient has not been established.

RADIATION

The ability of radiation to inhibit bone growth has been known by radiothera-pists for years. Irradiation prevents conversion of precursor cells to bone-forming cells. Early reports of irradiation in the treatment of myositis ossificans were often anecdotal. Now it appears that 1,000 rads at 200 rad/day immediately after total hip replacement is effective in preventing HO.[1,4] The location of HO formation in the neurologic patient cannot be predicted. Because radiation is relatively ineffective once HO is detected, its use in prevention of initial neurogenic HO may be limited. Presently, its effectiveness in this setting is not known.

Forceful Manipulation

The role of ranging joints involved with HO for maintenance or increasing joint motion is controversial. Some authors have suggested that ranging increases the amount of HO, whereas others have reported beneficial gains or maintenance of joint motion. A review of patients who underwent forceful manipulation under anesthesia demonstrated its usefulness in maintaining motion in most patients and actually increasing motion in others.[17] Manipulation is indicated in both traumatic and neurogenic HO. Head-injured patients frequently have spasticity, intolerance to pain, and voluntary muscle guarding. Consequently, anesthesia is usually required for manipulation. Examination under anesthesia allows differentiation of spasticity and true ankylosis. If spasticity is determined to be a major factor, treatment may be also directed toward it.

Large increases in motion are sometimes achieved under anesthesia, but motion may be gradually lost thereafter. If neurologic improvement continues, joint manipulation may be repeated as necessary. If the patient is remaining at a low level of neurologic recovery, repeated manipulations are not indicated. We have not manipulated a joint more than three times. Final arc of motion is closely related to the amount of neurologic recovery. Twenty-three of 28 joints (82%) gained motion at anesthesia. Eighteen joints (64%) maintained or gained further motion with rehabilitation. Review of the radiographs did not reveal an exacerbation of the ossific process.

Shoulder ankylosis is rare. Abduction range often persists, with loss of motion occurring in external rotation. At manipulation the elbow is flexed to 90°, and the arm is forcefully externally rotated. Mild gains in external rotation may be achieved, but a large gain is prevented by spastic internal rotator musculature. A pseudarthrosis line in the HO is frequently evident on the radiograph (Fig. 5).

Elbow joints with decrease in motion from anterior or posterior HO as well as traumatic HO respond to manipulation. Final range of motion is more dependent on the neurologic outcome and amount of new bone rather than on the location of the bone. Repeated manipulations are generally not indicated in the severely hemiplegic or persistently extended limb.

The elbow is flexed and extended maximally under anesthesia. If the elbow was initially positioned in flexion, it is placed in extension after manipulation. A circular plaster is then applied, which prevents the elbow from returning to the previous position and aids in control of pain and swelling. The cast is removed at 1 week, and a dropout cast or anterior-posterior splints are applied. Active and passive range-of-motion exercises may also begin. If the elbow was initially in extension, it is placed in flexion at manipulation and circular plaster applied. At 1 week, the cast is removed and active and passive range of motion is initiated. If ankylosis of the elbow seems inevitable, the elbow is placed in approximately 45° of flexion. This position allows some function during rehabilitation and prevents a significant flexion contracture. Surgical resection is simplified if indicated at a later date. If ankylosis occurs, the bone may be resected, and the muscles and joint capsule will not require surgery. We feel the elbow ankylosed at 45° degrees is optimum for the patient who remains at a low neurologic level. The average gain in motion in eight elbows was 47°.

The response to manipulation at the hip depends mainly on the neurologic outcome. Flexion to 90° may frequently be maintained with a small amount of flexion contracture. Loss of internal and external rotation motion is common. Traumatic injuries about the hip result in a mild-to-excessive amount of ectopic bone. With mild amounts of new bone, functional hip motion can be maintained with manipulation.

The hip is flexed and extended maximally under general anesthesia. Internal and external rotation is attempted with the hip and knee flexed at 90°. This is an excellent time to perform percutaneous phenol adductor nerve blocks if adductor spasticity is present. Knee manipulation may also be required if flexion contractures are present. A long leg cast may be necessary to prevent knee flexion contracture and corresponding hip flexion contracture. Placement of the hip in extension is indicated if copious HO is forming and ankylosis is inevitable. Resection of the HO will be technically easier at a later date because no contracture is present and soft tissue releases will not be necessary. Extension is also a desirable position in the low-level patient in ankylosis if predicted. The average gain in seven manipulated hips was 50°.

Surgery

Surgery is indicated for joint mobility, limb positioning, or sitting. Various operative procedures have been described.[17,32,33] Precise timing for surgery is infrequently mentioned but is determined in respect to the quiescent state, indicated by normal SAP levels, mature radiographic appearance, and baseline RNBI. Postoperative complications are common, especially in comparison to standard orthopaedic procedures.

The natural history of neurologic recovery is the best indicator for surgical excision, recurrence, and functional outcome. The majority of motor recovery occurs by 1.5 years. Excision in the patient with a rapid neurologic recovery may be undertaken when alkaline phosphatase level is normal and no spasticity is present. Surgery should be delayed longer than 1.5 years if the motor recovery is prolonged (Figs. 1A and 1B; 2A and 2B). Recurrence is common in the presence of normal or abnormal laboratory values in the neurologically compromised patient, and delaying excision because of abnormal laboratory values is unwarranted. Surgery is indicated for limb positioning in the neurologically compromised patient.

No studies currently available have defined the role of medical prophylaxis after resection. The stimulus to form HO has subsided in the normal recovery group, and medical prophylaxis may not be necessary for these patients. Because the neurologically compromised patient continues to form HO after resection, present prophylactic methods may be inadequate for this group. A mildly to moderately neurologically compromised patient should respond to prophylaxis after resection.

REFERENCES

1. Ayers DG, Evarts CM, Parkinson JR: The prevention of heterotopic ossification in high-risk patients by low-dose radiation therapy after total hip arthroplasty. J Bone Joint Surg 68A:1423–1430, 1986.
2. Bressler E, Marn C, Gore R, Hendrix R: Evaluation of ectopic bone by CT. Am J Roentgenol 148:931–935, 1987.
3. Connor JM, Evans DAP: Fibroplasia ossificans progressiva. The clinical features and natural history of 34 patients. J Bone Joint Surg 64B:76–83, 1982.
4. Coventry MB, Scanton PW: Use of radiation to discourage ectopic bone. J Bone Joint Surg 63A:201–208, 1982.
5. Fleisch H: Diphosphonates: History and mechanisms of action. Bone 3:279–287, 1981.
6. Flora L, Hassing GS, Cloyd GG, et al: The long-term skeletal effects of EHDP in dogs. Bone 3:289–300, 1981.

7. Freed JH, Hahn H, Menter MD, Dillion T: The use of the three-phase bone scan in the early diagnosis of heterotopic ossification (HO) and in the evaluation of didronel therapy. Paraplegia 20:208–216, 1982.
8. Garland DE: Clinical observations on fractures and heterotopic ossification in the spinal cord and traumatic brain injured populations. Clin Orthop 233:86–101, 1988.
9. Garland DE: A clinical perspective of common forms of acquired heterotopic ossification. Clin Orthop 263:13–29, 1991.
10. Garland DE: Surgical approaches for resection of heterotopic ossification in traumatic brain-injured adults. Clin Orthop 263:59–70, 1991.
11. Garland DE, Alday B, Venos KG, Vogt JC: Diphosphonate treatment for heterotopic ossification in spinal cord injury patients. Clin Orthop 176:197–200, 1983.
12. Garland DE, Alday B, Venos KG: Heterotopic ossification and HLA antigens. Arch Phys Med Rehabil 65:5531–5532, 1984.
13. Garland DE, Blum CE, Waters RL: Periarticular heterotopic ossification in head injured adults: Incidence and location. J Bone Joint Surg 62A:1143–1146, 1980.
14. Garland DE, Hanscom DA, Keenan MA, et al: Resection of heterotopic ossification in the adult with head trauma. J Bone Joint Surg 67A:1261–1269, 1985.
15. Garland DE, Miller G: Fractures and dislocations about the hip in head-injured adults. Clin Orthop 186:154–158, 1984.
16. Garland DE, O'Hollaren RM: Fractures and dislocations about the elbow in the head-injured adult. Clin Orthop 168:38–41, 1982.
17. Garland DE, Razza BE, Waters RL: Forceful joint manipulation in head-injured adults with heterotopic ossification. Clin Orthop 169:133–138, 1982.
18. Hunter T, Dubo HIC, Hildahl CR, et al: Histocompatibility antigens in patients with spinal cord injury or cerebral damage complicated by heterotopic ossification. Rheumatol Rehabil 19:97–99, 1980.
19. Keenan MAE, Kauffman DL, Garland DE, Smith C: Late ulnar neuropathy in the brain injured adult. J Hand Surg 13A:120–124, 1988.
20. Kjaersgaard-Andersen P, Schmidt SA: Indomethacin for prevention of ectopic ossification after hip arthroplasty. Acta Orthop Scand 57:12–14, 1986.
21. Larson JM, Michalski JP, Collacott EA, et al: Increased prevalence of HLA-B27 in patients with ectopic ossification following traumatic spinal cord injury. Rheumatol Rehabil 20:193–197, 1981.
22. Mendelson L, Grosswasser Z, Najenson T, et al: Periarticular new bone formation in patients suffering from severe head injuries. Scand J Rehabil Med 7:141–145, 1975.
23. Mielants H, Vanhove E, deNeels J, Veys E: Clinical survey of and pathogenic approach to para-articular ossifications in long-term coma. Acta Orthop Scand 46:190–198, 1975.
24. Minare P, Betuel H, Girard R, Pilonchery G: Neurologic injuries, paraosteoarthropathies, and human leukocyte antigens. Arch Phys Med Rehabil 61:214–215, 1980.
25. Orzel JA, Rudd TG: Heterotopic bone formation: Clinical, laboratory, and imaging correlation. J Nucl Med 26:125–132, 1985.
26. Puzas JE, Miller MD, Rosier RN: Pathologic bone formation. Clin Orthop 245:269–281, 1989.
27. Ritter MA, Gioe TJ: The effect of indomethacin on para-articular ectopic ossification following total hip arthroplasty. Clin Orthop 167:113–117, 1982.
28. Roberts JB, Pankratz DG: Surgical treatment of heterotopic ossification at the elbow following long-term coma. J Bone Joint Surg 61A:760–763, 1979.
29. Russell RGG, Smith R: Diphosphonates—Experimental and clinical aspects. J Bone Joint Surg 55B:66–86, 1973.
30. Sazbon L, Najenson T, Tartakovsky M, et al: Wide-spread peri-articular new bone formation in long-term comatose patients. J Bone Joint Surg 63B:120–125, 1981.
31. Schmidt SA, Kjaersgaard-Anderson P, Pederson NW, et al: The use of indomethacin to prevent the formation of heterotopic bone after total hip replacement. J Bone Joint Surg 70A:834–838, 1988.
32. Spielman G, Gennarelli TA, Rogers CR: Disodium etidronate: Its role in preventing heterotopic ossification in severe head injury. Arch Phys Med Rehabil 64:539–543, 1983.
33. Weiss S, Grosswasser A, Ohri A, et al: Histocompatibility (HLA) antigens in heterotopic ossification associated with neurological injury. J Rheumatol 6:88–91, 1979.

DAVID J. KOLESSAR, MD
MARY ANN E. KEENAN, MD

SURGICAL MANAGEMENT OF UPPER EXTREMITY DEFORMITIES FOLLOWING TRAUMATIC BRAIN INJURY

From the
Department of Orthopaedic
  Surgery (DJK, MAEK)
Albert Einstein Medical Center
  and
Department of Physical Medicine
  and Rehabilitation (MAEK)
Temple University School of
  Medicine
Philadelphia, Pennsylvania

Correspondence to:
Mary Ann E. Keenan, MD
Department of Orthopaedic
  Surgery
Albert Einstein Medical Center
5501 Old York Road
Philadelphia, PA 19141

Spasticity with resultant joint contractures accompanies numerous neurologic disorders in adults. Traumatic brain injuries have become a leading cause of disability, outweighing that of spinal cord injury, stroke, cerebral palsy, or multiple sclerosis.[23,26] These victims can be faced with life-long debilitating loss of function, residual spasticity, and impaired motor control.[12,23] Most are young men injured during motor vehicle accidents, and the vast majority of them will survive to live a normal lifespan.[1,14,23,28] Advances in prehospital care, rapid transport to defined trauma centers, and a progressively better understanding of medical physiology in treating polytraumatized patients have reduced mortality rates of traumatic brain injury patients, creating a growing population.[2,3,16]

Following craniocerebral trauma, loss of upper-motor neuron control may lead to muscle spasticity with resultant deformity or extremity posturing. Spasticity results from loss of normal inhibition of the stretch reflex and the feedback system responsible for maintaining muscle tone. When the normal inhibition from an intact upper motor neuron is lost, the lower motor neuron stretch reflex arc goes unchecked in its activity.[4,9,30a,35] This abnormal and prolonged muscle hypertonicity can lead to muscle-tendon unit contractions and, over time, fixed contractures. Certainly, any limb allowed to remain in a fixed position for a prolonged period will develop

KOLESSAR, KEENAN

contractures of muscle-tendon units, ligaments, and joint capsules. In an attempt to avoid contractures, spasticity is conventionally treated with limb mobilization, muscle stretching, antagonistic muscle strengthening, corrective positioning, static and dynamic splinting, serial casting, and medications to aid muscle relaxation.[4,6,15,27,30] Adjunctive treatments have included electrical muscle stimulation of antagonistic muscles and serial lidocaine, marcaine, or phenol motor nerve blocks.[4,10,30a]

Refractory spasticity and fixed contractures involving the extremities can cause a multitude of problems for the traumatic brain injury patient, including severe functional deficits, limb-positioning difficulties with use, skin breakdown over pressure points, pain, disfigurement, hygienic problems, and need for intensive nursing care.[4,15] Treatment of spasticity is indicated when it persistently interferes with activities of daily living, both functional and hygienic. When pain is disabling from spasticity or contractures and has not responded to conventional treatment, surgical intervention can proceed provided spontaneous recovery of the limb function is no longer expected (Table 1).[4,15,18,32]

The timing of reconstructive surgical procedures is important. Traumatic brain injury patients can experience spontaneous functional recovery over an 18-month period following injury.[9,17] Functional neurologic recovery in patients with head trauma parallels that of stroke victims, although the time frame is different. Neurologic recovery following stroke generally has plateaued by 6 months. In patients who sustain traumatic brain injury, recovery can continue for up to 18 months.[11,13,14,20,21,33,34]

During this period of neurologic recovery, definitive surgery is avoided because the degree of spasticity may change with continued neurologic improvement. Reconstructive surgery performed on patients still in the recovery phase or who show continued functional improvement gives unpredictable results. On occasion, troublesome fixed contractures may develop prior to neurologic stabilization, necessitating surgical intervention once conventional measures fail. Conversely, if a patient's neurologic recovery continues beyond 18 months with conventional means of treatment, surgery should be delayed.[4,15]

In general, the goals of orthopaedic treatment are to increase joint range of motion, enhance potential function, decrease spasticity, and improve contractural deformities. In nonfunctional limbs, goals are to improve limb position, relieve pressure points, and facilitate nursing care and hygiene.[17,19] It is imperative that the goals of rehabilitation be established prior to surgery. They should be realistic and clearly understood by the patient, family, and the medical staff caring for the patient.

PREOPERATIVE EVALUATION

The upper extremity evaluation in traumatic brain injury patients should be comprehensive. Categorization for potentially functional or nonfunctional extremities needs to be determined based on cognitive and communicative skills, presence of

TABLE 1. Indications for Surgery

1. Improve function	5. Prevent pressure sores
2. Relieve pain	6. Facilitate nursing care
3. Improve hygiene	7. Comesis
4. Facilitate limb positioning	

motor control, and hand sensibility.[21,23] A thorough physical examination is performed with attention to position and capacity of spontaneous use with various activities. Motor control quality both proximally and distally need to be assessed. This can often be limited by the patient's inability to follow simple commands.

Intact sensation is essential for optimum upper-extremity function. Sensation with respect to pain, temperature, light touch, proprioception, and two-point discrimination are tested. All of these factors are important predictors of function, especially the ability of two-point discrimination of less than 10 mm.[25]

Upon evaluating these patients, one should not automatically attribute their reduced range of motion solely to spasticity or contracture. Possible causes of decreased arcs of motion can include numerous other disorders (Table 2).[19] Radiographs can rule out fracture, dislocation, and established heterotopic bone. Occasionally, a technetium bone scan is necessary to detect early heterotopic ossification.

Diagnostic nerve blocks using local anesthetics are extremely valuable in assessing a spastic limb and can easily be performed at bedside. Specific muscle contributions to deformities can often be defined by selective motor nerve blocks. Strength and volitional control of antagonistic muscles may also be determined. By blocking spastic muscle groups, volitional control of antagonistic muscles may be unmasked. Also, by temporarily eliminating pain and muscle tone, patient cooperation can be gained and the amount of fixed contracture more accurately demonstrated. Common upper extremity selective diagnostic blocks include brachial plexus, musculocutaneous nerve, radial nerve, median nerve blocks at the elbow, and median and ulnar nerve blocks at the wrist (Fig. 1).[19]

Dynamic electromyography (EMG) can provide detailed information of specific muscles during a functional activity. Demonstrating muscle phasic activity at rest and during specific tasks using multichannel analogue tape permits identification of overactive or out-of-phase muscle activity. A standard classification system is used to describe the patterns seen in dynamic EMG (Table 3).[23,31] Indwelling wire electrodes are used to provide individual muscle tracings necessary when evaluating fine movements of the upper extremity and hand. Adding goniometric tracing and event markers to EMG recordings allows interpretation of muscle activity in relation to specific tasks, such as grasp and release.[6,17,23,25]

The upper extremity spasticity pattern most frequently exhibited is that of flexion, with shoulder adduction and internal rotation, elbow flexion, and flexion of the wrist and fingers, and thumb-in-palm deformity. In the presence of significant spasticity, functional deficits can result from loss of proximal muscle control and the inability to position the hand in space. Distally, extrinsic or intrinsic spasticity or contracture impedes coordinated movements of the hand, digits, and thumb required for grasping, pinching, and releasing. Pain can often accompany these contractures. Severe spasticity or contracture also leads to hygienic problems of the axilla, antecubital fossa, and palm, resulting in skin irritation and maceration. Constant finger pressure and nails being flexed into the palm can breed infection.

TABLE 2. Etiologies for Limitation of Range of Motion

1. Increased muscle tone	5. Pain
2. Myostatic contracture	6. Lack of cooperation secondary to
3. Heterotopic ossification	diminished cognition
4. Undetected fractures or dislocations	7. Peripheral nerve injury

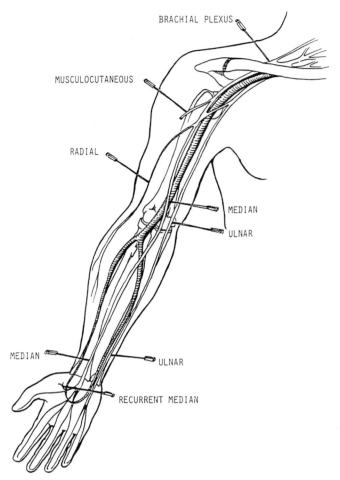

FIGURE 1. Locations of common diagnostic or therapeutic nerve-block sites of the upper extremity.

TABLE 3.   Classification of Dynamic Electromyographic Activity*

Class	Description
I	Normal phasic activity
II	Premature prolonged activity
IIIA	Mildly prolonged activity
IIIB	Moderately prolonged activity
IIIC	Severely prolonged activity
IV	Continuous activity
V	Stretch response activity
VI	No activity

* Adapted from Keenan MA, Haider TT, Stone LR: Dynamic electromyography to assess elbow spasticity. *J Hand Surg* 15A:607–614, 1990.

Principles and goals of surgery in the upper extremity can be simplified to improving function or positioning of the hand in space for patients with some volitional control. For nonfunctional extremities of severely spastic limbs, proper hygiene care of the axilla, antecubital fossa, and palm as well as facilitation of nursing care can be achieved. Any volitional control of a muscle or group of muscles must be preserved. Muscle-tendon lengthenings are used to preserve function and correct deformity. Release of severely spastic muscles or marked contractures are more commonly performed for hygiene problems, positioning difficultites, and pressure sores. Transfers are occasionally performed, but in general are unpredictable in spastic muscles. Bone operations are usually limited to excision of mature heterotopic ossification or wrist arthrodesis.[4,24a,34]

DEFINITIVE SURGICAL PROCEDURES

Shoulder

Deformity of the shoulder is usually characterized by internal rotation with adduction of the arm. This internal rotation and adduction is due to spasticity of the pectoralis major, subscapularis, latissimus dorsi, or teres major muscles. Surgical intervention is indicated when spastic contracture interferes with more distal function, causes severe pain, impedes dressing, or prevents axillary hygiene. Through examination of the arm in abduction, external rotation allows palpation of all but the subscapularis muscle. Therefore, with the arm at the side, external rotation of the humerous will evaluate subscapularis spasticity or contracture. Dynamic EMG may aid in identifying specific involved muscles. Functional shoulders may need only the pectoralis major and subscapularis muscles released. Nonfunctional or diffusely involved shoulder may require release of all four muscles mentioned earlier.[4,34]

The technique used in performing a shoulder release involves a 5- to 8-cm incision made over the insertion of the pectoralis major, which is easily identified and released. The subscapularis is then exposed and isolated from the shoulder capsule and released near its insertion on the humerus. The shoulder joint capsule is left intact to prevent the formation of intraarticular adhesions or anterior instability. The latissimus dorsi and teres major can then be released if found to be contributing to the deformity or residual contracture. Their release is performed through the interval between the short head of the biceps and deltoid muscles (Fig. 2). Drains are placed in dead space created. An aggressive mobilization program is instituted as soon as wound healing and patient comfort permit.[4,6,24a,34]

Elbow

At the elbow, the deformity is usually one of flexion contracture due to spasticity of the brachioradialis, biceps, and brachialis muscles. Smooth control of elbow flexion and extension is frequently impaired, limiting the patient's performance when good hand control is present. Dynamic EMG recordings have revealed that the brachioradialis muscle dominates in spasticity, and the biceps and brachialis are affected to a lesser degree.[20,23] After lidocaine block of the musculocutaneous and radial nerves, the proportion of deformity contributed by spasticity and contracture may be more accurately portrayed.

A functional elbow release is performed by a proximal myotomy of the brachioradialis muscle combined with a Z-lengthening of the biceps tendon and fractional myotendinous lengthening of the brachialis muscle. This is performed

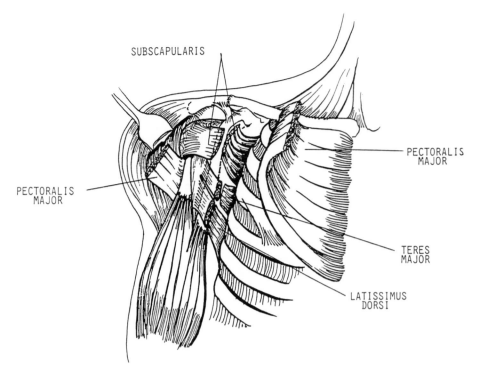

SUBSCAPULARIS

PECTORALIS
MAJOR

PECTORALIS
MAJOR

TERES
MAJOR

LATISSIMUS
DORSI

FIGURE 2. Shoulder muscles that may require release include pectoralis major, subscapularis, teres major, and latissimus dorsi.

through an S-shaped incision on the anterolateral aspect of the elbow (Fig. 3).[4,6,20,34] Postoperatively, the extremity is casted in 45° of flexion for 4 weeks, followed by night splints for an additional 4 weeks and an active therapy program.

In the nonfunctional elbow, both degree and duration of deformity are considered. If the flexion deformity is 120° or less, the brachioradialis and biceps muscles are released in conjunction with lengthening of the brachialis muscle. For long-standing deformities greater than 120°, a complete release of the brachialis muscle may be necessary. Musculocutaneous neurectomy has been advocated by some authors,[6,34] but this procedure does not eliminate the severe spasticity of the brachioradialis muscle, which is innervated by the radial nerve. Furthermore, late recurrence of spasticity in both the biceps and brachialis muscles has been seen after neurectomy. This recurrence is thought to be attributed to anatomic variation in the proximal motor branches exiting from the musculocutaneous nerve.[8] Ulnar nerve symptoms may necessitate its decompression and anterior transposition.

Severe rigid flexion contractures of the elbow can be approached through a lateral incision, which augments approximation of skin edges as the elbow is extended. The interval between the biceps and brachioradialis is developed. The radial nerve is identified and protected. The brachioradialis can be released by subperiosteal dissection from the humerus and from its attachment along the lateral intramuscular septum or division through the muscle belly itself. The biceps

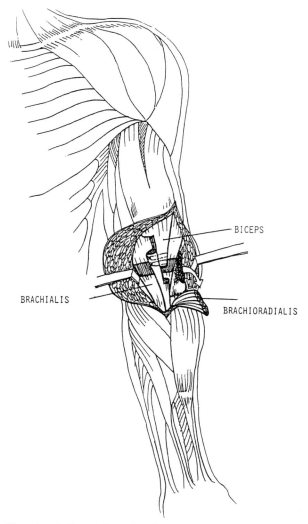

FIGURE 3.   Functional elbow release involves myotomy through the proximal portion of the brachioradialis, combined with a Z-lengthening of the biceps tendon and fractional myotendinous lengthening of the brachialis muscle.

tendon is tenotomized. Access to brachialis is then provided, and transection of the tendinous fibers and/or muscle belly is performed as needed (Fig. 4). Complete extension of the elbow is usually limited by the neurovascular structures. Drains and a posterior splint are applied.[4,6,34] Further correction of residual contracture is achieved by weekly serial-casting techniques.[24a]

Wrist

Flexion of the wrist and fingers result from spasticity of forearm wrist flexors and digital flexors. Impairments result from the inability to position the hand in

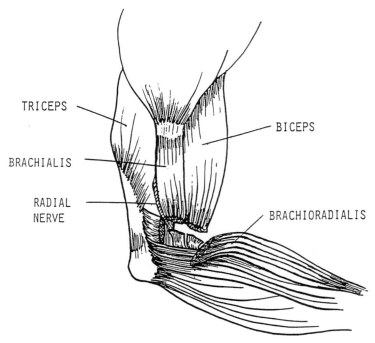

TRICEPS

BICEPS

BRACHIALIS

RADIAL
NERVE

BRACHIORADIALIS

FIGURE 4. Release of elbow flexors in severe flexion deformity and contracture.

space and problems with opening the hand to grasp or release. Hygiene in the palm can become a problem due to the chronically clenched fist. Median neuropathy has also been reported.[29]

In the functional extremity with a wrist flexion deformity, grasp may be weak because finger flexors are not at their optimal resting length; thus, lengthening of the wrist flexors should be performed. Prior to wrist flexor tendon lengthening or release, determination as to whether a patient will be able to extend his or her fingers once the wrist deformity is corrected needs to be addressed. When extrinsic finger flexors are spastic or contracted, finger extension may be impossible when the wrist is held in neutral or extension. Therefore, evaluation of the digits preoperatively, with the wrist held in the corrected position, allows proper assessment. If digital extrinsic muscles are contracted as well, lengthening of these at the time of wrist flexor lengthening should be considered.[4,30,33]

In the nonfunctional wrist, release of the wrist flexors will improve hygiene. Complete release of all wrist and finger flexors should be avoided because a resultant wrist extension deformity will occur. One may consider wrist arthrodesis to maintain correction; otherwise, a volar splint is necessary to prevent recurrent wrist flexion due to gravity.[4,6,24a,34]

Fingers

The inability to extend the fingers creates a situation of functional compromise and hygienic problems. In the functional hand, fractional lengthening of the finger flexors at the myotendinous junction has been effective.[4,21,33,34]

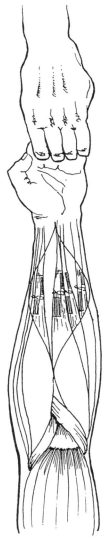

FIGURE 5.   Fractional lengthening of the flexor tendons by passive extension after Z-lengthening at the myotendinous junctions.

This technique uses an incision made on the volar aspect of the forearm. The palmaris longus tendon is divided. The flexor carpi radialis and flexor carpi ulnaris tendons are transected for Z-lengthening if a wrist flexion deformity is present. Lengthening of the flexor digitorum superficialis and profundus tendons is performed by incising the flexor tendons in a "Z" at the myotendinous junction and then passively extending the digits, allowing the tendons to slide distally.[21,34] Tendons are usually lengthened 1 to 2 cm and may be sutured in this position, but we have stopped using these Z-lengthenings and have encountered more uniform attitude of the fingers (Fig. 5). Wrist flexor Z-lengthenings are performed with the wrist brought to 20° of extension. The flexor pollicis longus often requires a similar lengthening procedure. Postoperatively, we begin the patient on an immediate hand therapy and range-of-motion program. Night splints may be fabricated for comfort with the wrist in 20° extension, metacarpophalangeal joints flexed 60°, and interphalangeal joints extended.[4,21,24a,34]

For the nonfunctional hand, the above procedure may improve hand position and hygiene. More often, greater lengthening is needed to correct the more severe contracture. The flexor digitorum superficialis to profundus tendon transfer is another option. Originally described by Braun et al.,[7] this procedure is reserved for patients lacking volitional control who have failed attempts to control hand position by nonoperative means. This procedure allows a greater degree of lengthening than by fractional technique, but it does sacrifice the function of the flexor digitorum profundus tendons. This technique has been modified from Braun's original description because of the variations in tension of digital flexors that developed in some patients treated.[4,24]

In this procedure, a longitudinal incision is made over the volar forearm. The distal portion of the incision is extended over Guyon's canal to access the motor branch of the ulnar nerve. The neurovascular structures are identified and protected. The palmaris longus tendon is divided. The four flexor digitorum superficialis tendons are identified just proximal to the transverse carpal ligament and sutured together "en masse" to form a single tendon unit (Fig. 6A). The tendons are then sharply transected distal to the suture and retracted proximately, exposing the flexor digitorum profundus tendons. These four profundus tendons are also sutured en masse at the most proximal juncture and transected proximal to the suture (Fig. 6B).[4,24] Capsular contractures of the metacarpophalangeal and proximal interphalangeal joints are usually correctable by passive extension of the digits. The flexor pollicis longus tendon should be examined because it frequently requires lengthening at this point. A Z-plasty or fractional lengthening technique may be used. The hand is then placed in the desired position, usually 20° of dorsiflexion at the wrist, 20° of flexion at the metacarpophalangeal and proximal interphalangeal

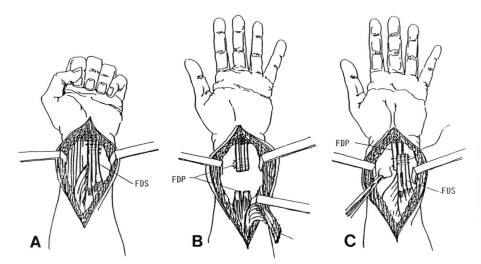

FIGURE 6. The flexor digitorum superficialis (FDS) to flexor digitorum profundus (FDP) "en masse" transfer used for severely contracted finger flexor deformities in the nonfunctional hand.

joints of the digits. Now, the proximal portion of the flexor digitorum superficialis tendon mass is sutured to the distal portion of the flexor digitorum profundus mass in the desired position (Fig. 6C).

If Z-lengthening of the flexor carpi radialis and ulnaris tendons has been necessary, they are reanastomosed at this time. It is recommended that a neurectomy of the motor branch of ulnar nerve be performed routinely in conjunction with this transfer. This step controls intrinsic spasticity and can be performed by extending this incision just distal to Guyon's canal. Once isolation of the motor branch is achieved and confirmed with a nerve stimulator, a 1-cm segment of nerve is excised.[4,24,24a]

Intrinsic Muscle Spasticity or Contracture

Intrinsic spasticity or contracture often exists concomitantly with extrinsic finger flexor deformity and is masked by their myotonic overpowering. Intrinsic muscle deformity should be addressed at the time of extrinsic flexor deformity correction; otherwise, an intrinsic plus deformity may result postoperatively. In the nonfunctional, clenched-fist deformity, neurectomy of the motor branch of the ulnar nerve is performed at the time of extrinsic finger flexor lengthening. Concomitant adductor pollicis spasticity will be relieved, and both hygienic and cosmetic appearance will improve. This will avoid an intrinsic plus deformity postoperatively; an intrinsic minus deformity has not been seen as a problem.

Intrinsic contracture release is performed on the lateral bands of the extensor hood mechanism at the level of the proximal phalanx. Here, the lateral bands are identified and a triangular section from the palmar fibers excised.[4] A neurectomy of the motor branch of the ulnar nerve is also performed to prevent late recurrent deformity secondary to spasticity of the interossei.[4,24a,34]

Thumb-in-Palm Deformity

A thumb-in-palm deformity frequently accompanies the clenched-fist deformity from extrinsic digital flexor spasticity. Because the thumb is pulled into the palm, it is unable to function dynamically for grip or as an opposing post for the fingers. In more severe cases, hygienic problems in the palm and thenar areas occur. The offending muscles can include flexor pollicis longus, flexor pollicis brevis, abductor pollicis brevis, opponens pollicis, adductor pollicis, and the first dorsal and palmar interossei muscles. Once conservative measures have failed (i.e., phenol blocks of the recurrent motor branch of the median nerve and ulnar nerves), surgical treatment is indicated. Preoperative evaluation is complicated because of the variable degrees of involvement of the muscles mentioned earlier. Physical examination, selective diagnostic lidocaine nerve blocks, and dynamic electromyographs are essential.[4,6,24a]

Interphalangeal joint flexion deformity is caused by flexor pollicis longus spasticity. Intrinsic spasticity can be eliminated by median and ulnar nerve blocks at the wrist to isolate flexor pollicis longus spasticity. Treatment can consist of fractional or Z-lengthening of the flexor pollicis longus tendon by using a technique similar to that described for extrinsic finger flexor lengthening. If an excessive fixed flexion contracture of the interphalangeal joint exists or if excessive flexion occurs during pinch, stabilization of the joint in less flexion by arthrodesis will both improve grasp and pinch functions in functional patients and facilitate hygiene. This procedure usually requires simultaneous flexor pollicis longus lengthening. The interphalangeal joint of the thumb is fused in approximately 10° of flexion.[4,6,22]

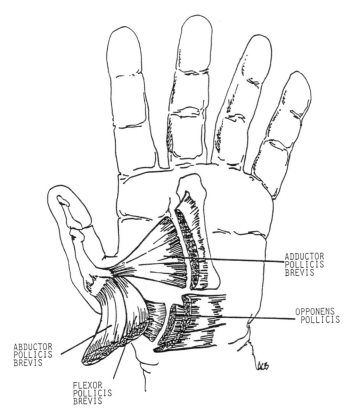

ADDUCTOR
POLLICIS
BREVIS

OPPONENS
POLLICIS

ABDUCTOR
POLLICIS
BREVIS

FLEXOR
POLLICIS
BREVIS

FIGURE 7.   Surgical release of thenar muscles for thumb-in-palm deformity.

Thumb intrinsic spasticity may involve the adductor pollicis, the first dorsal and palmar interossei, and the thenar muscles. Identifying the offending muscles is necessary for proper surgical release. Adductor pollicis spasticity causes flexion at the metacarpophalangeal joint, whereas spasticity of the first dorsal interosseous results in narrowing of the thumb web space. Lidocaine blocks of the ulnar nerve will decrease these deformities, and dynamic EMG studies will help further identify those offending muscles.[4-6]

Thenar muscle spasticity or contracture can involve the flexor pollicis brevis, abductor pollicis brevis, and the opponens pollicis muscles. Involvement is usually evident by palpation over the thenar muscle mass, which reveals spasm, and can be confirmed by lidocaine block of the median nerve or by dynamic EMG testing.

Surgical release of the thenar muscles can be performed by origin releases through a palmar incision along the thenar crease. The flexor tendons and neurovascular bundles are retracted toward the ulna. Once the origins of the adductor pollicis, flexor pollicis brevis, and abductor pollicis are identified, they are released and allowed to retract radially to eventually scar down in a new location, thus preserving their function while avoiding an overcorrection or hyperextension deformity (Fig. 7).[4-6] The distal thumb contracture is remedied by flexor pollicis longus lengthening in the forearm. Stabilization of the interphalangeal joint of the thumb by arthrodesis is recommended and beneficial in pinch strength. Postoperatively, a thumb spica cast is worn for 4 weeks, followed by an active therapy program.[24a]

SUMMARY

Spastic upper extremity deformities following traumatic brain injury can result in significant disability. Medical personnel from various specialties must join in the care of these complex patients. An understanding of neuromuscular spasticity is essential for optimizing treatment strategies. Once more conservative management techniques have been exhausted, surgical correction of spastic limb deformities can still yield successful and rewarding results for patients, families, and medical personnel.

ACKNOWLEDGMENTS

Medical illustrations were done by Anthony C. Berlet, MD. We are grateful to Dolores M. Smith and Sandra Q. McCarthy for their assistance in preparing this manuscript.

REFERENCES

1. Anderson DH, McLaurin RL: The National Head and Spinal Cord Injury Survey. J Neurosurg 53:S1–43, 1980.
2. Baxt WG, Moody P: The impact of advanced prehospital emergency care on the morality of severely brain-injured patients. J Trauma 27:365–369, 1987.
3. Baxt WG, Moody P: The differential survival of trauma patients. J Trauma 27:602–606, 1987.
4. Botte MJ, Keenan MA: Reconstructive surgery of the upper extremity in the patient with head trauma. J Head Trauma Rehabil 2:34–45, 1987.
5. Botte MJ, Keenan MA, Gellman H, et al: Surgical management of spastic thumb-in-palm deformity in adults with brain injury. J Hand Surg 13A:306–307, 1988.
6. Botte MJ, Waters RL, Keenan MA, et al: Orthopaedic management of the stroke patient: Part II—Treating deformities of the upper and lower extremities. Orthop Rev 17:891–910, 1988.
7. Braun RM, Vise GT, Roper B: Preliminary experience with superficialis-to-profundus tendon transfer in the hemiplegic upper extremity. J Bone Joint Surg 56A:466–472, 1974.
8. Flatow EL, Bigliani LU, April EW: An anatomic study of the musculocutaneous nerve and its relationship to the coracoid process. Clin Orthop 244:166–171, 1989.
9. Garland DE, Keenan MA: Orthopaedic strategies in the management of the adult head-injury patient. Phys Ther 63:2004–2009, 1983.
10. Garland DE, Lucie SR, Waters RL: Current uses of open phenol nerve blocks for adult acquired spasticity. Clin Orthop 165:217–222, 1982.
11. Garland DE, Rhoades ME: Orthopedic management of brain injured adults. Clin Orthop 131:111–122, 1978.
12. Goldstein M: Traumatic brain injury: A silent epidemic [editorial]. Ann Neurol 27:327, 1990.
13. Groswasser Z, Cohen M, Costeff H: Rehabilitation outcome after anoxic brain damage. Arch Phys Med Rehabil 70:186–188, 1989.
14. Heiden JS, Small R, Caton W, et al: Severe head injury and outcome: A prospective study. In Popp AJ (ed): Neural Trauma. New York, Raven Press, 1979, pp 181–193.
15. Herz DA, Looman JE, Tiberio A, et al: The management of paralytic spasticity. Neurosurgery 26:300–306, 1990.
16. Jacobs LM, Sinclair A, Beiser A, et al: Prehospital advanced life support: Benefits in trauma. J Trauma 24:8–13, 1984.
17. Jordan C: Current status of functional lower extremity surgery in adult spastic patients. Clin Orthop 233:102–109, 1988.
18. Kasdon DL: Controversies in the surgical management of spasticity. Clin Neurosurg 33:523–529, 1986.
19. Keenan MA: The orthopedic management of spasticity. J Head Trauma Rehabil 2:62–71, 1987.
20. Keenan MA: Management of the spastic upper extremity in the neurologically impaired adult. Clin Orthop 233:116–125, 1988.

21. Keenan MA, Abrams RA, Garland DE, Waters RL: Results of fractional lengthening of the finger flexors in adults with upper extremity spasticity. J Hand Surg 12A:575–581, 1987.

22. Keenan MA, Abrams RA, Garland DE, Waters RL: Results of the fractural lengthening of the finger flexors in adults with upper extremity spasticity. J Hand Surg 12A:575–581, 1987.

23. Keenan MA, Haider TT, Stone LR: Dynamic electromyography to assess elbow spasticity. J Hand Surg 15A:607–614, 1990.

24. Keenan MA, Korchek JI, Botte MJ, et al: Results of transfer of the flexor digitorum superficialis tendons to the flexor digitorum profundus tendons in adults with acquired spasticity of the hand. J Bone Joint Surg 69A:1127–1132, 1987.

24a. Keenan MAE, Kozin SH, Berlet AC: Manual of Orthopaedic Surgery for Spasticity. New York, Raven Press, 1993, pp 3–68.

25. Keenan MA, Perry J: Evaluation of upper extremity motor control in spastic brain-injured patients using dynamic electromyography. J Head Trauma Rehabil 5:13–22, 1990.

26. Kraus JF, Black MA, Hessol M, et al: The incidence of acute brain injury in a defined population. Am J Epidemiol 119:186–201, 1984.

27. McCollough NC: Orthotic management in adult hemiplegia. Clin Orthop 131:38–46, 1978.

28. Meals RA: Denervation for the treatment of acquired spasticity of the brachioradialis. J Bone Joint Surg 70A:1081–1084, 1988.

29. Orcutt SA, Kramer WG, Howard MV, et al: Carpal tunnel syndrome secondary to wrist and finger flexor spasticity. J Hand Surg 15A:940–944, 1990.

30. Ough JL, Garland DE, Jordan C, et al: Treatment of spastic joint contractures in mentally disabled adults. Orthop Clin North Am 12:143–151, 1981.

30a. Parziale JR, Akelman E, Herz DA: Spasticity: Pathophysiology and management. Orthopaedics 16:801–811, 1993.

31. Samilson RL, Morris JW: Surgical improvement of the cerebral palsied upper limb: Electromyographic studies and results of 128 operations. J Bone Joint Surg 46A: 1203–1216, 1964.

32. Sharkey PC: Medical and surgical management of spasticity. Clin Neurosurg 28:589–596, 1981.

33. Waters RL: Upper extremity surgery in stroke patients. Clin Orthop 131:30–37, 1978.

34. Waters RL, Keenan MA: Upper extremity surgery in stroke. In Chapman M (ed): Operative Orthopaedics. Philadelphia, JB Lippincott, 1988, pp 1449–1458.

35. Yarkony GM, Sahgal V: Contractures: A major complication of craniocerebral trauma. Clin Orthop 219:93–96, 1987.

MICHAEL S. PINZUR, MD

LOWER EXTREMITY COMPLICATIONS FOLLOWING TRAUMATIC BRAIN INJURY

From the
Gait Analysis Laboratory
Department of Orthopaedic
  Surgery
Loyola University Medical Center
Maywood, Illinois

Correspondence to:
Michael S. Pinzur, MD
Department of Orthopaedic
  Surgery
Loyola University Medical Center
2160 South First Avenue
Maywood, IL 60153

The role of the orthopaedic surgeon in the initial care of patients following traumatic brain injury (TBI) is generally limited to fracture management. Functional outcome in TBI patients is optimized when fracture care is approached with the same dedication as for the polytraumatized, neurologically intact patient. Acute injury care is best supervised by a traumatologist with consultation from medical specialists as dictated by the specific organ systems involved. Too often, rehabilitation is overlooked and functional outcome underestimated during this period of life and limb salvage, leaving patients with long-term severe joint contractures that increase their disability and complicate their rehabilitation. We have found that early intervention by a rehabilitation team is invaluable to ensure institution of appropriate therapies, including splinting, casting, positioning, and nerve blocks intended to maximize the potential for a good outcome. The orthopaedic surgeon becomes involved again as a member of the rehabilitation team when the patient plateaus in his or her recovery or when spastic deformity impairs further progress.

PRINCIPLES OF FRACTURE CARE

Both early and late outcome in TBI patients with fractures is enhanced by early mobilization. Traction, cast immobilization, and prolonged bedrest may lead to deconditioning, muscle atrophy, osteoporosis, hypercalcemia, soft tissue contractures, and decubitus ulcers. Long bone and spinal fractures should be treated aggressively, with a minimum of external immobilization and enforced bedrest. Traction as a rule is avoided in these patients due to the difficulty in maintaining fracture alignment secondary to muscle spasticity and poor compliance. The weight and bulkiness of enclosing casts limit the patient's mobility, and the patient may be unable to inform the physician of a tight or poorly contoured cast.

Methods of open reduction and rigid internal fixation should be employed to accomplish early mobilization and unencumber the patient. Many fractures that would ordinarily be treated with closed techniques should be treated surgically to enhance these goals.[2,3,4]

SPASTICITY MANAGEMENT

The second early role of the orthopaedic surgeon is the management of spastic deformities, including supervision of appropriate positioning, joint ranging and serial casting, as well as guiding early physical and occupational therapies in weight-bearing status, range-of-motion limitations, and the diagnosis of missed orthopaedic injuries. Splinting the ankle at a neutral position is not sufficient to prevent the development of an equinus contracture. Functional joint ranging by acute care nurses multiple times daily, in addition to twice-daily ranging by physical therapists, will greatly augment appropriate splinting and prevent static joint contracture.

When range of motion is unsuccessful, then serial inhibitory casting of the ankle and knee in a functional position will prevent contracture and dampen the stretch reflex. Anesthetic nerve blocks of the posterior tibial or sciatic nerve prior to casting relieve pain and allow for maximum correction of the deformity.

TIMING OF FUNCTIONAL ORTHOPAEDIC INTERVENTION

Early intervention should be reversible and is generally limited to nerve blocks with long-acting local anesthetics or phenol. Although phenol nerve blocks are easily performed percutaneously, occasionally open blocks may be warranted to avoid injecting mixed nerves with large sensory contributions. Surgical intervention in spastic TBI patients is generally delayed until the patient achieves his or her maximum spontaneous motor recovery, which usually occurs at approximately 18 months following injury. Alternatively, rather than use a fixed calendar to plan intervention, we attempt to assess improvement versus time (Fig. 1). When the patient reaches a plateau in functional progress or when the deformity impedes further progress, intervention can be considered. Invasive procedures in this population should be an adjunct to a standard functional rehabilitation program, not an alternative.

SPASTICITY MODEL

The deformities seen in TBI patients are either dynamic, static or, more often, a combination of both. Dynamic deformity is produced by muscle hypertonicity. Under anesthesia, or following a diagnostic anesthetic nerve block, the spastic deformity can be fully corrected by passive movement. Static deformity is a result of fixed contracture produced by connective tissue cross-linking in collagen within muscles, ligaments, and joints. Static contracture cannot therefore be corrected under anesthesia. With the combination of dynamic and static deformity, only the dynamic component can be corrected under anesthesia. Radiographs should be taken of the hip, knee, and ankle joints in TBI patients with contracture to rule out heterotopic ossification as a cause of the joint range-of-motion limitation.

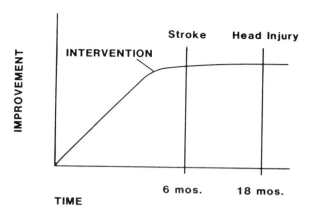

FIGURE 1. Intervention should be considered when patients either reach a plateau in functional improvement or when their dynamic deformity impedes the rehabilitation effort. We have rarely intervened in the stroke patient before 6 months and in the TBI patient before approximately 15 to 18 months following brain insult.

The phenomenon of spasticity is a complex disorder characterized neurologically by loss of descending inhibition, afferent excitation, and uncovering of more primitive motor patterns. For example, the newborn has reflexic activity but lacks the higher brain inhibitory centers to modulate these activities, as evidenced by the startle response. As the child grows and matures, he or she develops integration and modulation of these primitive motor patterns, which gradually mature into gross and, eventually, selective motor control. TBI damages these inhibitory pathways by diaschisis or shear and uncovers the characteristic synergic patterns of muscle activity associated with spasticity. Rehabilitation strives to re-educate and unmask alternative inhibitory modulatory controls, both during the period of spontaneous recovery and when the neurologic recovery plateaus.

When planning intervention, we use a simple agonist-antagonist muscle imbalance model. In normal movement, we assume smooth balance between the muscles on both sides of a joint. For example, when we grasp an object, balanced muscle activity occurs between wrist, finger flexor, and extensor muscle groups, with relatively greater activity of the flexors during grasp activities. The spastic patient has a loss of this balance between opposing muscle groups. Due to the imbalance, patients will cocontract and assume an unbalanced, poorly functional position and consequently will not be able to perform the task.

In our model for intervention, we use the length-strength characteristics of the involved muscle groups. There is an optimum muscle length for achieving the greatest force of contraction. If we surgically lengthen a muscle, we place it at a less advantageous position in its length-strength relationship, thus weakening its force. By lengthening the agonist muscle that is producing the dynamic deformity, the deforming motor force, as well as the stretch reflex, is weakened. Motor balance across the joint is thus achieved by weakening the agonist-deforming motor force and potentially augmenting the antagonist with a tendon transfer.

Early intervention should be minimal and reversible, taking advantage of spontaneous recovery. Late intervention at the completion of spontaneous recovery, on the other hand, should create dynamic motor balance.

GOALS FOR INTERVENTION

When it has been decided that surgical intervention is appropriate, one must consider the goals of treatment. Surgery can be performed for functional or nonfunctional goals. Contracture releases are generally nonfunctional surgeries limited to custodial or chair-bound patients with limited rehabilitation potential. Contracture releases are usually indicated to improve hygiene or wheelchair positioning or to relieve pain.

When surgery is considered to improve function, patients should be screened for cognitive deficits, motivation, and body-image awareness.[10,11] Patients should be out of a confusional state and possess short-term memory and the capacity for new learning. In addition to specific cognitive strengths, motivation is necessary for patients to use functional gains and participate in their rehabilitation program. Body-image awareness is essential for surgical intervention to become meaningful and potentially beneficial. Patients who do lack the awareness of a limb, i.e., neglect or its position in space should undergo therapy directed toward improving these deficits before surgical intervention is considered.

EVALUATION

Keenan et al.[5] have shown that balance is the best predictor of a patient's ability to ambulate following a stroke. In addition to balance, patients must achieve limb stability and muscle power to achieve limb advancement.[1] Many TBI patients will be able to regain the ability to walk, but their gait pattern will be energy demanding due to a combination of static and dynamic deformities.

Patients must be examined in the functional, i.e., standing, position. For example, one cannot prescribe a brace intended to correct a dynamic deformity after examining a sitting patient. Observations by the patient's therapist or family may also provide valuable information. In patients who regain their ambulation capacity, there is a consistent pattern of alteration in the hip-knee-ankle axis. We found a common pattern, characterized by ankle equinus at initial floor contact, i.e., "heel strike," knee hyperextension at midstance, and increased hip flexion at terminal stance. The magnitude of this dynamic deformity pattern varied with the severity of the brain insult (Fig. 2).[12,13]

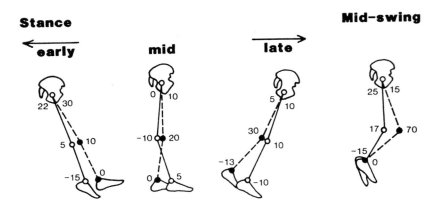

FIGURE 2.   These stick figures represent the average positions of the hip, knee, and ankle in a group of adult-acquired hemiplegic patients recorded using an electrogoniometer during walking. The dotted lines represent the position of hip, knee, and ankle in the normal unaffected limb, and the solid lines represent the hemiplegic limb. From Pinzur MS, Sherman R, DiMonte-Levine P, Trimble J: Gait changes in adult onset hemiplegia. *Am J Phys Med* 66:228, 1987; with permission.

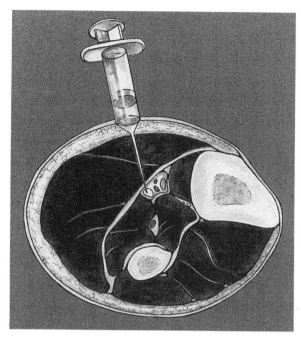

FIGURE 3. Posterior tibial nerve block is performed 7 cm distal to the popliteal flexion crease along a perpendicular line dropped from the proximal apex of the popliteal fossa.

We can define the correction of the dynamic deformity by diagnostic anesthetic posterior tibial nerve block (Fig. 3).[7,10,11] Posterior tibial nerve block is performed 7 cm distal to the popliteal flexion crease along a perpendicular dropped from the proximal apex of the popliteal fossa.

DYNAMIC ELECTROMYOGRAPHY

We recommend dynamic, i.e., walking, electromyography (EMG) in all patients as a planning tool prior to surgery. Although many motion-analysis laboratories use fine-wire intramuscular electrodes, we have found that surface electrodes are acceptable for decision making. It is unlikely that individual neurologically related muscles within a muscle compartment will fire at clinically different times during the gait cycle, so surface EMG is sufficient for surgical planning. By using muscle groups, the motor points for recording are relatively simple to identify (Fig. 4).[12] The EMG records the phasic electrical activity of the muscle groups, not muscle strength or force, and appears to amplify and improve clinical examination.

NONSURGICAL TREATMENT

The mainstay of treatment for the dynamic ankle equinus component of this gait deviation is to achieve ankle stability in neutral position during initial floor contact (i.e., heel strike) and stance, as well as floor clearance during swing phase.

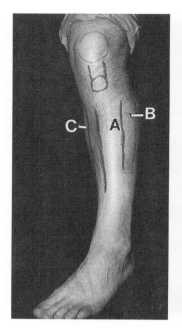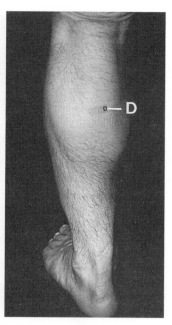

FIGURE 4. Superficial motor points for the anterior tibial (*A*), peroneal (*B*), posterior tibial (*C*), and gastrocnemius and soleus muscles (*D*). From Pinzur MS, Sherman R, DiMonte-Levine P, et al: Adult-onset hemiplegia: Changes in gait after muscle-balancing procedures to correct the equinus deformity. *J Bone Joint Surg* 68A:1249, 1986; with permission.

An adjustable ankle-foot orthosis, with available ankle dorsiflexion and a plantar flexion stop at neutral, is often used during the recovery period, followed by a rigid ankle-foot orthosis once the patient has plateaued in his or her recovery. We have sometimes found the dynamic equinus force to be sufficiently powerful that patients may well "walk out" of their brace (Fig. 5).[9,11] T-straps, increased trim lines, or rigidity are then added to the orthosis in an attempt to control the deformity, but these may not achieve satisfactory correction and maintenance of the ankle at neutral position during the stance phase. It is essential to achieve ankle stability without equinus deformity, because correction of the ankle equinus during stance generally corrects the apparently compensatory hyperextension deformity at the knee and hyperflexion deformity at the hip.[12]

If the diagnostic posterior tibial nerve block is successful in correcting the dynamic deformity, we proceed with percutaneous posterior tibial phenol nerve block with or without an ankle-foot orthosis.[7] Although dysesthesias appear to be common with phenol nerve blocks in the upper extremity, we have not experienced this morbidity in the lower extremity. To ensure accurate placement of the phenol, Moore and Anderson[8] have elected to accomplish this technique surgically by the direct exposure and injection of the motor branches. Motor balancing surgery is considered when the phenol nerve block's effect dissipates and no longer adequately corrects the dynamic deformity. We have found such patients to be "nonbraceable."

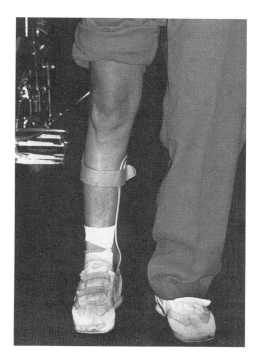

FIGURE 5. The dynamic ankle equinus in this young woman could not be controlled with a rigid ankle-foot orthosis, even following addition of a T-strap. She was considered "nonbraceable" and underwent motor-balancing surgery. From Pinzur MS: Functional surgery in stroke and head injury. *Complications Orthop* (May/Jun):73–77, 1990; with permission.

SURGICAL TREATMENT

Foot and Ankle Deformities

Ankle equinus is the most readily apparent and common disorder that we see in the TBI patient population. When orthotic management has not been successful or when patients have either static ankle equinus or nonbraceable dynamic ankle equinus that does not easily correct with percutaneous phenol or recurs following open posterior tibial nerve block, we recommend motor-balancing surgery to correct the ankle equinus and secondarily correct the hip and knee disorders.

Taking advantage of the length-strength characteristics of muscle, we treat the equinus deformity by Hoke percutaneous tendo-Achilles lengthening (Fig. 6). Overlengthening of the Achilles tendon leads to a "crouched" gait pattern, with knee flexion and ankle dorsiflexion during stance. This reverse deformity is potentially more disabling than equinus and can be avoided by combining percutaneous tendo-Achilles lengthening with 6-week postoperative immobilization in a walking cast with the ankle positioned at neutral. This allows the gastrocnemius-soleus muscle group to "find" the appropriate dynamic functional length.[9,12] These patients almost universally have a concomitant varus component, i.e., equinovarus. The dynamic varus-producing force in adults is the result of out-of-phase tibialis anterior muscle activity during stance.[12,15] This is different from the force in

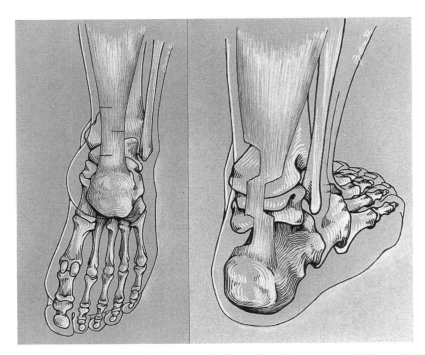

FIGURE 6. *Left,* Tendo-Achilles lengthening is performed percutaneously through three small stab wounds, leaving the tendon sheath intact. *Right,* By lengthening the spastic muscle within the tendon sheath, patients can set the correct balanced muscle length by walking in a short-leg walking cast with the ankle positioned at neutral. From Pinzur MS: Functional surgery in stroke and head injury. *Complications Orthop* (May/Jun):73–77, 1990; with permission.

children, in whom the varus-deforming force is generally the tibialis posterior muscle. This dynamic varus deformity is corrected either by split or complete lateral transfer of the tibialis anterior muscle.[9,12] If hindfoot varus is observed and dynamic EMG confirms out-of-phase swing phase activity of the posterior tibialis muscle as well, a fractional musculotendinous lengthening of the posterior tibialis muscle is performed at the time of tendon transfer. When we performed follow-up motion analysis in these patients, we found that although not normal, the energy-inefficient dynamic hip and knee deformities were greatly improved (Fig. 7).

Another method of treatment for this disorder is electrical stimulation of the overpowered ankle dorsiflexors, with superficial or implanted electrodes stimulating the peroneal nerve. This system is triggered by a heel-switch transmitter. Although adequate, the presently available systems are generally too "gadget intensive" for these patients.[17]

Occasionally, patients will develop a reverse dynamic pes valgus deformity, which may also be associated with a hypertonic, or tight, tendo-Achilles. With time, the midfoot becomes hypermobile and pronated. This "break" of the midfoot, with the talus displacing medially and plantarward, produces a type of "rocker-bottom" foot. If not severe, this dynamic deformity can be treated with a custom-corrective neutral orthotic in the shoe or an ankle-foot orthosis. If the

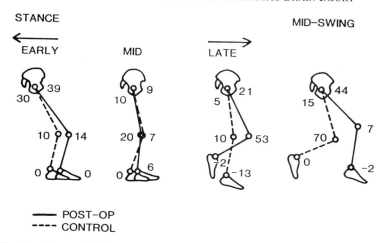

STANCE   **MID–SWING**

FIGURE 7. These stick figures represent the walking pattern in a group of adult-acquired hemiplegics following surgical correction of their dynamic equinus. Note that the energy-inefficient knee hyperextension and hip flexion were generally improved. From Pinzur MS, Sherman R, DiMonte-Levine P, et al: Adult-onset hemiplegia: Changes in gait after muscle-balancing procedures to correct the equinus deformity. *J Bone Joint Surg* 68A:1249, 1986; with permission.

midfoot has not become unstable or if the dynamic EMG reveals deforming peroneal muscles, they can be lengthened at their musculotendinous junction.[18] If the midfoot has become unstable, a subtalar fusion or triple arthrodesis is required to correct the deformity.

When the ankle equinus is corrected, the length between origin and insertion of the toe flexor muscles is lengthened, unmasking a dynamic, or fixed, spastic flexion deformity of the great toe and hammer or claw toe deformities of the lesser toes. This situation is avoided in most patients by lengthening of the flexor hallucis longus and brevis muscles through the harvesting incision for the tibialis anterior tendon insertion, and by percutaneous release of the flexor digitorum longus through plantar incisions at the level of the proximal phalanx of the lesser toes. If the joint deformities persist following motor-balancing surgery, the toe deformities should be considered as a neurologic claw toe deformity. If these deformities cannot be adequately accommodated in a shoe, we treat both the great toe and lesser toe flexion deformities with interphalangeal joint fusion. The great toe is stabilized with ASIF screw technique, and the lesser toes with smooth pin fixation.

Knee Deformities

Following correction of dynamic ankle equinus, a small number of patients will continue with knee extension or hyperextension during preswing that persists into the stance phase of gait. This so-called stiff-legged gait pattern is energy-inefficient due to the difficulty in clearing the floor with an extended knee. Waters et al.[16] have shown that the dynamic deformity in these patients is due to muscle imbalance overpowering of the quadriceps muscle group during preswing. It can be treated with distal and/or proximal release of the rectus femoris muscle, if it can be determined by dynamic EMG that the rectus femoris and vastus intermedius muscles are active during preswing and early swing phases of gait.[16] This must be distinguished from the normal short burst of rectus femoris activity during pre-swing acting in a muscle that acts on two joints (hip and knee) preventing hyperextension of the trailing limb. Patients are allowed to begin postoperative ambulation as tolerated.

Dynamic knee flexion deformity is treated with fractional muscle lengthening of the semimembranosis and release of the biceps and semitendinosus muscles to achieve dynamic balance.[6] When the knee flexion deformity has a static component, a modification of the Yount release used for pelvic obliquity in polio is performed.[14] The tensor fascia femoris functions as a hip flexor and knee extensor, so two small incisions can be used to perform a proximal and distal release. The distal incision is placed just proximal to the lateral femoral condyle. The iliotibial band is sharply transected, and a periosteal elevator is used to release several inches of the lateral intermuscular septum. A second small incision is made just distal to the anterior superior iliac spine and carried posteriorly for approximately 2 to 3 cm, where the anterior one-half of the muscle fascia of the tensor fascia femoris is released. Postoperatively, the patient is treated with serial long-leg cylinder walking casts to complete the correction. This procedure will generally also achieve correction of 30° of hip flexion contracture.

Because of early intervention, we now rarely see knee flexion contractures approaching 90° in this patient population. When the fixed static component of the knee flexion contracture approaches 90°, soft tissue release is not adequate. Patients develop pressure ulcers over the patella from the corrective casts, even when the casts are fully padded. In addition, the neurovascular structures may not be able to tolerate such severe stretching. For these reasons, we recommend a femoral wedge osteotomy if the patient is a potential walker as the most reasonable method of functional rehabilitation.

Hip Deformities

"Scissoring," i.e., hip adductor spasticity, is an energy-inefficient gait pattern caused by spastic hip adductor muscles. This scissoring causes the knees to bump into each other during limb advancement and may impede perineal hygiene. Some patients substitute their adductor muscles for limb advancement, so this dynamic deformity is first assessed by diagnostic anesthetic obturator nerve block before treatment with percutaneous phenol nerve block. When nerve blocks are not sufficient, the scissoring can be improved with percutaneous release of the adductors without the need for a obturator neurectomy. Postoperatively, patients start an aggressive physical therapy program and use a hip abduction splint when in bed for 6 weeks.

We try to avoid performing hip flexor releases, as this technique will generally compromise ambulation potential by eliminating the motor for limb advancement. Hip flexor release is necessary for positioning in the nonambulatory patient and to prevent recurrent knee flexion deformities.

REFERENCES

1. Botte MJ, Waters RL, Keenan MA, et al: Orthopaedic management of the stroke patient. Orthop Rev 17:637, 1988.
2. Garland DE, Jones RC, Kunkle RW: Upper extremity fractures in the acute spinal cord injured patient. Clin Orthop 233:110, 1988.
3. Garland DE, Rieser TV, Singer DI: Treatment of femoral shaft fractures associated with acute spinal cord injuries. Clin Orthop 197:191, 1985.

4. Garland DE, Saucedo T, Rieser TV: The management of tibial fractures in acute spinal cord injury patients. Clin Orthop 213:237, 1986.
5. Keenan MA, Perry J, Jordan C: Factors affecting balance and ambulation following stroke. Clin Orthop 182:165, 1984.
6. Keenan MA, Ure K, Smith CW, Jordan C: Hamstring release for knee flexion contracture in spastic adults. Clin Orthop 236:221, 1988.
7. Khalili AA, Bettes HB: Peripheral nerve block with phenol in the management of spasticity. JAMA 200:1155, 1967.
8. Moore TJ, Anderson RB: The use of open phenol blocks to the motor branches of the tibial nerve in adult acquired spasticity. Foot Ankle 11:219, 1991.
9. Perry J, Waters RL: Surgery. In Instructional Course Lectures, The American Academy of Orthopaedic Surgeons, vol 24. St. Louis, CV Mosby, 1975, pp 40–44.
10. Pinzur MS: Surgery to achieve dynamic motor balance in adult acquired spastic hemiplegia: A preliminary report. J Hand Surg 10A:547, 1985.
11. Pinzur MS: Functional surgery in stroke and head injury. Complications Orthop (May/Jun):73–77, 1990.
12. Pinzur MS, Sherman R, DiMonte-Levine P, et al: Adult-onset hemiplegia: Changes in gait after muscle-balancing procedures to correct the equinus deformity. J Bone Joint Surg 68A:1249, 1986.
13. Pinzur MS, Sherman R, DiMonte-Levine P, Trimble J: Gait changes in adult onset hemiplegia. Am J Phys Med 66:228, 1987.
14. Speed JS, Smith H: Ankylosis and deformity. In Speed JS (ed): Campbell's Operative Orthopaedics. St. Louis, CV Mosby, 1949.
15. Waters RL, Frazier J, Garland DE, et al: Electromyographic gait analysis before and after operative treatment for hemiplegic equinus and equinovarus deformity. J Bone Joint Surg 64A:284, 1982.
16. Waters RL, Garland DE, Perry J, et al: Stiff-legged gait in hemiplegia: Surgical correction. J Bone Joint Surg 61A:927, 1979.
17. Waters RL, McNeal DR, Faloon W, Clifford B: Functional electrical nerve stimulation of the peroneal nerve for hemiplegia. J Bone Joint Surg 67A:792, 1985.
18. Young S, Keenan MA, Stone LR: The treatment of planovalgus foot deformity in the neurologically impaired adult. Foot Ankle 10:317, 1990.

EUFROCINA S. TOMAS, OTR
MAUREEN FORTE UNDZIS, BS, OTR
EILEEN A. SHORES, BS, OTR
MARILYN R. SIDLER, MA, OTR

NONSURGICAL MANAGEMENT OF UPPER EXTREMITY DEFORMITIES AFTER TRAUMATIC BRAIN INJURY:

The Rancho Los Amigos Comprehensive Treatment Program

From the
Adult Brain Injury Occupational
 Therapy Department
Rancho Los Amigos Medical
 Center
Downey, California

Correspondence to:
Maureen Forte Undzis, OTR
Adult Brain Injury Program
Rancho Los Amigos Medical
 Center
7601 East Imperial Highway
Downey, CA 90242

Abnormal muscle tone and movement are complications affecting the adult traumatic brain injury (TBI) patient, posing significant obstacles to function. These complications are often in addition to a myriad of other residual deficits that compromise functional outcome. The occupational therapist's challenge is to maximize the patient's potential by facilitating upper-extremity control so the patient may once again participate in purposeful and meaningful activities within the physical and social environment to which he or she will return.

This chapter focuses on the presence of abnormal muscle tone or hypertonicity in the upper extremities and its influence on movement. Key elements in the evaluation are highlighted, and a sequenced treatment progression is described through five phases to normalize upper-extremity tone and movement. This coordinated treatment approach discusses the timing and sequencing of serial casting, motor-point or nerve blocks, and surgical procedures and how these are organized within a movement reintegration program.

This chapter is based upon the combined skills and expertise of occupational therapists and orthopedic surgeons at Rancho Los Amigos Medical Center who have developed a comprehensive treatment program that enables severely injured TBI patients to regain functional use of their upper extremities. A recent retrospective review of 36 patients treated in our program found that the mean length of coma was 55.8 days (SD = 41.79), with a range of 0 to 150 days. Initial Glasgow coma scores placed this group in the severely brain-injured category. The average time from the date of injury to admission at Ranchos Los Amigos Medical Center was 3 months. These patients presented with severe hypertonicity and contractures, usually in more than one limb. Their mobility and function were significantly compromised, and of the 36 patients reviewed at admission 72% were dependent in their self-care skills.[15,26] Taking into consideration the evaluation factors and following the treatment progression described in this chapter, these patients made significant gains in upper extremity control and function. All achieved at least an assisted level of self-care, and in some cases, independence, in self-care and selected home and community skills.

EVALUATION

Patient and family evaluation is an ongoing process throughout the course of rehabilitation. Establishing baseline evaluation information is critical to setting treatment priorities and predicting functional outcomes. This evaluation includes careful consideration of the following interrelated factors.

Time Interval Since Injury. Spontaneous recovery occurs during the first 18 months after injury. Conservative treatment measures are implemented for managing the upper extremity during this period. Surgical procedures are considered 18 to 24 months after the date of injury, when functional gains are no longer obtained from conservative treatment.[6,8,18,20,21,25,28,35]

Number of Extremities Involved. The number of extremities involved and the degree of impairment help set treatment priorities. For example, when serial casting is proposed for a patient with bilateral upper extremity involvement, casting is delayed in the least involved arm to leave a site for monitoring vital signs or intravenous tube placement.

Complications. Early identification of complications is necessary for prioritizing clinical treatment. Among the more common complications are pain, heterotopic ossification,[19] peripheral nerve injuries,[32] reflex sympathetic dystrophy, fractures,[21,24] and edema.

Postural Abnormalities. Poor head, neck, and trunk control lead to abnormal alignment and equilibrium. Axial alignment and trunk stability directly influence the quality of tone in the upper extremities and their emerging control. The trunk and extremities must be evaluated carefully and treated concurrently.

Upper Extremity Motor Control. Brunnstrom[10] describes control as no motion, patterned motion, motion deviating from pattern, selective motion with pattern overlay, and selective motion. Improved functional outcomes are expected when a patient's motor control is at least deviating from pattern.[1]

Severity of Tone. For discussion purposes, the terms *abnormal tone, hypertonicity,* and *spasticity* are synonymous. Abnormal tone is classified using a three-category clinical scale based on resistance to stretch. Tone may be minimal, moderate, or severe. The severity of the patient's tone helps determine treatment alternatives.[39] The less severe the tone, the more conservative the treatment can be.

Sensory Impairments. Sensation integrity (sharp-dull, position sense, light touch, and object identification) is assessed to predict the patient's spontaneous use of the spastic upper extremity. When sensation is impaired or absent, the patient generally has difficulty incorporating the arm and hand in functional tasks.

Cognitive Impairments. Understanding the patient's cognitive level and what to expect at succeeding levels allows the therapist to select appropriate treatment activities, equipment, instructional materials, and a plan for follow-up.

Visual-Perceptual Deficits. An intact visual-perceptual system is important for the patient to function in the environment. The patient's visual-perceptual deficits must be identified in order to adapt and modify treatment strategies.[41]

Discharge Plans. Identifying the discharge setting and the ability of the family to provide support are essential to treatment planning.[42] Both admission and discharge conferencing with the patient, family, and therapy team will result in setting mutual realistic goals.

The following discussion focuses primarily on the postural abnormalities, hypertonicity, and movement dysfunction, although it should be understood that these impairments are not treated in isolation from the other important aspects of patient care. Recovery from a severe TBI varies from patient to patient and may begin or plateau at any phase.

PHASE I

At this early stage, the patients are at a low arousal level and movement is restricted by severe spasticity, range-of-motion (ROM) limitations, abnormal posturing, and contractures (Fig. 1). Consequently, they are unable to carryout any purposeful tasks. The goals at this time are to normalize tone, increase range of motion, correct deformities, and improve trunk alignment to enhance sensorimotor integration and movement.

Proper positioning at all times is fundamental to enhance movement. A high percentage of the patient's time is spent in bed or a wheelchair. Therefore, pillows, foam cutouts, lapboards, and arm troughs are used to help achive proper body alignment. Nerve or motor-point blocks and serial casting are considered to normalize tone, increase ROM, and correct existing deformities. Nerve blocks refer to the injection of a pharmacologic agent to either the motor point of the muscle or the nerve innervating that muscle group to anesthetize the nerve for hours (in diagnostic uses, e.g., lidocaine), or weeks (in therapeutic uses, e.g., phenol) (*see* Chapter 7 by Stone and Shin). Nerve blocks are used when spasticity is graded as moderate or severe.[28,29]

Serial casting is an effective technique to increase lost ROM caused by the deforming force of spasticity on soft tissue.[12] Casting a spastic or contracted joint maintains a slow stretch to the muscle while decreasing afferent excitation.[38] When multiple joints are involved, proximal joints are casted first, progressing distally. The emphasis of stretch is placed on one or two joints at a time to achieve better positioning and prevent further deformities. Prior to application of the cast, the therapist positions and mobilizes the patient's upper extremity for better alignment. The upper extremity is passively placed in maximum pain-free range and then casted in that position. Casting is more effective when applied immediately after the neurolytic block, rather than waiting a day or more.[5,40,44] When a neurolytic block is not necessary, lidocaine may facilitate pain-free casting and greater range.

During the serial casting program, patients are started in mat activities incorporating sensory integration and neurodevelopmental treatment principles to assist them in gaining normal movement patterns. Goals include improved head control and trunk stability, followed by mobility, separation of movement between upper and lower trunk, and isolated shoulder movement. Passive mobilization of

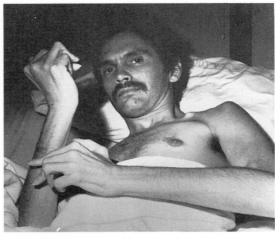

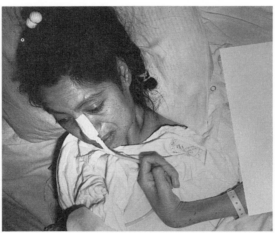

FIGURE 1.   Phase I. Severe abnormal tone and joint contracture limit the patient's ability to move.

the scapula and trunk may be necessary prior to mat activities to prepare the patient for movement.

PHASE II

At phase II, the patient is less restricted by abnormal tone and contractures. Better trunk alignment is attained by placing the upper extremities in a weight-bearing position on a stable surface (Fig. 2). This is critical in gaining proximal motor control. The patient has now relearned more normal movement and is better able to respond to simple verbal commands, but he or she still requires tactile input.

The treatment emphasis at this phase is to facilitate improved postural alignment and proximal control. Proximal stability and mobility are essential for upper extremity function; therefore, initial treatment must be focused on facilitation of

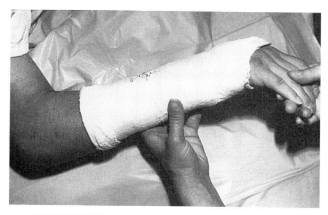

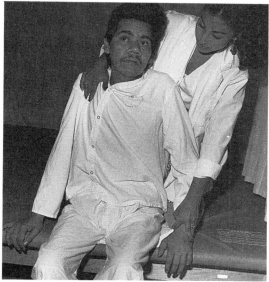

FIGURE 2. Phase II. Short arm serial cast (*top*) and upper extremities placed in a weight-bearing position on mat (*bottom*).

shoulder and scapular control. The scapula is often retracted and depressed. The shoulder exhibits adduction and internal rotation. Less typical, yet not uncommon, variations from this pattern are found. For example, the scapula may be protracted and elevated. Stability in the shoulder girdle is necessary for the patient to use the upper extremities in simple function, i.e., as a weight-bearing support during weight shift and transfers. This controlled weight bearing activates normal patterns of movement in the upper extremity, such as elbow extension and cocontraction. The process of gaining ROM in all upper-extremity joints and decreasing spasticity is continued at this phase. At this point, the last stages of serial casting may still be in progress. Once the maximum ROM is achieved, the cylindrical cast is bivalved and made into a splint. Tolerance to the splint is gradually increased to maintain the increased ROM. The splint can be worn at night, during the day, or both when the patient is not in therapy. There are various customized inhibitory splints based on neurodevelopmental treatment principles that are beyond the scope of this chapter. Additional nerve blocks may still be needed to further decrease spasticity. The decision regarding which specific muscle groups to block is made jointly by the physician and occupational therapist.[7,22,23,31,36,37]

Treatment choices in phase II are based on the following neurodevelopmental treatment principles:

1. Motor control is more effectively gained proximal to distal;
2. Development of gross motor control is a prerequisite for effective fine-motor control;
3. Control of movement patterns into and out of static postures is necessary for function; and
4. Repetition and variation of motor patterns is necessary for integration to occur.

Physical progress depends on normalization of postural tone, reintegration of primitive reflexes, and redevelopment of normal automatic movement.[2,4,13,14,16,17,27]

Physical modalities may be used to augment the treatment program. For the patient who has a low pain threshold with minimum spasticity but still requires ROM, the continuous passive motion machine may be preferred to manual ranging (Fig. 3). Its consistent, predictable, and rhythmic properties assist in decreasing edema, reducing adhesions, increasing ROM, and joint mobility. This leads to increased spontaneous movement and ultimately better functional use. To facilitate motor control, neuromuscular electrical stimulation may also be incorporated.[3] Neuromuscular electrical stimulation serves four purposes: (1) increase ROM, (2) strengthen muscle, (3) reeducate muscle, and (4) decrease spasticity by reciprocal inhibition. Neuromuscular electrical stimulation programs can easily be combined with functional tasks to augment the quality of the patient's movement and to allow the patient to complete the demands of the task.[3,45,46]

At this stage, the patient begins participation in gross motor functional tasks, realizing that he or she still has diminished capacity to process sensory information rapidly. Thus, the patient requires much structure and verbal cuing, as well as tactile input to regain normal movement patterns for gross motor tasks.

PHASE III

Phase III of recovery is characterized by the patient's emerging active use of the distal upper extremity in gross movement for simple functional tasks (supporting, stabilizing, holding, pointing) (Fig. 4). This improvement occurs providing the patient has improved cognitively and can attend and complete multistep directions involving overlearned and familiar tasks.

The treatment goal at this phase is guiding the patient to integrate the upper extremity into functional activities while maintaining postural control. Increasing and maintaining the ROM achieved are continued to allow the patient to efficiently perform functional tasks. During normal movement, a person moves in whole patterns or normal synergies. The patient relearns a repertoire of these normal components of movement to allow for greater participation in activities of daily living. Trunk control is critical in facilitating normal movement patterns to develop. These foundation skills are important preliminary steps in normalizing overall spasticity.[17]

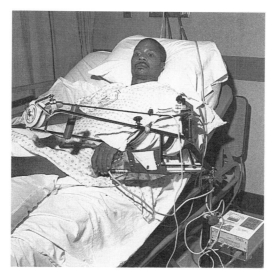

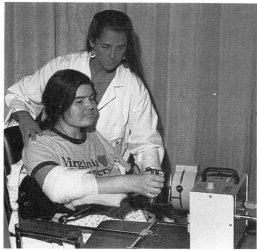

FIGURE 3. Phase II. Elbow continuous passive motion machine (*top*) and hand and wrist continuous passive motion machine (*bottom*).

Strength and endurance remain limited at this stage. Therefore, adaptive equipment, including splints, suspension slings, suspension feeder, and lapboards, are incorporated to support the trunk and upper extremities. Commercially available or custom-designed splints made from thermoplastic materials are selected to suit individual patient needs.[11]

Proper positioning, ranging, casting, and weight-bearing activities prepare the patient to participate actively in movement. The therapist builds on earlier sensory and postural facilitation to promote body scheme and motor planning.

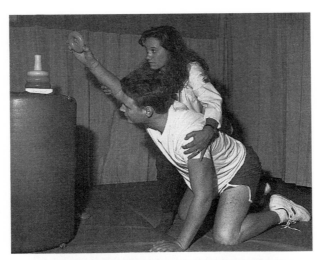

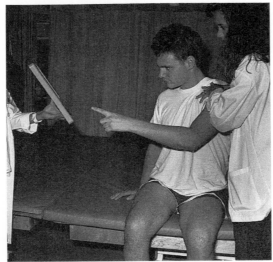

FIGURE 4. Phase III. *Top,* Functional range is achieved, but the patient requires assistance for trunk stability. *Bottom,* The patient is using involved upper extremity movement to communicate by pointing.

If shortened tendons and ligaments continue to interfere with function or hygiene management 18 months after the injury, surgery may be considered. The purposes of the surgery would be to lengthen shortened tendons and ligaments that interfere with functional ability or hygiene care (*see* Chapter 14 by Kolessar and Keenan).[9,30,33,34]

PHASE IV

At phase IV, the patient has achieved good trunk stability and mobility and now progresses to functional activities, such as hygiene, grooming, and dressing without requiring his or her upper extremities for trunk support (Fig. 5). The patient consistently incorporates the involved upper extremity or extremities in these activities as a stabilizer and for some limited manipulation. With verbal cueing, he or she is able to actively correct postural alignment and subtle movement abnormalities in the upper extremity. The patient may still be using splints at this time for functional use and positioning. Cognitively, the patient begins to gain insight into his or her deficits.

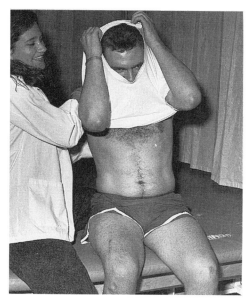

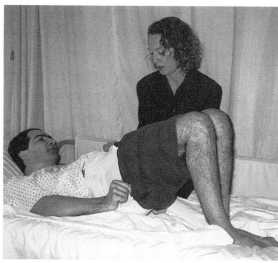

FIGURE 5.   Phase IV. The patient engages in self-care but still requires tactile and verbal input to maintain trunk alignment and efficient use of upper extremities.

The treatment goal is to increase spontaneous, automatic, controlled, normal movements in the upper extremity during more complex and physically challenging activities. Treatment will therefore focus on improving upper-extremity control during transitional movements (i.e., from sitting to standing) and in activities performed from the wheelchair or standing if the patient is able.[43]

Patients are still closely observed while performing activities. Self-care activities are structured in order to help the patient perform them in the most normal way possible. Verbal and tactile cues are given to the patient, either to reinforce normal movement patterns or to extinguish abnormal movement. For example, during a transfer, if the patient hikes the shoulder and leans toward one side, the therapist provides verbal and tactile cues to relax that shoulder and promote symmetrical weight bearing.

As the patient's activity level increases and basic self-care goals are achieved, other therapeutic activities are incorporated to enhance the patient's hand function. Activities such as crafts, computer software tasks with large switches and gross-grasp joysticks, table games, and adapted sports serve to enlarge the patient's experience. Using occupational therapy principles of graded activities, the tasks are modified to match a patient's cognitive and physical ability, still providing a challenge to improve on these abilities. The benefits of using meaningful, purposeful activity are paramount in helping patients integrate normal components of movement and sensory awareness. As a result of this approach, patients generalize newly learned motor patterns to other tasks and develop more refined levels of movement for increasingly complex activities of daily living.

PHASE V

At this phase, the patient has good trunk stability and mobility and is also able to coordinate and isolate upper extremity movements in all joints in various planes and directions with little or no influence of hypertonicity (Fig. 6). Cognitively, the patient may be more aware of his or her limitations and more accepting of compensatory strategies. The patient now spontaneously corrects improper positioning and abnormal patterns of movements or posturing. However, limitations are still present in fine-motor coordination, speed, endurance, timing, and accuracy of skilled motor tasks.[43] For example, this limitation is often observed in the patient laboring to button a shirt, tie shoe laces, or regain the rhythm of cursive writing.

The treatment goals at this stage are to increase the timing, speed, and accuracy of upper extremity movements for activities of daily living. Endurance and dynamic mobility are important in self-care and in advanced home and community skills, which are also emphasized at this phase.

Individualized progressively resistive weight programs or crafts (woodwork, macrame, leather, ceramics, or copper tooling) are used to increase both strength and dexterity. To further improve the patient's upright endurance and dynamic balance, work positions are varied from sitting to standing within a wide variety of individualized tasks (i.e., occupational therapy projects, work simulated tasks, or home chores). Also at this phase, the patient participates in therapy groups providing peer interaction to further reinforce use of the advanced motor skills. An example is a sensorimotor integration group, which incorporates modified sports-like activities to facilitate adaptive physical responses.

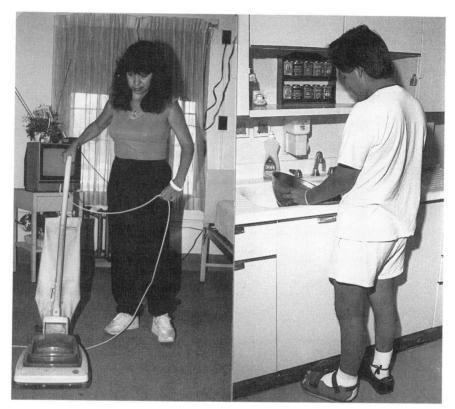

FIGURE 6.   Phase V. Patients are able to perform complex activities of daily living.

CONCLUSIONS

Abnormal muscle tone and movement are complications affecting the TBI patient and his or her ability to resume meaningful life tasks. The severity varies from patient to patient and stage of recovery. Treatment therefore must be individualized. Family involvement is vital for success in an intensive therapy program. Throughout this process, family and staff must understand the patient's emotional, cognitive, and physical limitations. Each family decides to what extent they can participate in augmenting treatment. Their involvement can provide carry-over of treatment and enhance the recovery potential.

The comprehensive treatment program described in this chapter has been developed over a number of years with patients recovering from TBI at Rancho Los Amigos Medical Center. Our clinical experience has convinced us that no one treatment approach is capable of addressing the complex needs of this patient population. To optimize functional outcome, treatment is viewed as a dynamic continuum requiring ongoing assessment of patient's needs and responses to chosen interventions (i.e., occupational therapy, nerve or motor-point blocks, serial casting, or surgery). The planning, timing, sequencing, and implementation of this program owe its success to a close interdisciplinary collaboration acknowledging the central position of patient and family.

REFERENCES

1. Andric M: The hemiplegic arm: Reach out and take control. In Stroke Rehabilitation: State of the Art. Downey, CA, Professional Staff Association of Rancho Los Amigos Medical Center, 1984.
2. Ayres J: Sensory Integration and Learning Disorders. Los Angeles, Western Psychological Services, 1973.
3. Benton L, Baker LL, Bowman BR, et al: Functional Electrical Simulation: A Practical Clinical Guide, 2nd ed. Downey, CA, Professional Staff Association of Rancho Los Amigos Medical Center, 1981.
4. Bobath B: Adult Hemiplegia: Evaluation and Treatment, 3rd ed. London, Butterworth-Heinemann, 1991.
5. Booth BJ, Doyle M, Montgomery J: Serial casting for the management of spasticity in the head-injured adult. Phys Ther 63:1960–1966, 1983.
6. Botte MJ, Keenan MA: Reconstructive surgery of the upper extremity in the patient with head trauma. J Head Trauma Rehabil 2:34–45, 1987.
7. Botte MJ, Keenan MA: Percutaneous phenol blocks of the pectoralis major muscle to treat spastic deformities. J Hand Surg 13A:147–149, 1988.
8. Botte MJ, Keenan MA, Gellman H, et al: Surgical management of spastic thumb-in-palm deformities in adults with brain injury. J Hand Surg 14A:174–182, 1989.
9. Botte MJ, Keenan MA, Korchek J, Waters RL: Modified technique for the superficialis-to-profundus transfer in the treatment of adults with spastic clenched fist deformity. J Hand Surg 12A:639–640, 1987.
10. Brunnstrom S: Movement Therapy in Hemiplegia: A Neurophysiological Approach. Hagerstown, MD, Harper & Row Medical Department Publishers, 1970.
11. Callahan AD, McEntree P: Splinting proximal interphalangeal joint flexion contracture: A new design. Am J Occup Ther 40:408–413, 1986.
12. Cruickshank DA, O'Neill DL: Upper extremity inhibitive casting in a boy with spastic quadriplegia. Am J Occup Ther 44:552–555, 1990.
13. Davis P: Steps to Follow: A Guide to the Treatment of Adult Hemiplegia. Berlin, Springer-Verlag, 1985.
14. Davis P: Right in the Middle: Selective Trunk Activity in the Treatment of Adult Hemiplegia. Berlin, Springer-Verlag, 1990.
15. Dougherty PM, Radomski MV: Clinician's Guide to Program Evaluation: Occupational Therapy Practice 2. Gaithersburg, MD, Aspen Publishers, 1991, pp 38–45.
16. Eggers O: Occupational Therapy in the Treatment of Adult Hemiplegia. Gaithersburg, MD, Aspen Publication, 1984.
17. Fisher B, et al: Neurodevelopmental Treatment Approach to Adult Hemiplegia: Manual for Certification Course. Downey, CA, Rancho Los Amigos Medical Center, Los Amigos Research and Education Institute, 1990.
18. Garland DE (ed): Orthopedic management. J Head Trauma Rehabil 2:13–26, 1987.
19. Garland DE, Blum CE, Waters RL: Periarticular heterotopic ossification in head injured adults. J Bone Joint Surg 62A:1143–1146, 1980.
20. Garland DE, Hanscom D, Keenan MA, et al: Resection of heterotopic ossification in the adult with head trauma. J Bone Joint Surg 67A:1261–1269, 1985.
21. Garland DE, Keenan MA: Orthopedic strategies in the management of the adult head-injured patient. J Am Phys Ther 63:2004–2009, 1983.
22. Garland DE, Lilling M, Keenan MA: Percutaneous phenol blocks to motor points of spastic forearm muscles in head-injured adults. Arch Phys Med Rehabil 65:243–245, 1984.
23. Garland DE, Lucie SR, Waters RL: Current uses of open phenol nerve block for adult acquired spasticity. Clin Orthop 2:217–222, 1980.
24. Garland DE, Rhoades ME: Orthopedic management of brain-injured adults. Clin Orthop 131:111–122, 1978.
25. Garland DE, Thompson R, Waters RL: Musculocutaneous neurectomy for spastic elbow flexion in non-functional upper extremities in adults. J Bone Joint Surg 62A:108–112, 1980.
26. Guide For the Use of the Uniform Data Set for Medical Rehabilitation: The Functional Independence Measure Research Foundation. Buffalo, State University of New York, School of Medicine, Department of Rehabilitation Medicine, 1987.
27. Kamm K, Thelen E, Jensen JL: A dynamic systems approach to motor development. Phys Ther 70:763–774, 1990.
28. Keenan MA: The orthopedic management of spasticity. J Head Trauma Rehabil 2:62–71, 1987.
29. Keenan MA: Management of the spastic upper extremity in the neurologically impaired adult. Clin Orthop 233:116–125, 1988.

30. Keenan MA, Abrams R, Garland DE, Waters RL: Results of fractional lengthening of the finger flexors in adults with upper extremity spasticity. J Hand Surg 12A:575–581, 1987.
31. Keenan MA, Botte MJ: Technique of percutaneous phenol block of the recurrent motor branch of the median nerve. J Hand Surg 12A:806–807, 1987.
32. Keenan MA, Kauffman D, Garland DE, Smith C: Late ulnar neuropathy in the brain-injured adult. J Hand Surg 13A:120–124, 1988.
33. Keenan MA, Korchek J, Botte MJ, et al: Results of transfer of the flexor digitorum superficialis tendons to the flexor digitorum profundus tendons in adults with acquired spasticity of the hand. J Bone Joint Surg 69A:1127–1132, 1987.
34. Keenan MA, Romanelli R, Lunsford B: The use of dynamic electromyography to evaluate motor control in the hands of adults who have spasticity caused by brain injury. J Bone Joint Surg 71A:120–126, 1989.
35. Keenan M, Stone L: Proceedings of the Third International Symposium, Neuro-Orthopedic Management of the Traumatic Brain Injured Adult. Downey, CA, Los Amigos Research and Education Institute, 1990.
36. Keenan M, Tomas E, et al: Percutaneous phenol block of the musculocutaneous nerve to control elbow flexor spasticity. J Hand Surg 15A:340–346, 1990.
37. Keenan M, Todderud E, Henderson R, Botte M: Management of intrinsic spasticity in the hand with phenol injection or neurectomy of the motor branch of the ulnar nerve. J Hand Surg 12A:734–739, 1987.
38. MacKay-Lyons M: Low-load, prolonged stretch in treatment of elbow flexion contractures secondary to head trauma: A case report. Phys Ther 69:292–296, 1989.
39. Occupational Therapy Evaluation Guide for Adult Hemiplegia. Downey, CA, Los Amigos Research and Education Institute, 1991.
40. Rehabilitation of the Head Injured Adult: Comprehensive Physical Management. Downey, CA, Professional Staff Association of Ranchos Los Amigos Medical Center, Los Amigos Research and Education Institute, 1979.
41. Siev E, Freishat B, Zoltan B: Perceptual and Cognitive Dysfunction in the Adult Stroke Patient. Thorofare, NJ, Slack, 1986.
42. Slater B, Kendricken M, Zoltan B: A Positive Approach to Head Injury: Guidelines for Professionals and Families. Thorofare, NJ, Slack, 1987.
43. Stroke Rehabilitation: State of the Art. Downey, CA, Professional Staff Association of Rancho Los Amigos Medical Center, Los Amigos Research and Education Institute, 1984.
44. Upper Extremity Sensory Evaluation: A Manual for Occupational Therapists. Downey, CA, Los Amigos Research and Education Institute, 1985.
45. Zablotny CM: Using neuromuscular electrical stimulation to facilitate limb control in the head-injured patient. J Head Trauma Rehabil 2:28–33, 1987.
46. Zablotny CM, Andric M, Gowland C: Serial casting: Clinical applications for the adult head-injured patient. J Head Trauma Rehabil 2:46–52, 1987.

INDEX

Entries in **boldface type** signify complete articles.

Aberrant regeneration, of oculomotor nerve, 481–482
ACTH. *See* Corticotropin
Adnexa, trauma to, 492–493
Affective disorders, 594, 597–599
Aggression, 594, 596–597, 604
Agitated state, 585–586
Alkaline phosphatase, serum, in heterotopic ossification, 612–613
Alzheimer's disease, 594, 600
Amino acids, excitatory, 467
Amitriptyline
    in aggression, 596–597
    side effects of, 566–567
Amnesia, post-traumatic, 462–464, 519, 583–587, 594
Androgens, 573
Angiography, cerebral, 443
Ankle deformity, 538
    nonsurgical management of, 641–643
    plantar flexor, 547–548
    surgical management of, 643–645
Ankle-foot orthosis, 642–643
Ankle sprain, 512, 514
Anomia, 595
Anosmia, 582
Anosognosia, 588
Antibody, to botulinum toxin, 550–551
Anticonvulsants, side effects of, 531
Antidiuretic hormone. *See* Arginine vasopressin
Antiepileptic drugs, 468–470
Antiepileptogenic agents, 466
Antiperoxidant, as anticonvulsant, 467
Anton's syndrome, 481
Anxiety disorder, 594, 599, 604
Aphasia, 464, 595, 598
Arginine vasopressin, 571–575, 578–579
Arteriovenous fistula, 443
Arteriovenous glucose difference, 454–455
Arteriovenous oxygen difference, 453–454
Asterixis, 524
Athetosis, 522
Attentional disturbance, 585–588, 593–594, 604
Autoregulation, of cerebral blood flow, 447–448
Axillary nerve lesions, 510

Background headache, 604
Baclofen, side effects of, 594
Balance exercises, 564–565
Balint's syndrome, 481, 588
Ballismus, 521–522

Behavioral therapy, 596
Benign paroxysmal positional vertigo, 559–562
Bipolar disorder, 598–599
Blepharospasm, 551
Blindness, cortical, 479–481, 487
Blindsight, 480
Blow-out fracture, of orbit, 482, 487, 493–497
Bone scan, in heterotopic ossification, 613–614
Botulinum toxin
    antibodies to, 550–551
    complications of use of, 551–552
    history of, 548–549
    mechanism of action of, 550
    mouse assay of, 549–550
    nerve block with, 530, 548–553
    pharmacology of, 549–550
    synthesis of, 549
    technical considerations in use of, 552–553
Brachial plexopathy, 508–510
Brachial plexus block 625–626
Brainstem auditory evoked potentials (BAEP), 457–458
Brainstem injury, 443, 482
Bupropion, side effects of, 596
Burn injury, exposure keratitis in, 488
Buspirone, in aggression, 597

Canalicular system of eye, intubation of, 492
Capgras syndrome, 585–586
Carbamazepine
    in affective disorders, 598–599
    in aggression, 597
    in Klüver-Bucy syndrome, 589
    in post-traumatic epilepsy, 468–469
    side effects of, 469
Carotid-cavernous fistula, 483
Carpal tunnel syndrome, 506–507
Casting, serial, 651, 653–659
Central vertigo, 559, 562, 566–567
Centrocecal scotoma, 479
Cerebral blood flow (CBF)
    autoregulation of, 447–448
    cerebral metabolism and, 446, 448, 453
    monitoring of, 446–453
    normal physiology, 447
    perfusion pressure and, 445
    systemic arterial pressure and, 448–449
Cerebral compliance, 444
Cerebral metabolism
    cerebral blood flow and, 446, 448, 453
    monitoring of, 453–454

Cerebral perfusion pressure, 445
Cerebral sequelae, post-traumatic monitoring
    of, **441–460**
    cerebral blood flow, 446–453
    cerebral metabolism, 453–455
    electrophysiologic, 455–458
    intracranial pressure, 444–446
    radiology, 442–443
Cervical vertigo, 562
Chelator, as anticonvulsant, 467
Chemical denervation, **527–558**. *See also* Nerve
    block
Chloral hydrate, for sedation, 597
Chorea, 521–522
Classification of brain injury, 527–531
Claw hand deformity, 504
    Claw toe deformity, 645
Clenched-fist deformity, 542, 633–635
Clonazepam
    in aggression, 597
    in post-traumatic epilepsy, 468–469
Clozapine, side effects of, 596
Cluster headache, 604, 607
Cognitive impairment, 593–596, 604, 651
Cognitive levels, 584
Cognitive retraining, 594–595
Color vision, loss of, 480–481
Coma, 464, 584–585
Communication disorder, 594–595
Compartment syndrome, 505, 512
Computed tomography (CT), 442–443
    in heterotopic ossification, 614
    for monitoring cerebral blood flow, 450–451
Concussion, 479, 519, 605
Confusional state, 585
Continuous passive motion machine, 654–655
Contracture
    lower extremity, 637–646
    upper extremity, 623–635, 649–659
Contrecoup contusion, 478–479, 519
Contusion, 442, 519–520
    contrecoup, 478–479, 519
    coup, 519
    focal cortical, 527–528
Cornea, protection of, 488
Cortical blindness, 479–481, 487
Corticotropin-releasing hormone (CRH), 571, 573
Corticotropin (ACTH), 571, 573, 575, 578
Cortisol, 573, 578
Coup contusion, 519
Craniomandibular dysfunction, 604
Cubital tunnel syndrome, 504, 506

Dacryocystorhinostomy, 492–493
Dantrolene, side effects of, 594
Dehydroepiandrosterone, 573
Delirium, post-traumatic, 585, 587
Delusions, 585, 599
Dementia, 599–600
Dementia pugilistica, 521

Depression, 594, 597–599, 604
Desipramine, in depression, 598
Detrusor sphincter dyssynergia, 549
Diabetes insipidus, central, 578–579
Diazepam, side effects of, 566–567, 594
Diffuse axonal injury, 520, 527–529, 582
    diagnosis of, 583
    neurobehavioral disorders in, 583–587
    recovery from, 583
Diphenhydramine, for sedation, 597
Diplopia, 494–496
Disconnection syndrome, 595
Doppler monitoring, of cerebral blood flow,
    452–453
Double vision, 482
Dry eye, 492
Dural shunt fistula, 483
Duret hemorrhage, 528
Dysarthria, 595
Dyskinesia, 519
Dysthyroid ophthalmopathy, 488
Dystonia, 522–523, 529–530, 549, 551

Ectropion, 496–497
Elbow
    heterotopic ossification about, 613–617, 620
    dislocation/fracture of, 504–505
    flexion deformity of, 540–542, 552
    surgical management of, 625, 627–629
Electroencephalography (EEG), 455–456, 606
    burst-suppression, 456
    cassette ambulatory, 467
    focal abnormalities in, 455, 464
    generalized abnormalities in, 455–456, 464
    prediction of seizures, 466–467
Electromyography (EMG), 504
    in lower extremity deformity, 641–642
    in upper extremity deformity, 625–626
Electronystagmography, 606
Emerging independence, 585, 587
Emotional incontinence, 596
Emotional lability, 596
Encephalopathy, traumatic, 521
Endocrine disorders, post-traumatic, **569–580**
Enophthalmos, 495–496
Entropion, 497
Enucleation, 498–500
Epidural hematoma, 520, 606
Epilepsy, post-traumatic, 456, 461, 605
    epileptic psychosis, 599
    incidence of, 461
    prevention of, 466–468
    risk factors for, 467
    treatment of, 468
Erb's paralysis, 509
Estrogen, 573
Ethosuximide, in post-traumatic epilepsy,
    468–469
Ethylhydroxydiphosphonate, in heterotopic
    ossification, 618–619

Evoked potentials, 456–458
Exposure keratitis, 487–492
Extraocular muscle lesion, 494–495
Eye. *See also* Visual disorders
    dry, 492
    prosthetic, 499–500
Eyelid, impaired closure of, 485–492

Facial nerve lesions, 511
Facial trauma, 486
    fixation of facial fractures, 496–497
    midfacial, 496
Family dynamic interruption, 605
Felbamate, 468
Femoral fracture, 512
Femoral nerve block, 547
Femoral nerve lesions, 512
Fiberoptic catheter, monitoring intracranial
    pressure with, 446
Fibrodysplasia ossificans progressiva, 612
Finger flexion deformity, 542–544, 552
    surgical management of, 625, 630–633
Flail extremity, 504, 508–510
Fluoxetine
    in aggression, 597
    in depression, 598
Fluphenazine, side effects of, 596
Focal brain contusion, 588–589
Focal cortical contusion, 527–528, 583
Focal dystonia, 522–523, 530, 549
Focal hypertonicity, 530–531
Follicle-stimulating hormone (FSH), 571, 573,
    575–577
Foot deformity
    foot drop, 512–513
    surgical management of, 643–645
Forced duction test, 495
Forceful manipulation, in heterotopic
    ossification, 620–621
Forearm fracture, 508
Fourth-nerve palsy, 482–483
Fracture care, lower extremity, 637–638
Fregoli syndrome, 586
Froment's sign, 504
Frontal convexity syndrome, 588
Frontal lobe lesions, 594
Frontal lobe syndrome, 588–589
Frontal sinus fracture, 496

Gabapentin, 468
Gait pattern, 640–641
    in adult onset hemiplegia, 640, 645
    crouched, 643
    scissoring, 646
    stiff-legged, 645
Galloping tongue, 524
Galveston Orientation and Amnesia Test, 585
Gaze stabilization exercises, 564
Generalized dystonia, 530
Generalized hypertonicity, 530–531

Generalized myoclonus, 524
Gilles de la Tourette syndrome, 523
Glaucoma, low-tension, 476
Glucose difference, arteriovenous, 454–455
Glutamate receptor antagonists, 467
Gold weight implantation, in eyelid, 490–491
Gonadotropin-releasing hormone (GnRH), 571,
    573
Great toe flexion deformity, 645
Growth hormone (GH), 570–572, 575, 578
Growth hormone-releasing hormone (GHRH),
    570–571

Hallucinations, 585, 599
Haloperidol, in aggression, 597
Hammer toe deformity, 645
Headache syndrome, post-traumatic, **603–609**
    assessment of, 606
    clinical features of, 603–605
    pathophysiology of, 605
    treatment of, 606–607
Heme compounds, tissue injury caused by, 467
Hemidystonia, 522–523
Hemifacial spasm, 549
Heterotopic ossification, **611–622,** 625
    diagnosis of, 612–614
    genetics and predisposition to, 612
    location of, 614–617
    neurogenic, 611
    peripheral nerve injury and, 503–504
    prevalence and onset of, 612
    treatment of, 618–621
Hip
    adductor deformity of, 538, 544–546
        surgical management of, 646
    extensor deformity of, 538, 546–547
    flexor deformity of, 544
    fracture/dislocation of, 512
    heterotopic ossification about, 613–616,
        620–621
Homonymous hemianopia, 480
Hormonal disturbance, post-traumatic, **569–580**
Horner's sign, 510
Humeral fracture, 507–508
Hydrocephalus, 531
Hygroma, 531
Hyperarousal, 585–586
Hyperemia, 448
Hypertonicity
    early versus late, 530
    generalized versus focal, 530–531
    management using chemical denervation,
        527–558
    upper extremity, 649–659
Hypogonadism, 576
Hypothalamus, **569–580**
    anatomic evaluation of, 570
    assessment of function of, 574–576
    function after head trauma, 576–579
    lesions in head trauma, 569–570

Hypothalamus *(cont.)*
  normal function of, 570–574
Hypoxic-ischemic injury, 529, 583
  boundary-zone, 529
  diagnosis of, 587–588
  diffuse, 529
  neurobehavioral disorders in, 587–588

Indomethacin, in prevention of heterotopic
  ossification, 619
Infarction, 480, 522, 527–528, 587
Inferior gluteal nerve block, 546–547
Inferior rectus injury, 494–495
Intellectual/social competence, 585, 587
Intention, disturbances of, 529
Intention tremor, 524
Interpersonal situations, impaired awareness of,
  594
Intracranial hematoma, 442, 462–464
Intracranial pressure
  elevations of, 444–445, 476
  measurement and control of, 444–445
  monitoring of, 443–446
  normal physiology, 444
Intracranial pressure-volume relationship,
  444
Intrinsic muscle spasticity, surgical management
  of, 633
Iron salts, tissue injury caused by, 467

Keratitis, exposure, 487–492
Kindling, 467
Kleine-Levin syndrome, 600
Klumpke's paralysis, 509
Klüver-Bucy syndrome, 586, 589
Knee
  deformities of, surgical management of,
    645–646
  extension deformity of, 547, 645
  flexion deformity of, 547, 553, 646
  heterotopic ossification about, 617

Labyrinthitis, 566
Lacrimal dysfunction, 492, 496
Lactate-glucose index, 454
Lamotrigine, 468
Language disorder, 594–595
Lateral geniculate nucleus, 477
Lateral pectoral nerve block, 539
Lewy body, 520
Lidocaine, in hypertonic disorders, 530
Lightheadedness, 604
Limb positioning, 503–514
  heterotopic ossification and, 611–612
  lower extremity, 637–646
  upper extremity, 623–635, 649–659
Lithium, in manic disorder, 598
Lorazepam, in aggression, 597
Lower extremity, fracture care, 637–638

Lower extremity deformity, post-traumatic,
  637–647
  evaluation of, 640–641
  goals for intervention in, 639–640
  spasticity management, 638
  spasticity model, 638–639
  timing of orthopaedic intervention, 638–639
  treatment of
    nerve blocks, 544–548
    nonsurgical, 641–643
    surgical, 643–646
Lower subscapular nerve block, 540–541
Lumber plexus, blocking of, 544–545
Lumbosacral plexopathy, 513
Luteinizing hormone (LH), 571, 573, 575–577

Magnetic resonance imaging (MRI), 443
Mania, 594, 598
Manipulation, forceful, in heterotopic
  ossification, 620–621
Maprotiline, side effects of, 596
Mass effect, 442–443
Mat activities, 651–652
Maxillary fracture, 496
Medial frontal syndrome, 588
Medial pectoral nerve block, 539
Median nerve block, 542–543, 625–626
Median nerve lesions, 506–507, 538
Memory deficit, 593–594
Meniere's disease, postconcussional,
  559
Meralgia paresthetica, 512
Metacognition, 594
Methyldopa, side effects of, 594
Middle cerebral artery rupture, 523
Migraine headache, 604, 606
Molindone, side effects of, 596
Monitoring. *See* Cerebral sequelae
Monteggia fracture, 508
Mood disturbance, 604
Motor tic, 523
Movement disorders
  drug-induced, 531
  post-traumatic, **519–526**, 529
Multifocal dystonia, 530
Multifocal myoclonus, 524
Multi-modality evoked potentials (MMEP),
  457–458
Muscle tone, disorders of, 529–530
Musculocutaneous nerve block, 542–543,
  625–626
Mute responsiveness, 584–585
Myoclonic dystonia, 522
Myoclonus, 524
Myofascial pain syndrome, 607

Nadolol, in aggression, 597
Nasoethmoidal fracture, 496
Neck pain syndrome, 604
Negative myoclonus, 524

Nerve block, 651
  botulinum toxin, 548–553
  diagnostic, 606, 625
  indications for, 537–538
  for lower extremity deformities, 544–548, 638
  phenol. *See* Phenol neurolysis
  preparation for, 538
  principles of, 538–539
  for upper extremity deformities, 539–544
Nerve conduction studies, 504
Nerve injury, peripheral, post-traumatic, **503–518**
Neuralgia, 604, 607
Neurobehavioral disorders, post-traumatic
  biologic and psychosocial factors in, 581–582
  in diffuse axonal injury, 583–587
  early neurobehavioral sequelae, **581–591**
  in focal brain contusion, 588–589
  in hypoxic-ischemic injury, 587–588
  late neurobehavioral sequelae, **593–602**
  pathophysiology of, 582–583
  stages of recovery, 582–583
Neuroendocrine disorders, post-traumatic, **569–580**
  assessment of, 574–576
Neuromuscular electrical stimulation, 654
Nortriptyline, in depression, 598
Nuchal segmental dystonia, 522
Nystagmus, 560–566

Obsessive-compulsive disorder, acquired, 594
Obturator nerve block, 544–546, 646
Obturator nerve lesions, 513
Oculomotor misdirection syndrome, 481
Oculomotor nerve lesion, 481–482
Ophthalmic artery spasm, 478
Ophthalmoplegia, 482–483
Ophthalmoscopy, indirect, 497–498
Optic nerve atrophy
  injuries and mechanisms of, 475–479
  primary, 475–476
  secondary, 475–476
Orbit
  blow-out fracture of, 482, 487, 493–497
  blunt trauma to, 477–478, 493–497
  penetrating injury to, 477
Orbital-frontal syndrome, 588
Organic aggressive syndrome, 596–597
Organic delusional syndrome, 599
Organic hallucinosis, 599
Organic personality syndrome, 599
Oromandibular dystonia, 549
Ossification, heterotopic. *See* Heterotopic ossification
Overt Aggression Scale, 596
Oxygen difference, arteriovenous, 453–454
Oxytocin, 571, 574

Palpebral spring insertion, for paralyzed eyelid, 490–492
Panic disorder, 594, 599, 604

Parakinesia, 522
Paraldehyde, for sedation, 597
Parkinsonism, post-traumatic, 519–521, 586, 588
Parkinson-plus syndromes, 521
Parkinson's disease, 520–521
Paroxysmal choreoathetosis, 522
Pelvic fracture, 504, 513
Perceptual deficit, 595
Perceptual-motor disorder, 594
Perilymphatic fistula, 559, 562
Peripheral nerve injury, post-traumatic, **503–518,** 625. *See also* specific nerves
  diagnosis of, 504
  fracture and, 503
  heterotopic ossification and, 503–504
Peroneal nerve lesions, 512–513
Personality disorder, 589
Pes valgus deformity, reverse dynamic, 644–645
Petrous fracture, 559
Phalen's sign, 506
Phenobarbital
  in seizure prevention, 466–467
  side effects of, 469, 594
Phenol neurolysis, 530, 642. *See also* Nerve block
  chemistry of, 534
  complications of, 535–537
  concentration of phenol, 534
  history of, 531–532
  intramuscular procedure, 533–534
  intravenous procedure, 532–533
  in lower extremity, 638
  paravertebral procedure, 533
  pathophysiology of, 534–535
Phenytoin
  in post-traumatic epilepsy, 468–469
  in seizure prevention, 466–468
  side effects of, 469
Phonic tic, 523
"Pie in the sky" visual impairment, 479
Pituitary, **569–580**
  anatomic evaluation of, 570
  anterior necrosis of, 569–570
  anterior pituitary hormones, 570–573
  assessment of function of, 574–576
  function after head trauma, 576–579
  lesions in head trauma, 569–570
  normal function of, 570–574
  posterior pituitary hormones, 570–574
  symptoms and signs of insufficiency, 575–576
Plantar adductor deformity, 553
Plantar flexor deformity, 552–553
Plexopathy
  brachial, 508–510
  lumbosacral, 513
Positioning of patient, 651
Positive myoclonus, 524
Positive visual phenomenon, 481
Positron-emission tomography (PET)
  in behavioral disturbances, 606
  monitoring cerebral metabolism, 454–455

Posterior cerebral artery syndromes, 528
Posterior interosseous nerve lesions, 508
Posterior tibial nerve block, 547–548, 641–642
Post-traumatic stress disorder, 586, 594, 599
Postural tremor, 524
Precocious puberty, 577
Primidone, side effects of, 594
Progressive supranuclear palsy, 521
Prolactin, 571, 573, 575, 577–578
Propranolol
    in aggression, 597
    side effects of, 594
    in tremor disorders, 524
Prosopagnosia, 480–481, 595
Prosthetic eye, 499–500
Pseudo-Argyll Robertson sign, 481
Pseudopsychopathic syndrome, 588
Pseudoretarded syndrome, 588
Pseudo-von Graefe's sign, 481
Psychosis, post-traumatic, 594, 599
Psychosocial function, preinjury, 582
Ptosis, 492–493, 497
"Punch-drunk" state, 521

Radial nerve block, 541–542, 625–626
Radial nerve lesions, 507–508
Radiation therapy, in prevention of heterotopic
    ossification, 619
Radiology
    in head trauma, 442–443
    in heterotopic ossification, 614
Radionuclide bone scan, in heterotopic
    ossification, 613–614
Rancho Los Amigos
    Comprehensive Treatment Program, **649–661**
    Scale of Cognitive Levels, 584
Rebound headache, 607
Reduplicative paramnesia, 585–586
Reflex myoclonus, 524
Retinal detachment, 477, 487, 497–498
Retrobulbar hemorrhage, 478
Retrobulbar injection, 477–478
Riddoch's phenomenon, 480
Rigidity, 529–530

Scapular notch fracture, 510
Schizophrenic-like symptoms, 599
Sciatic nerve block, 547, 638
Sciatic nerve lesions, 512
Sedation, of agitated patient, 586
Segmental dystonia, 530
Seizure
    drug-induced, 596
    electroencephalography in, 456
    post-traumatic, **461–473,** 605
        classification of, 461–462
        early, 461–462, 465–466
        generalized, 464–465
        late, 461–466
        long-term control of, 469–470

Seizure (cont.)
    post-traumatic (cont.)
        partial, 464–465
        prevention of, 466–468
        risk factors for, 462–464
        treatment of, 468
        type of, 464–466
Semont maneuver, 560
Sensation, in upper extremity, 625, 650
Sensorimotor integration, impaired, 529
Sensorimotor integration group, 658
Sensory nerve action potential (SNAP), 510, 512
Sensory pathways, assessment of, 456–458
Serotonin, in post-traumatic delirium, 587
Shoulder
    adduction deformity of, 538–540
        nonsurgical management of, 653
        surgical management of, 625, 627
    dislocation/fracture of, 504, 508, 510
    heterotopic ossification about, 615, 618, 620
Silicone encircling band, for eyelid, 490
Single-photon emission computed tomography
    (SPECT), monitoring cerebral blood
        flow, 451–452
Sixth-nerve palsy, 483, 566
Skull films, post-traumatic, 442
Skull fracture, 562–563
    basilar, 442
    depressed, 442, 462–464
Sleep disturbance, 586, 604–606
Somatosensory evoked potentials (SSEP),
    457–458
Somatostatin, 570–571
Spasmodic dysphonia, 549, 551
Spasticity, 529–530, 549
    lower extremity, 637–646
    upper extremity, 623–635, 649–659
Speech disorder, 594–595
Sphenoid fracture, 475, 478
Spinal headache, 604
Spinal nerve block, 544
Splinting, upper extremity, 654–657
Status epilepticus, 462, 466
Stereopsis, loss of, 480–481
Stimulants, in diffuse axonal injury, 586
Styloid process trauma, 604
Subarachnoid bolt, monitoring intracranial
    pressure with, 446
Subarachnoid hemorrhage, 443
Subcortical hemorrhage, 527–528
Subdural hematoma, 455, 463, 520, 522, 606
Subdural hemorrhage, 443, 531
Substance abuse, preinjury, 582
Suicide, after brain injury, 598–599
Sumatriptan, 606
Suprascapular nerve lesions, 510
Sympathetic ophthalmia, 499
Syndrome of inappropriate antidiuretic
    hormone secretion (SIADH), 578–579
Systemic arterial pressure, cerebral blood flow
    and, 448–449

Tardy ulnar palsy, 504, 506, 611–612
Target-specific tremor, 524
Tarsal tunnel syndrome, 514
Tarsorrhaphy, 489–490
Tears
    artificial, 492
    crocodile, 511
    excessive, 492
Temporal bone fracture, 511, 562
Temporal lobe injury, 596
Temporal lobe syndrome, 588–589
Temporolimbic syndrome, 589
Tendo-Achilles lengthening, 643–644
Testosterone, 573, 577
Tethered median nerve stress test, 506
Thioridazine, in aggression, 596
Third-nerve palsy, 482–483
Thoracodorsal nerve block, 540
Thumb-in-palm deformity, surgical
    management of, 625, 633–635
Thyroid-stimulating hormone. *See* Thyrotropin
Thyrotropin (TSH), 571–573, 575, 577
Thyrotropin-releasing hormone (TRH),
    571–572
Tibial nerve block, 547–548, 638
Tibial nerve lesions, 514
Tic disorders, 523
Tinel's sign, 506
Tolerance tests, 574–575
Torticollis, 522, 549
Trazodone, in aggression, 597
Tremor, 524

Ulnar fracture, 508
Ulnar nerve block, 542–543, 625–626
Ulnar nerve lesions, 504–506, 538
Ultrasound, Doppler, monitoring cerebral
    blood flow, 452–453
Unresponsive vigilance, 584–585
Upper extremity, flail, 508–510
Upper extremity deformity
    evaluation of, 650–651
    flexion deformity, 506–507
    nerve blocks in, 539–544
    nonsurgical management of, **649–661**
    range of motion in, 625
    surgical management of, **623–636**

Upper extremity deformity *(cont.)*
    surgical management of *(cont.)*
        definitive procedures, 627–635
        goals of, 624
        indications for, 624
        preoperative evaluation of, 624–627
        timing of, 624

Valproic acid
    in post-traumatic epilepsy, 468–469
    side effects of, 469
    in tremor disorders, 524
Vascular lesions, 443
Vegetative state, persistent, 584–585, 587
Ventricular catheter, monitoring intracranial
        pressure with, 445–446
Ventriculography, 443
Vertigo, **559–568**, 604
Vestibular adaptation, 566–567
Vestibular deficits, post-traumatic, **559–568**
    central, 566–567
    peripheral, 566–567
    unilateral, 562–567
Vigabatrin, 468
Visual agnosia, 481
Visual disorders, post-traumatic
    injuries and mechanisms of, **475–484**
    management and rehabilitation of, **485–502**
Visual evoked potentials (VEP), 457–458, 480,
        606
Visual pathways
    anatomy of, 476–477
    trauma to, 477–479
Visual-perceptual deficit, 651
Visuospatial disorder, 595

Wrist drop, 508
Wrist flexion deformity, 542–544, 552
    surgical management of, 625, 629–630

Xenon (stable) method, monitoring cerebral
        blood flow, 450–451
Xenon-133 methods, monitoring cerebral blood
        flow, 448–450

Zygomatic fracture, 496